Health promotion
Theory and practice

John Kemm
Ann Close

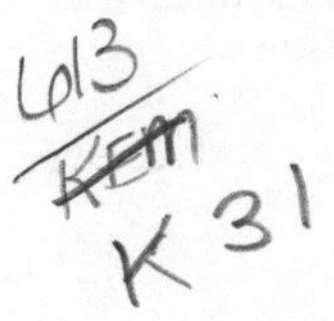

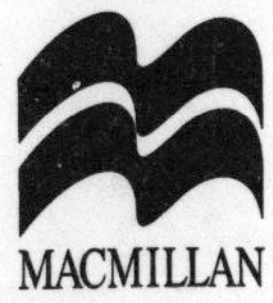

MACMILLAN

First published 1995 by
MACMILLAN PRESS LTD
Houndmills, Basingstoke, Hampshire RG21 6XS
and London
Companies and representatives
throughout the world

ISBN 0–333–57769–8

A catalogue record for this book is available from the British Library.

10 9 8 7 6 5 4 3 2
04 03 02 01 00 99 98 97 96

Printed in Great Britain by
Mackays of Chatham PLC
Chatham, Kent

Contents

Introduction

A reviewer of an early draft of this book accused us of being enthusiasts. We cheerfully plead guilty. We think health promotion is both worthwhile and enjoyable.

In writing this book we have tried to practise what we preach. Writing it has been an exercise in teamwork and we hope it is the better for the different professional backgrounds and the different blends of anarchy and discipline that we bring to it. We recognise that people promote health in many ways, ranging from the intimacy of individual patient care to the impersonality of national media campaigns. We accept the relevance to health of issues ranging in size from the micro issues of personal behaviour to the mega issues such as poverty or global warming. Ultimately, health is promoted by action but we try to cover both theory and practice because each enriches the other. We hope that all streams of thought in health promotion will find something useful in this book but that none will claim it as their exclusive property.

Using information is an important step in learning. We have therefore included in each chapter several Discussions/Activities which can be used for group work. There are no 'correct' answers to the questions and few 'incorrect' ones. We hope that thinking about these discussion points will help you make use of the material that you have read and clarify your own values and preferred ways of working.

In an effort to use gender-neutral language we have used 'they', 'them' and 'their' for the third person singular. This is grammatically incorrect but seemed preferable to the cumbersome 'he or she' or the barbarous 'he/she'. We also had difficulties in finding a word for the individuals whose health was being promoted. We have used 'patient' or 'client' for this purpose but neither word adequately conveys the sense of autonomy and partnership that ought to characterise health promotion.

We thank Mrs Pam Wills for typing the manuscript and Julie Wagstaff for help with the references. Finally we thank our long-suffering spouses for tolerating us while we laboured to produce this book.

John Kemm
Ann Close

Chapter contents

Tables and figures

Discussions/activities

1.1 Does prevention work?
1.2 Whose job is health promotion?
1.3 Health of the Nation targets

2.1 Who is healthy?
2.2 What is health promotion?
2.3 The right to make unhealthy choices

3.1 How healthy is your environment?
3.2 How healthy is your lifestyle?

4.1 How do we decide which theories to believe?
4.2 Which patients to educate?

5.1 Legislation about individual behaviour
5.2 Limitations on tobacco sales
5.3 Why are 'drugs' and alcohol treated differently?

6.1 Turning theory into practice
6.2 Educational approaches for different age groups

7.1 What influences a patient's health behaviour?
7.2 Motivating a family to adopt healthier dental behaviours

8.1 Obtaining better occupational health services
8.2 Writing to the press

9.1 Local health needs
9.2 Setting aims and objectives

10.1 Choosing outcome measures
10.2 Planning an evaluation

Acknowledgements

The following copyright owners are thanked for permission to reproduce figures:

Churchill Livingstone, for Figure 3.1 adapted from Morris J.N. (1975), *Uses of Epidemiology*, 3rd edition. Edinburgh: Churchill Livingstone.

Royal College of Physicians, for Figure 3.2 adapted from Expert Committee (1983), Obesity: a report of the Royal College of Physicians, *Journal of Royal College of Physicians* 17, 6–65.

President and Fellows of Harvard College, for Figure 4.4 adapted from Keys A. (1980), *Seven Countries: A Multivariate Analysis of Death and Coronary Heart Disease*. Cambridge MA: Harvard University Press.

Lancet Ltd. for Figure 4.5 adapted from Strom A and Jensen R.A. (1951), Mortality from circulatory disease in Norway 1940–45, *Lancet* i, 126–129.

Oxford University Press, for Figure 4.6 adapted from Doll R. and Peto R. (1981), *The Cause of Cancer.* Oxford.

Controller of HMSO, for Figure 5.1 adapted from Chief Medical Officer's report: *On the State of the Public Health for the Year 1988*. London: HMSO.

Kings Fund, Health Education Authority and London School of Hygiene and Tropical Medicine, for Figure 5.2 adapted from Smith A. and Jacobson B. (1991), *The Nation's Health* (revised edition). London.

Charles Slack Inc, for Figure 7.3 from Rosenstock I. in Becker M. (ed.) (1974), *The Health Belief Model and Personal Behaviour.* Thorofare NJ.

BMJ Publishing Group, for Figure 10.1 adapted from Nutbeam D., Smith C. and Catford J. (1990), Evaluation in health education: a review of progress, possibilities and problems, *Journal of Epidemiology and Community Health* **44**, 83–93.

BMJ Publishing Group, for Figure 15.1 adapted from Fullard E., Fowler G. and Gray M. (1987), Promoting prevention in primary care: a controlled trial of low technology low cost approach, *British Medical Journal* **294**, 1080–1082.

World Health Organisation, Regional Office for Europe, Copenhagen, for Figure 18.1.

Every effort has been made to trace all copyright holders but if any have been inadvertently overlooked, the publishers will be pleased to make the necessary arrangements at the first opportunity.

SECTION 1

Theory

CHAPTER 1

Introduction and history

GOAL

To appreciate the need for health promotion, its potential to help people be healthier and its organisational context.

OBJECTIVES

- to argue the case for health promotion
- to recognise the limitations of curative medicine and caring services
- to discuss the historical origin of health promotion and the new public health
- to describe the main organisations concerned with health promotion at a national and international level

THE CASE FOR HEALTH PROMOTION

Health promotion is the name given to all those activities which are intended to prevent disease and ill health and to increase well-being in the community. This obviously sounds a good idea but can it be done and does it work? In this chapter we look at some of the reasons why nurses and others should be doing health promotion and at some of its origins and achievements. In the next chapter we return to the question 'What is health promotion?'

Here are some examples of health prevention and promotion:

The conquest of smallpox Smallpox used to be one of the most feared of all diseases. Now it does not exist. The last case in the world occurred in Somalia in 1975. It was eradicated by a concerted campaign of vaccination of all contacts.

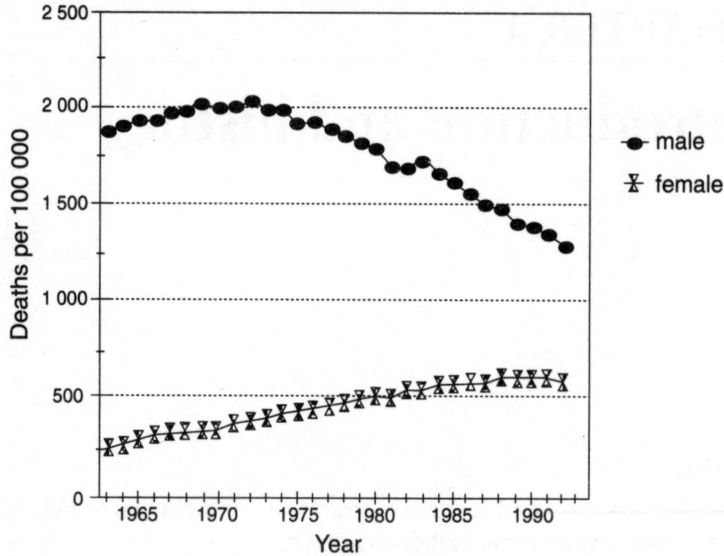

Figure 1.1 Death rates from lung cancer
Death rates from lung cancer in the UK in men aged 35–74 have been steadily falling for the last twenty years. The same period has seen a steady increase in death rates from lung cancer in women. The figures shown are age adjusted for reasons explained in Chapter 4 (see page 70).
Source Data from OPCS (Office of Population Censuses and Surveys), *Mortality in England and Wales,* Series DH2, Cause 1964–1992; London: HMSO.

Prevention of lung cancer Lung cancer is one of the diseases for which we do not have any very effective treatment. The most important cause is smoking. Today fewer men smoke and the number of cases of lung cancer in men has shown a marked decrease (see Figure 1.1). The frequency of lung cancer in women is still rising.

Prevention of heart disease The frequency of heart disease deaths has fallen markedly in the United States and is just starting to fall in this country (see Figure 1.2). One possible explanation for this fall is the effort that has been made to persuade people to give up smoking, eat less fat in their food, watch their blood pressure and take more exercise.

Prevention of chronic bronchitis and emphysema Chronic bronchitis and emphysema used to be much more common than they are now. The better air quality in our towns resulting from the

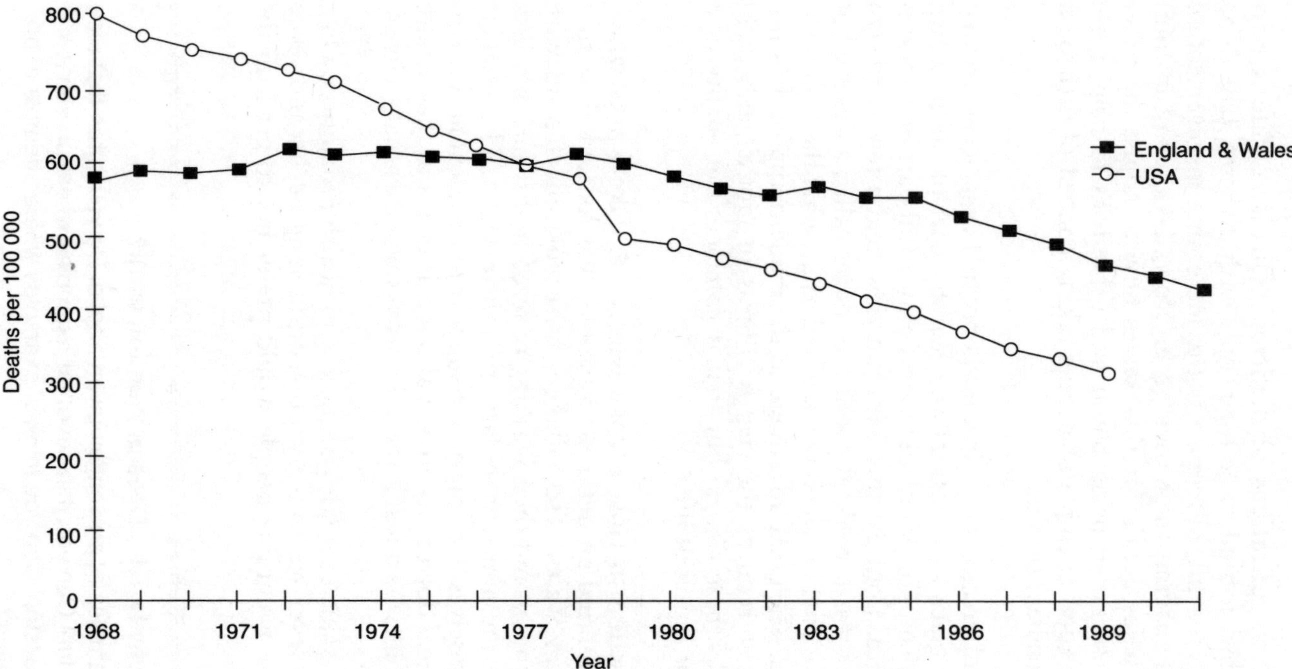

Figure 1.2 Death rates from heart disease
Death rates (age adjusted) from ischaemic (coronary) heart disease in men aged 35–74 have fallen dramatically in the USA over the past twenty years. Death rates in England and Wales showed very little change in the period covered by this figure though there is a suggestion that they had started to fall by the late 1980s. This trend is much more obvious for later years not covered here.
Source Data from British Heart Foundation (1994), *Coronary heart disease statistics 1993*; London.

Clean Air Acts as well as the reduction in smoking have played important parts in reducing the frequency of this disease.

Prevention of complications of diabetes Quality of life is now much better than it used to be for people with diabetes. One thing which has made a big difference is the increasing involvement of diabetics in managing their own care. Nowadays many insulin-requiring diabetics decide for themselves how to adjust their diet and insulin dose, often using blood and urine tests to help them. This is a very good example of people taking control of their own health with excellent results.

Management of pregnancy Nowadays pregnancy is being restored to its rightful place as a normal and healthy part of life in which mothers-to-be (supported by midwives) play a full part in decisions about their care. Contrast this with the view held a few years ago that pregnancy was a medical condition (never called a disease but treated just like one) in which women had to do what their obstetrician told them. The great advantage of the modern approach is not so much that it reduces the risk of illness in mother and child (though it does these things) but that it enhances the quality of a very important aspect of life.

Community action to close a coke works A coke works which permanently emitted an acrid black smoke was located close to a small village in Wales. The villagers were not only fed up with having their houses and their washing covered in dirt but they also suspected that the fumes were damaging their health. The villagers organised themselves with the active support of the local health visitors and the local doctors to protest about this threat to their health and quality of life. As a result the coke works was eventually closed.

These are just some examples of successful health promotion. On a more general level we can say prevention is good because even when a disease is curable people would prefer not to get it in the first place.

Discussion/Activity 1.1 Does prevention work?

Look at the examples of prevention given above. Do you agree that they are all successful? Can you think of other examples where prevention has been successful? Can you think of examples where attempts at prevention have failed?

CURING, CARING, PREVENTING

Health services and health care professions have always had a threefold task: curing, caring and preventing. Popular stereotypes have usually concentrated on curing disease or, when cure is not a realistic goal, caring for the sick person. The prevention of ill health and disease goes logically with curing and caring but has usually received less attention. Prevention is a rather inadequate word for this third part of health services since it should be about improving the whole quality of life not just preventing disease.

THE LIMITATIONS OF CURATIVE MEDICINE

Before the 20th century there were very few effective treatments for disease, and medical care made very little difference to the outcome (McKeown 1979). Then technical advances such as safer anaesthesia, better surgery, antibiotics, other modern medicines and blood transfusion changed the picture. At long last there were effective treatments. Conditions such as tuberculosis, appendicitis and perforated ulcer ceased to be death sentences. When these technical advances were combined with social reforms making health care available to all (for example the establishment of the National Health Service in the UK), the expectation was that disease would become rare and everyone would be healthy. The reality was somewhat different. Expenditure on health services increased, even more effective and usually even more expensive technologies were developed but disease remained obstinately common. Although many of the old diseases were controlled, their place seemed to be taken by others such as heart disease, cancer, arthritis and mental illness. It is this background that has led many to rediscover prevention.

REFOCUSING UPSTREAM

The idea of health promotion is often illustrated by the analogy of refocusing upstream. Someone was standing on a bridge when they saw a man in the river shouting for help and on the verge of drowning. The person on the bridge immediately jumped into the water and after a great battle with the current reached the drowning man. The rescuer pulled him to the shore, gave him mouth-to-mouth resuscitation and managed to revive him. No sooner had the first victim recovered than the rescuer heard another cry for help and was horrified to see another person floundering in the river. The rescuer was very tired but leapt in again and rescued the second victim. No sooner had they done this than they saw a third and fourth person in the river and then more and more. At great risk to themselves they spent the whole day fishing people out of the river and resuscitating them. Furthermore, despite their superhuman efforts many more could not be rescued and were drowned.

The point of this story is that although the rescuer was doing a great job rescuing people in desperate need of help, they never stopped to look upstream and find out why all these people were falling into the river. Maybe if they had done this and then done something to prevent the accidents (fencing the bridge, for example), their effort would have been more effective. Is there a parallel to be drawn with all our praiseworthy efforts to cure disease? Are there times when it would be better to think about why people get the disease in the first place and try to prevent it?

The concept of 'refocusing upstream' comes from experience in developing countries. Health workers in these countries found that their main task was treating disease in children. They made heroic efforts to cure the common infectious diseases and malnourishment which were so common but realised that they were only making a tiny impact on the problem. They also realised that while expensive treatment in hospitals made very little difference, cheap and simple measures such as more breast feeding, better weaning foods, clean water supplies and immunisation could prevent much of the disease against which they battled. Health workers in developed countries similarly need to ask themselves if the balance between caring, curing and prevention is right.

HEALTH GAIN AND 'LOW-HANGING FRUIT'

In making difficult choices about which health services should have top priority when all services are short of resources, we must aim to maximise health gain. Health gain is the amount that people's health is improved by our activities. It is all too easy to count the number of patients treated in hospital or the number of visits made by health visitors. It is much more difficult to count how much health gain has been produced by these activities. We know that some activities such as hip-replacement operations or drug treatment of tuberculosis produce excellent health gain and transform people's quality of life. We know that others use a large amount of money and nursing effort but produce little or no health gain (Welsh Office NHS Directorate 1990). Health promotion activity such as advising and helping people to give up smoking often produces a great deal of health gain for a small amount of resource.

Some health gains are easy to obtain, others will be very difficult. Before concentrating on the difficult health gains it makes sense to ensure that we have made the easy health gains. Before worrying about giving smoking advice to all the people who are not in contact with health services we might make sure that every patient who comes to the health clinic receives appropriate advice and help. This principle of doing the easy things first is often referred to as 'gathering the low-hanging fruit'.

THE ECONOMICS OF HEALTH PROMOTION

Some politicians have enthusiastically adopted health promotion on the grounds that prevention is cheaper than cure. It costs hundreds of thousands of pounds to care for a child severely damaged by congenital rubella. Immunisation with measles, mumps, rubella vaccine (MMR) costs only a few pounds and will protect a woman from ever having children with this disease.

While there are striking examples of this sort, it is a mistake to think that effective prevention will remove the need for curing and caring services. Prevention might bring financial benefits but the economic calculations are complex (Cohen and Henderson 1988). Prevention could in the long run cost more because it allows people to live to an older age when they may need more health services. The main argument for prevention is that it is better for people, not that it is cheaper.

A SHORT HISTORY OF HEALTH PROMOTION

Every ancient school of medicine has included teaching on how people could protect their health. Hippocrates in ancient Greece wrote on the importance of diet and exercise. Traditional Chinese medicine includes extensive advice on how to stay healthy and avoid disease. The papyri from ancient Egypt include instructions for healthy living.

THE SANITARY REVOLUTION

The modern history of health promotion starts in the 19th century (Table 1.1). At this time very high death rates and high frequencies of disease and disability were features of cities such as London, Liverpool, Manchester and Birmingham, and life in the country was not much better. People realised that this was not inevitable, that much of the disease was caused by unhealthy living conditions and that these could be improved. The changes which resulted from this realisation are often called the 'sanitary revolution' and are the foundation of public health as we know it.

Great Victorians such as Chadwick and Simons in London, Rowntree in York, and Duncan in Liverpool (Chave 1984) first described the appalling conditions in which the poor lived and then lobbied local and national government to get them improved. The results of their efforts were impressive (Brockington 1965). Sewers were built, clean water supplies were provided, housing was improved, conditions of work in factories became less terrible, schools and hospitals were founded. This improvement of the environment was coupled with the appointment of medical officers of health (MOHs) and sanitary inspectors. New legislation gave these officials powers to seek out health hazards in the environment and take action to correct them.

In addition to improving the buildings and infrastructure of towns, the sanitary reformers had another aim. They believed that disease was encouraged by dirt, intemperance and lack of thrift. Their solution to these problems was education and self-improvement. Visitors went to the homes of the poor, and gave them educational tracts and advice on cooking, cleaning, housecraft and caring for children. The approach could even be described as holistic for the visits were often combined with Christian evangelistic activity (Aveson 1987).

NURSING AND HEALTH PROMOTION

While Victorian cities were being rejuvenated by the sanitary reformers, Florence Nightingale introduced new standards of cleanliness and order – first in the army hospitals of the Crimea and then at St Thomas' Hospital in London. While she is rightly famed for insisting that nurses should be trained in the skills of curing and caring, she and other early leaders of the profession also emphasised the educational and preventive tasks of the nurse (Woodham-Smith 1953). The health promotion component of nursing has been repeatedly restated by the profession. The most recent legislation on training of nurses, midwives and health visitors (HMSO 1989) states that preparation programmes should enable students to identify 'health-related learning needs of patients and clients, families and friends and to participate in health promotion'. The required competencies were expanded in curriculum guidelines for project 2000 programmes and each branch programme has to prepare students in health promotion and the prevention of illness in a variety of settings (UKCC 1989).

HEALTH VISITING

In 1862 the Manchester and Salford Ladies Sanitary Reform Society decided to employ women to visit the poor in their homes in order to promote health and hygiene (Aveson 1987). This is conventionally considered to be the start of health visiting. As more and more local authorities employed women for this purpose there was much debate as to whether they were to be more like sanitary inspectors or mothers' friends (Davies 1987). By the early part of this century the role had narrowed down to concentrate mostly on promoting the health of mothers and young children. Other aspects of the health of the home environment became the responsibility of the sanitary inspectors. The core of the health visiting task was educational, helping mothers to acquire child-rearing skills. More recently health visitors have expanded their role to take an interest in all members of the home but the fundamental nature of the task remains health promotion.

THE NEW PUBLIC HEALTH

This phrase has been coined to describe the renewed interest in a communal effort to improve health by bringing together environ-

Table 1.1 Some milestones in health promotion

1840–70	The time when the sanitary revolution was most active.
1842	Edwin Chadwick publishes report on the sanitary condition of the labouring population of Great Britain. This highlights the appalling conditions in which most people are living.
1844	First meeting of the Health of Towns Association – this becomes a highly active lobby group demanding improved conditions in towns.
1846	First medical officer of health (MOH) appointed (Dr Duncan in Liverpool).
1848	Public Health Act allows all municipal boroughs to appoint MOHs. Second MOH appointed (Sir John Simons in London).
1862	Manchester and Salford Ladies Sanitary Reform Society employ first health visitors.
1890	Manchester is first borough to employ health visitors.
1892	First school nurse appointed by London School Board.
1896	First meeting of Women Sanitary Inspectors' Association. (This body, after several name changes, became the Health Visitors' Association in 1962.)
1902	Central Midwives' Board established.
1912	County and borough councils take over the functions of the old Poor Law authorities.
1944	Education Act finally makes free secondary schooling available to all.
1946	National Health Service Act leads to establishment of NHS in 1948.
1956	Clean Air Act makes way for steps to reduce air pollution.
1968	Health Education Council (HEC) established.
1981	WHO council adopts Health for All strategy.
1984	WHO launches the Healthy Cities project.
1985	HEC abolished. Replaced by the Health Education Authority.
1988	Acheson Report on public health in England suggests that Directors of Public Health (successors to MOHs) should issue an annual report on the health of their districts.
1992	Health of the Nation published. For the first time government sets out health targets for the nation.

mental improvement, personal preventive measures and therapeutic interventions (Ashton and Seymour 1988). In other words, to rethink the principles of the old public health which were so successful one hundred years ago and to apply their modern counterparts to the health problems of today.

SELF-HELP GROUPS

Self-help groups such as Alcoholics Anonymous, the Cystic Fibrosis Association, the Alzheimer's Disease Society, the Ileostomy Association and the Cystitis Association are other examples of new thinking about health care. What these groups all have in common is that they are run for and by patients or relatives of patients with these problems. They aim to inform their members about living with these conditions and help them take control of their own lives. This is a long way from the traditional model of medicine, with the compliant patient unquestioningly following the instructions of health professionals. It is however an example of health promotion in action and most nurses and doctors welcome this development since they realise that people get better care when they are fully involved in decisions about themselves (Brearley 1990; Richardson 1991).

DISTRICT HEALTH PROMOTION DEPARTMENTS

Nearly every health district now has a health promotion or health education department that supports health education throughout the district. These departments were mostly established in the 1970s following major reorganisation of the National Health Service and local government (Ewles 1993). Staff in these departments will do some or all of these things:

- give or loan health education materials such as posters, leaflets, videos, etc.
- provide training to other professionals such as nurses, midwives, doctors and teachers to help them develop their skills and knowledge in health promotion
- provide advice, information and resources to other professionals working in health education
- work directly with the public to give them the information they need to make healthy choices and live healthy lives
- organise local events and campaigns

Health promotion departments often put a lot of their effort into helping other professions incorporate health promotion into their work rather than working directly with the public. The advantage of working indirectly through others is that it should be possible to influence many more people.

THE HEALTH EDUCATION AUTHORITY

The Health Education Authority (HEA) is a special health authority and has its head office in London. Its task is:

- to advise the government on health promotion
- to support other organisations, health professionals and other people who provide health education to the public
- to provide information and advice directly to members of the public

These are some of the things the HEA does:

- produce national advertising campaigns (posters, television, radio, newspapers and magazines)
- design, produce and distribute health education materials (leaflets, posters, etc.)
- co-ordinate programmes such as LAYH (Look After Your Heart) and national events such as National No Smoking Day, Drinkwise Day, Low Fat Fortnight, etc.
- provide training and professional development for professionals working with the public

The HEA does these things in England. There are corresponding bodies in Wales, Scotland and Northern Ireland.

As a special health authority the HEA is accountable to the Department of Health. This has the advantage of making it easier for the HEA to influence policy but it also has the disadvantage of limiting the HEA's freedom to comment on the health effects of government policy. The HEA replaced the Health Education Council, which, as a quango (Quasi Autonomous Government Organisation), was less directly accountable to the government and sometimes annoyed ministers by criticising aspects of their policy.

THE WORLD HEALTH ORGANISATION

The World Health Organisation (WHO) was founded in 1945 and is an agency of the United Nations. It promotes co-operation for health between national governments. Its first task was to help war-ravaged countries rebuild health care services and combat the epidemic diseases that were threatening the whole world. While still concerned with the infectious diseases that affect so many, WHO has become increasingly involved in the control of chronic diseases such as heart disease, cancer and mental illness.

WHO has channelled support for health programmes from rich to poor countries. It is a framework for agreement on health regulations for travellers and (with the Food and Agricultural Organisation) food standards. It promotes meetings between health workers and publishes authoritative summaries on health problems and ways of tackling them. It evaluates both traditional and modern health technologies so that countries can make best use of the technologies that are available to them (WHO 1988).

The conquest of smallpox is probably the greatest achievement of WHO. But programmes on tuberculosis, yaws, schistosomiasis, leprosy, malaria, diarrhoeal disease and protein energy malnutrition have all reduced the burden of disease.

The headquarters of WHO is in Geneva. WHO is divided into six regions, one of which is the European region, with its headquarters in Copenhagen. WHO has been criticised for being bureaucratic and wasteful but it is probably no more flawed than other human organisations. The vision behind it is exciting and it has been responsible for some notable contributions to the health of the world.

HEALTH FOR ALL

Health for All by the year 2000 was adopted as WHO policy by the 34th World Health Assembly in 1981. The European office of WHO developed this, laying out 38 Health for All targets for member states (WHO 1985). Health for All has come to be a shorthand phrase for a whole approach to health:

- adding life to years
- adding years to life

This means increasing life expectancy (the number of years that people live) and improving the quality of life enjoyed during those years of life. Five general principles are characteristic of the Health for All approach:

1. equity
2. empowerment
3. participation
4. emphasis on primary care
5. multidisciplinary interagency working

Equity means fairness and implies that everyone should have similar opportunities to enjoy health. **Empowerment** means giving people control over their own health. **Participation** means involving people in the planning and running of the services they use and the decisions that effect their community. An **emphasis on primary care** means providing services close to the people who need to use them. **Multidisciplinary interagency working** means all who serve the community working together for the good of that community. These are big ideas and will all be discussed further in later chapters.

MULTIDISCIPLINARY INTERAGENCY WORKING

The many things that influence our health are discussed in Chapter 3 but it immediately becomes clear that health does not depend only on health services or nurses and doctors. Our health and enjoyment of life are influenced by social workers, teachers, environmental health officers, policemen, engineers who build houses, sewers and roads, retailers who sell the products we use, government officers, politicians and many others (Figure 1.3). The wide range of activities which make up health promotion needs a correspondingly wide range of skills. This means that health promotion has to be a team activity and nurses have to work with many other disciplines. No single profession has a monopoly of health promotion wisdom or is equipped to perform all the necessary tasks. Accepting the need to work with others may at times be uncomfortable but it is essential if we are to be effective in improving health (DoH 1993).

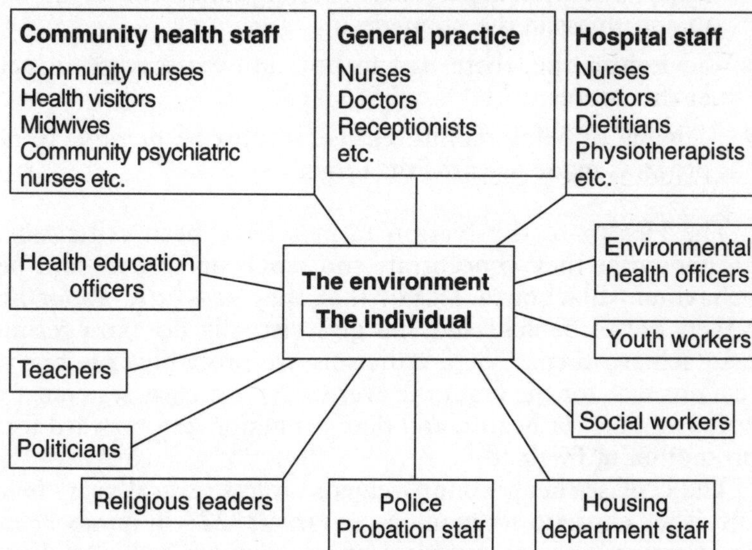

Figure 1.3 Who are the health promoters?
There is a wide range of different people whose activities promote health.

Discussion/Activity 1.2 Whose job is health promotion?

Look at the list of professions in Figure 1.3. Can you think of any other professions which ought to be added to the diagram? What contribution has each profession to make to health promotion?

HEALTH OF THE NATION

Health of the Nation is the title of a white paper published by the government in 1992. The document is important because for the first time ever the government was committing itself to a specific series of health targets for England (corresponding documents were also prepared for Scotland, Wales and Northern Ireland). These targets, covering five areas, together with some risk factors are summarised in Table 1.2. The targets were said to be 'challenging but achievable'.

Before publishing *Health of the Nation* the government had invited comments on a draft set of proposals, and hundreds of organisations and individuals had taken the opportunity to give their views. Several of the target areas suggested in the draft proposals were omitted from the final version. The criteria on which the final targets were chosen were that they should be:

- important health problems, i.e. common causes of death or major illness in the population
- achievable, i.e. there had to be a known way of reducing the health problem
- capable of being monitored, i.e. it must be possible to measure progress made towards the target

The Health of the Nation targets have been criticised on the grounds that they concentrate too much on disease and personal behaviour (Blackburn 1993), that they say little about how the targets are to be achieved and give virtually no extra resources to help achieve them. These criticisms are probably true but the fact remains that for the first time ever we have a clear statement of government aims for health, and that is a major step forward for health promotion in England.

The USA set health improvement targets several years before the UK. They chose to set many more targets (226 in number) and they are described in considerable detail in a document called 'Promoting health / preventing disease' (USDHHS 1980). Ten years later these objectives have been revised and modified in the light of experience (USDHHS 1990).

Table 1.2 Summary of Health of the Nation targets

A. Heart disease and stroke

- to reduce death rates from both coronary heart disease and stroke

	Target Reduction by year 2000	
	Under 65s (%)	65–74 (%)
CHD	40	30
Stroke	40	40

B. Cancer

- to reduce death rate for breast cancer in population invited for screening by at least 25% by year 2000
- to reduce incidence of invasive cervical cancer by at least 20% by year 2000
- to reduce death rate for lung cancer under age of 75 by at least 30% in men and 15% in women by year 2010
- to halt year on year increase in incidence of skin cancer by year 2005

C. Mental health

- to improve significantly the health and social functioning of mentally ill people
- to reduce suicide rate by year 2000 by at least 15% overall and by at least 33% in severely mentally ill people

D. Sexual health

- to reduce the incidence of gonorrhoea by at least 20% by 1995
- to reduce by at least 50% the rate of conceptions among the under 16s by year 2000

E. Accidents

- to reduce death rates from accidents by year 2005 by at least 33% in people aged under 15, 25% in people aged 15–24 and 33% in people aged 65 and over

F. Risk factors – Smoking

- to reduce prevalence of smoking to no more than 20% in men and women by year 2000
- to reduce consumption of cigarettes by at least 40% by year 2000
- to ensure that at least 33% of women smokers stop smoking at the start of their pregnancy by year 2000
- to reduce prevalence of smoking in 11–15 year olds by at least 33% by 1994

G. Risk Factors – diet and nutrition

- to reduce by year 2005:
  average percentage of food energy derived from saturated fatty acids to no more than 11% of total food energy and from total fat to no more than 35% of total food energy
  proportion of men and women aged 16–64 who are obese to no more than 6% and 8% respectively
  proportion of men drinking more than 21 units of alcohol per week and women drinking more than 14 units per week to 18% and 7%, respectively

H. Risk factors – Blood pressure

- to reduce mean systolic blood pressure in the adult population by at least 5 mm Hg by 2005

I. Risk factors – HIV/AIDS

- to reduce percentage of injecting drug users who report sharing injecting equipment in the previous four weeks from 20% in 1990 to no more than 10% by 1997 and no more than 5% by year 2000.

Discussion/Activity 1.3 Health of the Nation targets

Look at the Health of the Nation targets in Table 1.2. What needs to be done in order to achieve these targets? How can nurses contribute? Do you think any of these targets ought not to have been chosen?

What other targets would you like to add to the list?

SUMMARY POINTS

Health promotion is effective in preventing disease and increasing well-being in society. Curative and caring health services have made major contributions to health but there is now a case for 'refocusing upstream' and putting more energy into prevention.

Health promotion has a long history but the Victorian 'sanitary revolution' was the first substantial health promotion effort in the United Kingdom. This period saw:

- ☐ recognition of the effect of the environment on health
- ☐ improvement of the environment, especially in cities
- ☐ foundation of public health
- ☐ foundation of modern nursing and health visiting

The early founders of nursing emphasised the nurse's health promotion role and this has been reconfirmed many times by nursing leaders.

Health promotion is supported by:

- ☐ district health promotion departments
- ☐ the Health Education Authority

The World Health Organisation has adopted the policy of Health for All 2000. The main principles are:

- ☐ equity
- ☐ empowerment
- ☐ participation
- ☐ emphasis on primary care
- ☐ multidisciplinary interagency working

Health of the Nation, published by the United Kingdom Government in 1992, sets out a series of national targets for health.

REFERENCES

Ashton J. and Seymour H. (1988). *The new public health*. Milton Keynes: Open University Press.

Aveson J. (1987). Biblewomen and sanitary ladies. *Health Visitor* **60**, 156–161.

Blackburn C. (1993). Wealth and the nations' health. *Health Visitor* **66**, 254–256.

Brearley S. (1990). *Patient participation: the literature*. Royal College of Nursing Research Series. London: Scutari.

Brockington C.F. (1965). *Public health in the nineteenth century*. London: Livingstone.

Chave S.P.W. (1984). Duncan of Liverpool – and some lessons for today. *Community Medicine* **6**, 61–71.

Cohen D.R. and Henderson J.B. (1988). Case studies in primary prevention. Chapter 5 in *Health prevention and economics*. Oxford: Oxford Medical.

Davies C. (1987). Making history: the early days of the HVA. *Health Visitor* **60**, 145–148.

DoH (Department of Health) (1992). *Health of the Nation: a strategy for health in England*. London: HMSO.

DoH (Department of Health) (1993). *Health of the Nation: working together for better health*. London: HMSO.

Ewles L. (1993). Paddling upstream for 50 years: the role of health education officers. *Health Education Journal* **52**, 172–181.

Faculty of Community Medicine (1986). *Health for All 2000: a charter for action*.

HMSO (1989). *Statutory instrument for nurses, midwives and health visitors No. 1455 Nurses, midwives and health visitors (Parts of the Register) Amendment (No. 2) Order*.

McKeown T. (1979). *The role of medicine: dream, mirage or nemesis*. Oxford: Blackwell.

Richardson A. (1991). Health promotion through self help: the contribution of self help groups. Chapter 19 in Bandura A. and Kickbusch I. (eds.), *Health promotion research: towards a new social epidemiology*. Copenhagen: WHO European Regional Publication series No. 37.

Symonds A. (1993). Tracing the tradition of health visiting. *Health Visitor* **66**, 175–176 and 204–206.

UKCC (1989). *UKCC requirements for the content of project 2000 programmes*. UKCC professional standards and development division PS&D/89/04 (B).

USDHHS (US Department of Health and Human Services) (1980). *Promoting health/preventing disease: objectives for the nation*. Washington DC: US GPO.

USDHHS (US Department of Health and Human Services), Public Health Service (1990). *Healthy people 2000*. Washington DC: US GPO.

Welsh Office NHS Directorate (1990). *NHS Wales: agenda for action 1991–1993*.

WHO (World Health Organisation) (1985). *Targets for Health for All*. European Health for All Series No. 1. Copenhagen: WHO Regional Office for Europe.

WHO (World Health Organisation) (1988). *Four decades of achievement: highlights of the work of WHO*. Geneva: WHO.

Woodham-Smith C. (1953). Florence Nightingale and health education. *Health Education Journal* **11**, 7–3.

FURTHER READING

Department of Health (1993). *Health of the nation: key area handbooks*. London, HMSO.

Coronary heart disease
Cancer
HIV/AIDS and sexual health
Mental illness
Accidents

CHAPTER 2

Some basic principles

GOAL

To understand the wide range of activities and philosophies that make up health promotion and consider the ethical implications of these activities.

OBJECTIVES

- to discuss the meaning of health, disease and ill health
- to identify the wide range of activities which make up health promotion
- to understand the relation of health education to health promotion
- to describe the different models that inform health promotion activity
- to discuss the health professional's mandate for health promotion
- to explore the ethical problems posed by health promotion

WHAT IS HEALTH?

Health is one of those words that everyone uses but whose precise meaning they find difficult to explain. Before we think further about health promotion we have to reach some shared understanding of what constitutes health.

The World Health Organisation's constitution (WHO 1946) defines health as 'a state of complete physical, mental and social well-being and not merely the absence of disease and infirmity'. What would a person in a state of complete physical, mental and social well-being be like? Physical well-being means that they would be free of all physical disease and free of aches, pains and other symptoms. Their joints, muscles, heart, lungs, liver, stomach and all their other organs would function well. They would be fit, strong and agile, with good eyesight and acute hearing. They would be able to resist infection and if they suffered injury they would recover quickly. Furthermore, there would be no indication that they were likely to develop any disease or infirmity in the future.

Mental well-being means that their mental function would be as good as their physical state. They would be intelligent, well-balanced, resilient and able to cope with the stresses of daily life. They would feel happy and at peace with the world and themselves.

Social well-being means that they would function well in society. They would relate well to their family and other members of society. They would have a role in society and would value and be valued by others.

This paragon of health would live in a situation which enhanced and protected their health. The physical environment would supply shelter, warmth and food. They would not be exposed to undue risk of infection or physical accident. The society in which they lived would give them affection and esteem but also enough challenge to keep them stimulated.

This description suggests that 'complete physical, mental and social well-being' is not a realistic goal for health promotion. Three important points can however be drawn from the WHO definition:

1. There is a lot more to being healthy than just being in good physical shape. We also have to think of mental and social function.
2. Absence of disease and infirmity is a necessary feature of health.
3. Health requires the presence of various features which are referred to as positive health.

Figure 2.1 shows some of the components of health.

Does it make sense to talk of healthy people who are confined to a wheelchair, healthy people who are blind or healthy people with mental handicap? According to the WHO definition of health it would make no sense but most nurses would find these terms meaningful.

A more practical definition of health recognises that people differ and have different limitations. Health is a state in which people are able to work towards attaining their 'realistic chosen and biologic potentials' (Seedhouse 1986).

This definition seems to be much more helpful than the WHO definition and suggests a goal that we can realistically hope to achieve.

DOES IT MATTER?

Whole books have been written on the single question 'What is health?'. Philosophers have studied it for years; religious teachers

	Absence of disease	Absence of ill health	Presence of positive health (well-being)
Physical health	Long life No physical disease Low-risk of disease Low-risk lifestyle	No physical symptoms No physical disability	Fitness Health-promoting lifestyle
Mental health	No psychiatric disease	No mental distress No mental disability	Self-esteem Mental ability Resilience
Social health	No social/family breakdown	No social/family frictions	Role in society Social support Sense of belonging

Figure 2.1 What is health?
Health has at least three components: absence of disease, absence of ill health and presence of positive health. Each of these can be identified in the fields of physical health, mental health and social health.

and political theorists contribute to the discussion; the practical experience of health workers adds further to our understanding. There is no simple answer and we cannot settle the issue in a few paragraphs (Pender 1987). Different people will always have slightly different ideas of what constitutes health.

Some have even concluded that the whole effort to define health is unhelpful and 'de-energising' (Ashton and Seymour 1988). Certainly every health promoter will have to work with other health promoters whose views on the nature of health differ slightly from theirs. There is a danger that obsessive concern with the meaning of 'health' can paralyse our activity and create sectarian divides between workers who should be co-operating. There will always be a wide range of activities that everyone agrees to be health promoting. We should get on with these tasks without waiting for agreement on all matters. At the same time we will be more effective health promoters if we frequently ask ourselves what it is we are trying to promote. In so doing we must not expect everyone else to reach the same answer or allow the debate to became an excuse for schism or inaction.

Discussion/Activity 2.1 Who is healthy?

Table 2.1 gives thumbnail sketches of eight people. They all have features which might be considered healthy and features which might be considered unhealthy. Which of these people do you consider to be the most healthy? Which of them do you consider to be the least healthy? What factors lead you to this conclusion?

Table 2.1 Eight thumbnail sketches of people in different states of health

Andy is a fit young man. He can run a marathon in three and a half hours. He feels well, is happily married, has an active social life and enjoys his job as a market gardener. He is profoundly deaf.

Beatrice lives in a flat on the sixth floor of a tower block with her two young children. She is separated from her husband and receives no support from him. She relies on benefits, is behind with the rent and has other debts. She is worried and unhappy and frequently visits her doctor complaining of tiredness and 'nerves'. The doctor is unable to find any physical disease to account for her symptoms.

Charles is a successful businessman. Every moment of his day is occupied. He spends most of his time working at the desk in his office or driving his car. Most weekends he plays a round of golf. He smokes ten cigars a day and drinks two or three bottles of whisky in a week. His firm pays for him to have a health screen and last time he was found to have raised blood pressure and a high blood cholesterol. Charles considers himself to be in the best of health.

Delia is 11 years old. She has Down's syndrome and her mental age is 5. She is very happy and has parents who adore her. She is attending a special school but is unlikely ever to be able to fully look after herself.

Emma is 30 and works as a solicitor. She fractured her spine in a riding accident and is now paraplegic. She has a wheelchair, a car and a house adapted to meet her needs. She is fiercely independent and leads a very full professional and social life.

Fred is 19 and lives with his parents on an inner-city estate. He left school at 16 and has never been able to get a job. He is bored and spends most of his time having a laugh with the lads. He has had several convictions for offences such as burglary and stealing cars. As a schoolboy he sometimes sniffed glue with his friends. He has recently started to experiment with smoking opiates. He is strong and physically very fit.

George is 25 and is having a wonderful time. He works in the city, has a good salary and lots of friends. He does not know it but he is HIV positive, having acquired the infection on a recent holiday overseas.

Hilda is 70 and is a cheerful soul. Her activity is limited by her rheumatoid arthritis, which has caused considerable deformity in her hands and makes walking rather painful. She manages to look after her house and herself. She lives alone apart from her cat but looks forward to Sunday evenings when her neighbours take her to church and Wednesdays when her daughter-in-law comes to see her. She spends most of her time listening to the radio. She considers herself very lucky to be 'so well for her age'.

DISEASE AND ILL HEALTH

Curative medicine is primarily concerned with diseases. A disease is a recognised complex of symptoms and physical signs which can in theory be explained by disordered working of mechanisms within the body. Tuberculosis, ischaemic (coronary) heart disease and a broken leg are all examples of diseases. Tests such as blood chemistry and X-rays often help with diagnosis of disease and demonstrating the underlying malfunction. However, all of us from time to time and some people for most of the time experience symptoms such as tiredness, backache, headache and anxiety. Often no recognisable 'disease' can be found to account for these symptoms. The term ill health is used to cover all these forms of distress which cannot be included within the concept of disease.

IMPAIRMENT, DISABILITY AND HANDICAP

The terms impairment, disability and handicap are used to describe the different ways in which disorders affect different people. Impairment describes the anatomical or physiological disorder, disability describes how it interferes with function, and handicap how it interferes with daily living (WHO 1980).

Thus two people might have the same impairment of damage to the cartilages in the knee joint but one might still be able to move the knee freely and so have no disability while the other might be unable to walk because of it and so have considerable disability. Similarly, two people with the same disability may experience very different degrees of handicap. If someone with a sedentary desk job has a stiff painful knee it may hardly interfere with their life at all and thus cause them no handicap. On the other hand, the same disability in a nurse working on a ward or in a ballet dancer would make it impossible for them to continue with their occupation and would therefore be a considerable handicap.

POSITIVE HEALTH

It is easy to accept that health is something more than the absence of disease and ill health, and to call that 'something more' 'positive health'. It is much more difficult to define positive health (Catford 1983; Kemm 1992).

Positive physical health includes aspects of fitness such as strength, stamina, suppleness and speed. Other things which could be included are the ability of the different organs to work harder (for example how much blood the heart can pump or how much air the lungs can take in and expel) and the ability of the body to resist infection. Positive mental health includes happiness, self-esteem, ability to solve problems, ability to adapt to mental stresses and so on. Positive social health includes, for example, having a role in society and being able to form social links.

Health promotion is often urged to pay less attention to the prevention of disease and ill health and to pay more attention to promotion of 'positive health'. In theory this is fine but finding practical ways of doing it is much more difficult.

WHAT IS HEALTH PROMOTION?

Health promotion includes all those activities which are intended to prevent disease or to promote positive health. Table 2.2 lists some of them and it can seen that the list is both long and varied (Tannahill 1985). It is clear that many different disciplines and professions have a part to play in health promotion and also that health promotion involves all levels of social organisation from national government to the individual citizen.

Table 2.2 Some health promotion activities

Making the environment safe	sewage disposal improving housing road engineering speed limits legislation for safe products safety-at-work legislation food hygiene
Individual protection	immunisation seat-belt legislation crash helmets protective clothing at work needle exchange schemes for injecting drug users
Health education (knowledge for health)	raising awareness of health issues helping people acquire the skills and knowledge for health
Making healthy choices easy	increased availability of 'healthy' products subsidies on 'healthy' products taxation on 'unhealthy' products (e.g. cigarettes)
Protection against anti-health	control of advertising banning certain products
Detecting problems at a stage where they are reversible	cervical screening breast cancer screening coronary risk factor assessment

MAKING THE ENVIRONMENT SAFE

One of the most effective ways of promoting health is to provide a living environment which is conducive to health. Provision of adequate methods of sewage disposal, supplying clean water, replacing bad housing with good, and careful road engineering all reduce the risk that an individual will suffer infectious disease or physical accident. These topics are discussed further in Chapter 3.

INDIVIDUAL PROTECTION

In addition to minimising environmental hazards, it is possible to increase the ability of the individual to resist such hazards. Immunisation against infectious disease is one obvious example. Children can be protected against diphtheria, pertussis (whooping cough), tetanus, polio, measles and rubella in this way. People visiting the tropics may be immunised against other diseases and take tablets to protect themselves against malaria. Use of seat belts in cars, crash helmets on motor cycles and head guards for cyclists are ways in which individuals can protect themselves against the consequences of an accident. In the workplace, protective clothing (goggles, ear protectors, hard hats, steel toecaps, etc.) can also reduce the risk that individuals will be damaged by their environment.

KNOWLEDGE FOR HEALTH

Many aspects of the way we live, such as our smoking, eating, drinking and exercise habits or use of health services, affect our chances of health. Helping people obtain knowledge about the things which influence their health may enable them to improve their health.

MAKING CHOICE AVAILABLE

Knowledge by itself is not enough. For example it is of little help to know that contaminated water is dangerous if the only supply available to you is not clean. In developed countries less obvious barriers may prevent people choosing healthier ways of living. If the local shop only sells foods that contain large amounts of fat and sugar and little fibre, then choosing a low-fat high-fibre diet may not be a realistic option. Not smoking, and drinking moderately, are difficult if it means being the odd one out among your friends. Making choice available is an important health promotion activity.

PROTECTION AGAINST ANTI-HEALTH

Minimising the effect of things which actively work against health is another part of health promotion. Banning advertising of health-damaging products such as tobacco is one example. Customs and police activity to limit the importation and selling of illicit drugs is another.

SCREENING

Many disease processes can be reversed if they are detected early, while treatment at a later stage may be less effective. The cervical screening programme aims to prevent cervical cancer by detecting the early indications of the disease. Other diseases whose worst effects can be prevented by screening programmes are breast cancer, glaucoma (raised pressure in the eye leading to blindness) and high blood pressure (which may lead to strokes). Screening is further described in Chapter 15.

Discussion/Activity 2.2 What is health promotion?

Look at Table 2.2 again. Can you think of other activities which could be classed as health promotion and added to the list? Are there any activities included in that table which you do not think should be classed as health promotion?

LEVELS OF PREVENTION

Disease prevention can take place at three levels:

Primary prevention Preventing the disease from ever happening. *Examples*: preventing road accidents by engineering safer roads, preventing polio by immunising children, preventing lung cancer by encouraging non-smoking.

Secondary prevention Detecting disease before it causes any symptoms – at a stage where it can be effectively cured. *Examples*: screening for breast or cervical cancer; identifying and counselling heavy drinkers.

Tertiary prevention Preventing recurrence of a disease which has been cured or preventing a disease causing complications or handicap. *Examples*: advising a patient how to modify their lifestyle after a heart attack so as to reduce the risk of recurrence; helping a diabetic patient avoid complications by keeping good control of their blood glucose levels.

MODELS OF HEALTH PROMOTION

Knowledge – attitude – behaviour (KAB)

Much early health education was based on the view that all that was necessary was to give people knowledge as to what behaviour would give them the best chance of health. It was then hoped that this increase in knowledge would lead to a change in attitudes to the behaviour which in turn would lead to a change in behaviour. Governments often seem to have a touching belief in the efficacy of giving knowledge.

There is now a mass of evidence that this model is not an adequate description of how most people think and behave. Often people behave in a way that is apparently uninfluenced by their beliefs. Changes in behaviour frequently precede changes in belief.

The KAB model is also criticised because it places too much emphasis on the behavioural choices of the individual and ignores all the external factors which constrain and influence those choices. The KAB model is often coupled with an emphasis on avoiding disease rather than promoting 'positive health'. This combination of emphasis on knowledge, individual responsibility and disease avoidance is often referred to as the 'medical model'.

While rejecting the crude KAB model we should not totally reject the importance of knowledge. Much of our behaviour may not be rational but there may be a few circumstances in which behaviour is to a small extent influenced by beliefs. Ajzen and Fishbein (1980) have suggested a model in which beliefs about the outcome of a behaviour and the values attached to those outcomes may predict behavioural intention. Furthermore, informed choice cannot be a reality for people if they do not have the information.

The empowerment model

The empowerment model seeks to increase individuals' ability to choose and to influence their environment. The aim is to equip individuals with the skills and information that will give them the power to take control of their own health. An essential part of the empowerment approach is value clarification – helping people be clear about what they really want.

This model is apparently value-free. Taken to extremes, this would mean that one would be unconcerned about how people chose to behave (illicit drug use, high risk sexual behaviour, and so on) as long as their choice was informed. In practice this approach is usually combined with the promotion of values such as valuing oneself and valuing others.

The community action model

This model stresses the many factors affecting health over which the individual has little control. It seeks to encourage individuals to act together as a community to demand changes in their environment to make it healthier (Watt 1986). For example they might act to stop a local factory emitting smoke which pollutes the air or act to reduce heavy traffic passing their homes.

In its extreme form, the community action model may be very demeaning to the individual, presenting them as no more than the helpless pawn of their environment, unable to make any individual decision.

THE USE AND ABUSE OF MODELS

It is clear that each model has some elements of truth, and Figure 2.2 attempts to draw these different ideas together. However, no model is an adequate guide for all situations (Caraher 1994). Nearly all problems require for their solution a combination of methods drawn from several models. If used eclectically, the different models are a helpful guide to the practice of health promotion (French and Adams 1986). It is sad that all too often models are abused by those who pretend that their particular model is the

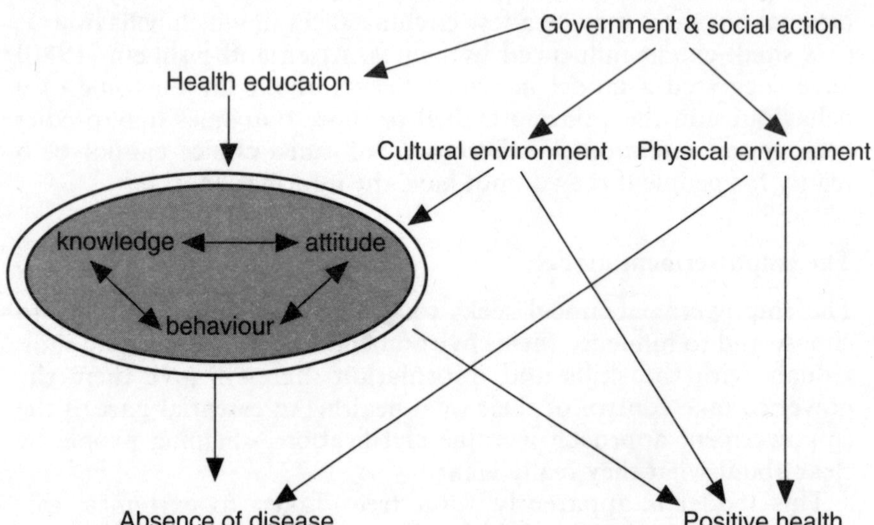

Figure 2.2 A composite model of health promotion
This model recognises that both individual action (lifestyle) and government and social action (cultural and physical environment) are important.

whole and only truth and attack advocates of any other model as misguided or mischievous.

HEALTH EDUCATION

Health education is one very important method of health promotion. It is an eclectic discipline based in education but informed by other disciplines including social psychology and even marketing.

Health education tasks include raising awareness of issues, influencing people's agendas, helping them clarify their values and helping them acquire knowledge and skills. A very ambitious health education programme may even try to influence motivations or modify attitudes. Health education uses a wide variety of methods. These are described in Chapters 6, 7 and 8.

PROFESSIONAL AND PRIVATE ROLES IN HEALTH PROMOTION

Health promotion potentially involves almost all areas of human activity. There is no doubt that having an atom bomb (or any other sort of bomb) dropped on you is very bad for your health. Equally there is no doubt that the activities of political parties have both good and bad effects on the health of populations. Does this mean that health promoters should campaign for disarmament or work for the political party that they believe will be most beneficial for health?

In order to resolve awkward questions such as these we have to distinguish between the professional and the private roles of the health worker. As private citizens, health promoters have just the same rights and duties as any other citizen, and they are as free to decide how to work for the common good as anyone else. In their professional roles as nurses, doctors, health promotion officers, teachers, environmental health officers and so on, they have responsibilities to their clients and their employers which limit the range of activities in which it is proper to engage (French 1990).

THE MANDATE FROM THE CLIENT

The health promoter's client may be an individual or a community. What is the implicit agreement between the patient and the health worker? The guiding principle must be respect for the patient's autonomy. The health promotion mandate is to offer information and give it to willing recipients. Nurses and other health workers have no mandate to force information on people who do not wish to have it. Deciding what information people want is one of the great skills of health education. It is difficult to decide how far the mandate from the client invites the nurse to challenge the client's value systems and beliefs when the nurse believes these to be incompatible with health.

THE MANDATE FROM THE EMPLOYER

For a few health care professionals the employer is the client but more usually it is a health authority or trust. For other health promoters it may be a local authority, an education authority or some other agency. Health promoters have to fit into and work within their employing organisations. The employer will probably have ideas as to the limits of the health promoter's mandate but these will need to be continually renegotiated.

There will be occasions when the duties to the employer appear to conflict with the duty towards the client.The decision to close a hospital or to build a new road, for example, will affect the health of people in their vicinity. Before the decision is made, the health care professional has a duty to make their beliefs known and to argue the case as forcefully as they can. But once a decision which might be harmful to health has been made, should it be accepted? Exceptionally there may be situations in which the organisational values are so incompatible with the health promoter's values that the only honest course is resignation. More usually the health promoter will find that they can best serve their clients by judicious compromise.

THE ETHICS OF HEALTH PROMOTION

Whose values?

The discussion of mandates and conflicting duties has introduced the question of the ethics of health promotion (Doxiadis 1990). In health promotion we are constantly faced with the question of whether it is morally right to do something. The first set of problems arises because health promotion is based on a set of values which may not be shared by all. The nurse values health highly and probably values some aspects of health more highly than others. Clients may well take a different view. Health promoters often discount future benefits such as being fit in old age only slightly, while most people discount future events a great deal. (Discounting means attaching less value to events which happen in the future than to events which happen now.) To what extent is the nurse health promoter justified in persuading others to accept their particular value system?

The problem of 'Whose values?' is one example of the general problem of the conflict between paternalism and autonomy. Paternalism is taking decisions on behalf of and in the best interests of others. Autonomy is allowing others to make their own decisions even when they harm themselves by so doing. A conflict between these two values frequently occurs in health promotion work.

Transfer of benefit

A second set of ethical problems arises from the fact that most health promotion activity can cause harm as well as good. Immunisation against pertussis (whooping cough) confers great benefit on the many children who would otherwise catch a disease which is unpleasant for nearly all and fatal for a few. However, there are also a very small but not negligible number of individuals who suffer reactions to the injection and are harmed by it, sometimes severely. Similarly, though less dramatically, if we advise people of the risks of smoking, then those who stop and feel better could be said to have benefited. However, those who merely feel guilty and worried but continue to smoke could be said to have been harmed by our activity. Even the simplest actions involve some harm. Does the benefit to the vast majority justify the harm to the very few?

Ethical responsibility cannot be avoided by arguing that health educators only offer information and it is up to the client whether they act upon that information. If our information influences the decisions made by a client then we must accept some responsibility for the consequences of giving that information. Nor can responsibility be avoided by doing nothing. If harm could have been avoided by giving information and we decided not to give that information then that harm is attributable to our lack of action. A decision to do nothing is just as much a decision as a decision to act, and we are equally accountable for the consequence of that decision.

The conflict between the principles of beneficence (doing good) and non-maleficence (doing no harm) frequently occurs in health promotion. Usually health promotion relies on a utilitarian philosophy that we should seek the greatest good for the greatest number. This implies that an action which causes some degree of harm can be justified if it also causes a larger amount of good. However, those who are harmed might take a different view, and how much benefit justifies a particular degree of harm?

There are many difficulties with this utilitarian approach. An action which does good to some people but also harms other people involves a 'transfer of benefit' or redistribution of health. How can that be justified? The situation is made more difficult by the fact that those who benefit by avoiding an unpleasant disease in the future cannot be identified and are unaware that they have benefited. On the other hand, those who are harmed are well aware of it and easily identifiable. A further problem is the 'paradox of prevention' which means that usually any health promotion activity benefits only a small fraction of those exposed to it (Kemm 1985). This 'paradox of prevention' is further explained in Chapter 4.

Discussion/Activity 2.3 The right to make unhealthy choices

You are nursing a 50-year-old man who has just had arterial reconstruction for small vessel disease in his legs. If the disease progresses it is very likely that the leg will have to be amputated in the future. It will almost certainly progress if the patient continues to smoke. The patient has smoked 60 cigarettes a day since he was 15. He has become very distressed by the repeated suggestions that he ought to give up smoking and has said very plainly that he does not want anyone to mention the subject again. Should his clearly stated wishes be respected?

EQUITY

Equity (or fairness) is a central value of health promotion. It seems fair that everyone should have an equal chance of being healthy and yet health is very unequally distributed. An inequality may be considered fair if, like the greater life expectancy of women compared with men, it arises from a fundamental biological characteristic. It may also be fair if, like the greater risk of dying run by people who go hang gliding, it arises from a freely chosen lifestyle. However most of the inequalities in health, such as those associated with class or ethnicity (described in Chapter 3), are neither biological nor chosen. They are the result of the physical and cultural settings in which people have to live and are therefore examples of inequity (Whitehead 1991).

The principle of equity might suggest that services such as health education should be equally distributed to all. However, if such services are equally distributed, the other inequalities in society are likely to result in the more favoured sections deriving most benefit and therefore in increased inequity of health. An alternative may be to concentrate services on the most deprived sections of society so that they receive the most benefit and inequity is reduced.

DISCRIMINATION AND EQUAL OPPORTUNITIES

Sometimes we may purposely discriminate in favour of one group in order to reduce inequity (for example concentrating health promotion effort in deprived wards of a city). On the other hand, there is always the risk of inadvertent discrimination against some groups. Careless use of language, inappropriate visual materials or unsuitable cultural contexts may all make health promotion activities irrelevant or offensive to certain groups (Mares, Henley and Baxter 1985). Choice of time or location may make activities inaccessible to many. All health promotion activities have to be scrutinised to ensure that they are not excluding people and in particular the very people who could derive most benefit from them.

SETTING AN EXAMPLE

In their health education role nurses may be called upon to counsel patients to give up smoking, moderate their drinking, take more exercise and control their body weight. Does this mean that the nurse has to do all these things? To be sure the health educator who smells of smoke while they advise others not to smoke lacks credibility. On the other hand, few of us are perfect and admitting to our own difficulties in following a healthy lifestyle may help us empathise with the client. This is discussed further in Chapter 7.

SUMMARY POINTS

Health is difficult to define but has physical, mental and social aspects. Health is more than the mere absence of disease and ill health.

Health promotion comprises all activities intended to prevent disease or promote well-being. It includes:

- ☐ making the environment safe
- ☐ protecting the individual
- ☐ knowledge for health
- ☐ making healthy choices available
- ☐ protection against anti-health forces
- ☐ screening

There are various models for health promotion:

- ☐ knowledge – attitudes – behaviour models
- ☐ empowerment
- ☐ community action

Each model has some elements of truth and none is an adequate guide for all situations.

Health education is an important part of health promotion.

Health promoters must distinguish their professional and private roles in health promotion. They need to consider the mandate from their client and from their employer.

Health promotion work raises many ethical issues:

- ☐ respecting autonomy of clients who do not share the health promoter's value sets
- ☐ not harming clients (non-maleficence)
- ☐ issues of equity

REFERENCES

Ajzen I. and Fishbein M. (1980). *Understanding attitudes and predicting social behaviour*. Englewood Cliffs NJ: Prentice-Hall.

Ashton J. and Seymour H. (1988). *The new public health*. Milton Keynes: Open University Press.

Caraher M. (1994). Health promotion: time for an audit. *Nursing Standard* 8 (No. 20), 32–35.

Catford J.C. (1983). Positive health indicators: towards a new information base for health promotion. *Community Medicine* 5, 123–132.

Doxiadis S. (1990). *Ethics in health education*. Chichester: John Wiley and Sons.

French J. (1990). Boundaries and horizons, the role of health education within health promotion. *Health Education Journal* 49, 7–10.

French J. and Adams L. (1986). From analysis to synthesis: theories of health education. *Health Education Journal* 45, 71–73.

Kemm J.R. (1985). The ethics of healthier eating. *Community Medicine* 7, 289–294.

Kemm J.R. (1992). Measuring health. In Norgan C., *Measurement of health in communities*. Cambridge: Cambridge University Press.

Mares P., Henley A. and Baxter C. (1985). *Health care in a multiracial Britain*. Health Education Authority / National Extension College. Cambridge.

Pender N.J. (1987). Towards a definition of health. Chapter 1 in *Health promotion in nursing practice*. Norwalk CT: Appleton and Lange.

Seedhouse D. (1986). *Health: the foundations for achievement*. Chichester: John Wiley and Sons.

Tannahill (1985). What is health promotion? *Health Education Journal* 44, 167–168.

Watt A. (1986). Health education and community development. *Journal of the Royal Society of Medicine* 79, Supplement 13, 20–24.

Whitehead M. (1991). Concepts and principles of equity and health. *Health Promotion International* 6, 217–220.

WHO (World Health Organisation) (1946). *Constitution*. Geneva: WHO.

WHO (World Health Organisation) (1980). *International classification of impairments, disabilities and handicaps*. Geneva: WHO.

FURTHER READING

Crawford R. (1980). Healthism and the medicalisation of everyday life. *International Journal of Health Services* 10, 365–388.

Downie R.S., Fyfe C. and Tannahill A. (1990). *Health promotion models and values*. Oxford: Oxford University Press.

Ewles L. and Simnett I. (1992). *Promoting health: a practical guide*. London: Scutari.

Tones K., Tilford S. and Robinson Y. (1990). *Health education: Effectiveness and efficiency*. London: Chapman and Hall.

CHAPTER 3

The determinants of health

GOAL

To understand that the individual's health is strongly influenced by their environment and their lifestyle and that these factors produce marked inequalities of health.

OBJECTIVES

- to understand that health is determined by the interaction of genetics, environment and lifestyle
- to identify the environmental factors that influence health
- to identify the lifestyle factors that influence health
- to discuss how an individual's lifestyle choices are constrained by their environment
- to describe the inequalities of health between social classes, between ethnic groups and between employed and unemployed

INTRODUCTION

There are three main factors which determine how healthy a person will be (Smith 1992):

- genetics
- environment
- lifestyle

It is helpful to think of these three things separately although they all interact and are not independent of each other.

Genetic endowment cannot be changed but how the individual is affected by their genes will to a large degree be influenced by the way they live their life. It is convenient to divide living conditions into environment and lifestyle. Environment refers to aspects of a person's surroundings such as their housing, their neighbourhood, the water they drink and the air they breathe. In general these are things over which individuals have little control. Lifestyle refers to aspects of the way people live over which they have some control, such as smoking, eating and drinking. The distinction between environment and lifestyle is not clear cut and in many situations people have little real choice over lifestyle issues. The environment has a major influence on lifestyle and the lifestyle can modify the effect of the environment.

Some of the major influences on health are listed in Table 3.1.

GENETICS

Everyone is born with a set of genetic material which controls their future growth and development and determines their potential. The maximum height to which a person can grow is determined by their genes, but they will not reach that height if they are malnourished or suffer repeated infections while they are growing. Some diseases such as thalassaemia (a failure to make red blood cells properly)

Table 3.1 Some factors that influence health

Genetic make up	
Basic needs	warmth and shelter food and water freedom from physical violence
Physical environment	housing drinking water / sewerage air quality food quality and safety roads transport noise workplace
Lifestyle	smoking eating drinking exercise illicit drug use safe sex practices use of medical services
Environmental constraints on lifestyle	availability of facilities (exercise, food choice in shops) peer pressure advertising cultural pressures education

and haemophilia (a failure of the blood to clot properly) are entirely genetically determined. There are many more diseases in which genetics have some influence but non-genetic factors are much more important. Examples of such diseases are diabetes, coronary heart disease, breast cancer and stomach cancer (Emery and Mueller 1992). Health promotion cannot alter genetics but it can help people to make the best of what their genes make possible.

ENVIRONMENT

The conditions under which a person lives have a major effect on how healthy they will be. The improvements in health which were seen in the early part of this century were largely due to an improved physical environment.

WHOLESOME DRINKING WATER

Many infectious diseases such as cholera, typhoid and polio are carried in water. The organisms that cause these diseases can get into drinking water if human excreta are not properly disposed of. One of the great achievements of the Victorians was to build sewage and water systems so that public supplies of drinking water became safe. Many countries in the third world still do not enjoy this benefit (Diamant 1992).

There is no room for complacency. Even in developed countries, water supplies are sometimes contaminated. There have been several recent outbreaks of infectious diarrhoea in children in the UK caused by Cryptosporidium. These were almost certainly due to contamination of the water supplies with this protozoal organism (DoH 1990).

Water must not only be free of disease-causing micro-organisms but it must also be free of other harmful substances (Monkley-Poole 1992). Even if the water coming to the house is pure, the water coming out of the tap may have quite high levels of lead and other toxic metals. This is because many houses still have lead piping from which toxic metals get into the domestic supply. In several areas of Britain the levels of nitrate in water are higher than allowed by EU standards. There is also concern that pesticides and herbicides used in agriculture may contaminate some water supplies.

RECREATIONAL WATER

Water is used not only for drinking but also for enjoyment. Swimming in the sea should be a healthy and pleasurable activity. However, a large number of UK beaches are heavily contaminated with sewage. In addition to exposing swimmers to risk of infection from faecal organisms, it is thoroughly unpleasant. Many rivers and canals are also heavily polluted so that virtually no plant or animal can survive in them. This too detracts from people's quality of life (Walker 1992).

HOUSING

Warmth and shelter are among the most basic needs of humans. People living in cold, damp housing are much more likely to develop asthma and respiratory infections. This is particularly true for children. Crowded housing increases the likelihood of transmission of infection between residents. Bad housing also predisposes to psychological illness. Poor design and poor maintenance greatly increase the risk of accidents within the home.

Many of our large cities had slum areas in which the housing conditions were terrible. These were largely replaced by modern buildings. Unfortunately the design of the new buildings was often little better than that of the old so that the problems of damp and cold were not solved. Worse still, the new buildings frequently broke up the close community, adding problems of isolation and loneliness. High-rise blocks in particular were often unsatisfactory when vandalism and poor maintenance of lifts left residents of upper floors virtually imprisoned in their homes (Coleman 1985). Thoughtful housing design fosters health not only by providing a safe physical environment but by fostering development of a real community in which the residents have meaningful control of their environment (Lowry 1989; Ineichen 1993).

AIR

The importance of air quality was dramatically illustrated in the London smogs of the 1950s, which caused a very large number of deaths (Figure 3.1). It has been suggested that air pollution exacerbates chronic bronchitis and asthma and plays a part in respiratory infections and possibly lung cancer. Children may be particularly vulnerable (Read 1991). Man-made pollutants in air include smoke particles, sulphur dioxide, oxides of nitrogen, and volatile organic compounds. Reactions of these in the atmosphere then produce acid aerosols and ozone. Coal- and oil-burning power plants, industry and domestic heating systems can produce very large quantities of particles and sulphur dioxide. Motor vehicles are important producers of nitrogen oxides and contribute to the formation of ozone (Anon 1991). The seriousness of the pollution produced by these sources depends very much on the ways in which fuel is used, the design and location of chimney stacks and the atmospheric conditions.

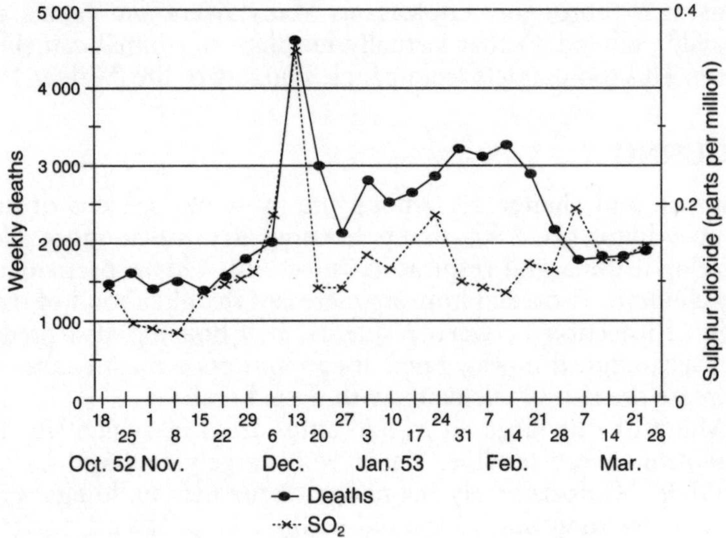

Figure 3.1 Deaths caused by the London smog, 1952
The figure shows the number of deaths per week in London in the winter of 1952/53. It also shows the concentration of sulphur dioxide in the air. Note the large peak in deaths in December which coincides with a peak in sulphur dioxide concentration. This occurred during one of the London 'smogs', a period in which atmospheric conditions produced a very large build-up of sulphur dioxide and other pollutants in the atmosphere.
Source Adapted from Morris J.N. (1974), *Uses of epidemiology*, 3rd edition; Edinburgh: Churchill.

Problems such as the London smog were largely due to domestic and industrial coal burning, which produced high levels of smoke particles and sulphur dioxide (see Figure 3.1). The Clean Air Acts have regulated the location of industry and the types of fuel which can be burnt. This has considerably improved air quality and smogs no longer occur in the UK. Air pollution due to road traffic (mostly nitrogen oxides, and volatile organic compounds) has got worse. Big cities such as Tokyo and Los Angeles experience photo-chemical smogs chiefly due to vehicle exhausts.

Air pollution is still a problem to those living near industrial zones. They may frequently complain of smell and nuisance from this cause. Even if this does not cause physical disease (and it probably does) it makes life unpleasant and damages mental well-being.

POLLUTION ON A GLOBAL SCALE

Recently we have become aware of air pollution on a larger scale. Some solutions such as taller chimney stacks may prevent local inconvenience but they only move the problem elsewhere. It has been suggested that sulphur dioxide vented from UK power stations is contributing to acid rain hundreds of miles away in Scandinavian countries.

Global warming due to the 'greenhouse effect' of carbon dioxide, methane and other gases in the atmosphere could change climate systems affecting the health of millions (McMichael 1993). Depletion of the ozone layer in the upper atmosphere by CFCs (chlorofluorocarbons) and other man-made gases, leading to reduced protection against natural ultraviolet radiation, could be followed by a greatly increased risk of skin cancers (WHO 1992).

LITTER AND GRAFFITI

You may be surprised to see this in a list of factors affecting health but there is no doubt that people are offended by litter and graffiti. These things probably do not cause physical disease but they interfere with people's enjoyment of their surroundings and harm their mental well-being. Litter and graffiti are not just problems in themselves, they are also symptoms of problems in society, indicating a feeling of alienation and lack of care for the environment in which we live.

TRANSPORT SYSTEMS

The influence of transport on health has to be viewed from the point of view both of those inside the vehicle and of those outside. Cars are convenient for their drivers, allow swift travel to the exact location and are warm, secure and generally safe. The negative effect on the driver's health of lack of physical exercise could largely be overcome by using the time saved in travel for recreational exercise. The health problems of cars relate largely to the rest of the community. Pedestrians and other road users are likely to suffer far more in a traffic accident than the occupants of any car involved. Furthermore, the environment is degraded by the need to construct roads with their attendant nuisance and health hazards of noise, dust and emissions (Wolff and Gilham 1991). The problems are particularly severe where traffic through residential areas is heavy. Even in developed countries such as the UK, it is a minority who benefit from car use. Thirty one per cent of households do not have use of a car (Central Statistical Office 1994) and even in families which do it is usually only one member of the family who has use of the car most of the time.

A similar analysis applies to the carriage of freight by road. Road transport may be convenient for the individual freight user who obtains fast delivery of their goods at low cost. The end consumer may also benefit by cheaper goods. However, the use of this mode of transport imposes significant costs on the rest of the community.

Public transport systems such as buses or trains impose a much lighter environmental burden on the community. On the other hand, travelling on such systems may be an unhealthy activity – as anyone using an overcrowded long-distance commuter route can testify. In addition, inadequate public transport systems force frustrated travellers to wait long periods in the cold and wet. This can damage both their mental and their physical health.

The pedestrian and cyclist might be considered to have a very healthy mode of transport (Friends of the Earth 1990; BMA 1992). They make minimal impact on the environment and improve their physical fitness at the same time. The disadvantage is that they are restricted in their choice of activities to those fairly near to them. Pedestrians and cyclists are also at risk from accidents. While modern cars give considerable protection to their occupants so they have a good chance of surviving accidents, pedestrians and cyclists have no such protection. The solution is to separate pedestrians and cyclists from vehicular traffic by providing separate walkways and cycle tracks. Very little progress has been made in providing such facilities for pedestrians and cyclists in Britain. Cycle helmets are also useful in giving some protection to cyclists.

This short discussion indicates that all forms of transport have health benefits for some people and harm the health of others. In the interests of health it is essential to have a balanced transport plan which maximises the benefits of transport, minimises the costs and fairly distributes both among the population.

THE WORKPLACE

Many people spend a great deal of their lives in their place of employment. Legislation covers not only those working with obvious hazards to health such as dangerous chemicals, machinery and processes, but all workers. The workplace must not be forgotten in the drive to make people's environment more conducive to health. Health in the workplace is described more fully in Chapter 17.

Discussion/Activity 3.1 How healthy is your environment?

Think of your home and neighbourhood or think of your hospital. How healthy an environment is it? What are the features that promote health? What are the features that damage health?

FOOD

In order to be healthy a person requires food which:

- supplies enough energy and nutrients
- is wholesome, i.e. free of pathogenic bacteria and free of natural or man-made toxins
- is nutritionally balanced

Adequate nutrients

A healthy diet has to supply enough energy, protein, vitamins, minerals and other essential nutrients to maintain the body and to support physical activity (Truswell 1992). It must also supply sufficient energy for growth in children, for foetal growth in pregnant women and for lactation in breastfeeding mothers. The commonest dietary problem in the world is not having enough food of any kind, leading to protein energy malnutrition. This is still depressingly common in developing countries and until the present century was not uncommon in this country. Where the diet supplies enough energy it may still be deficient in particular nutrients.

Table 3.2 list some of the diseases caused by vitamin or mineral deficiencies. Provided a person's diet supplies enough energy and is reasonably varied, they are very unlikely to develop these deficiencies. Infectious disease or other illness will increase the individual's need for nutrients and may precipitate deficiencies in people on a poor diet.

Wholesome food

Healthy food must be wholesome, that is to say free of harmful bacteria and other infectious organisms and free of toxic substances. Bacteria on food can cause disease either by multiplying inside the body after the food has been eaten (e.g. Salmonella) or by making toxins which cause symptoms when the food is eaten (e.g. Staphylococci or botulism). The raw material of food may be infected (e.g. meat from infected animals or eggs from infected birds) or the food may become infected during storage or prepara-

Table 3.2 Some diseases caused by nutritional deficiency

Nutrient	Disease
energy	protein energy malnutrition
vitamin C	scurvy
B vitamins	
niacin	pellagra
thiamin	beri-beri
folate	anaemia
vitamin D	osteomalacia, rickets
vitamin A	xeropthalmia, blindness
iodine	goitre, cretinism
iron	anaemia (usually associated with blood loss through gut)

tion. Fungal organisms also produce toxins which make food dangerous. Ergot poisoning used to be common in Europe and contamination of grain by aflatoxin (another fungal toxin) is still a common problem in parts of Africa. Strict supervision of all stages of food production is needed to keep it free of infection. Refrigeration and other methods of preserving and storing food have done a great deal to make food safer. Here are some ways of keeping food safe:

- good animal husbandry to reduce infection
- inspection at slaughterhouse to keep diseased animals out of food chain
- storage in proper conditions
- rejection of suspect food by caterer
- cooking at adequate temperature
- kitchen hygiene
- proper storage of prepared foods

Toxic substances – man-made or natural – in food can also be injurious to health. Some things such as toadstools are naturally poisonous. Other foods become contaminated with toxic substances from the environment in which they are produced. There was a major outbreak of heavy metal poisoning in Japan due to people eating fish from polluted water. Pesticides and other substances used during food production may still be present in the food when it is eaten. Rigorous quality control at all stages of the food chain is needed to ensure food is free of toxic substances.

LIFESTYLE

The word lifestyle is used to describe those aspects of the way a person lives over which they have some choice.

CHOOSING A BALANCED DIET

There is a strong suspicion that the way we eat plays a part in causing many of the diseases which are now common. Despite the fact that most people eat foods which are wholesome and supply enough nutrients, the balance of the diet increases their risk of disease. People in this country tend to eat a diet which is rich in fat, especially saturated fat, rich in refined carbohydrates such as sugar, and poor in dietary fibre and complex carbohydrate. It is suggested that if we reverse this trend, then diseases such as heart disease (DHSS 1984; James 1988), diabetes, hypertension (high blood pressure) and strokes would be less common. Table 3.3 summarises the recommendations of a recent expert committee.

MAINTAINING BODY WEIGHT

Being very overweight is associated with an increased risk of death and an increased risk of numerous diseases including heart disease, gallstones, diabetes, gout, arthritis and complications after any operation (Royal College of Physicians 1983). Being very underweight is also associated with an increased risk of death (see Figure 3.2). The old idea that being overweight was simply due to eating too much is a gross over-simplification but it is true that regulating body weight requires a balancing of energy intake (what we eat) and energy utilisation (exercise). Views about body weight are coloured by a host of cultural expectations and not a few unhelpful stereotypes. There is no doubt that many people have a profoundly unhealthy obsession with their weight and make themselves miserable by repeated attempts to lose weight by dieting. Thoughtless harping on the medical dangers of overweight may exacerbate this. There are however many people who would feel healthier if they managed to reduce their weight.

SMOKING

No single change would produce more benefit to the health of the country than if everyone stopped smoking (HEA 1991) but many

Table 3.3 Recommendations for healthy diet

- adjust energy intake to maintain 'ideal' body weight
- reduce percentage of energy derived from fat (and in particular from saturated fat)
- increase consumption of dietary fibres
- increase consumption of complex carbohydrates

Source National Advisory Committee on Nutrition Education (NACNE) (1983).

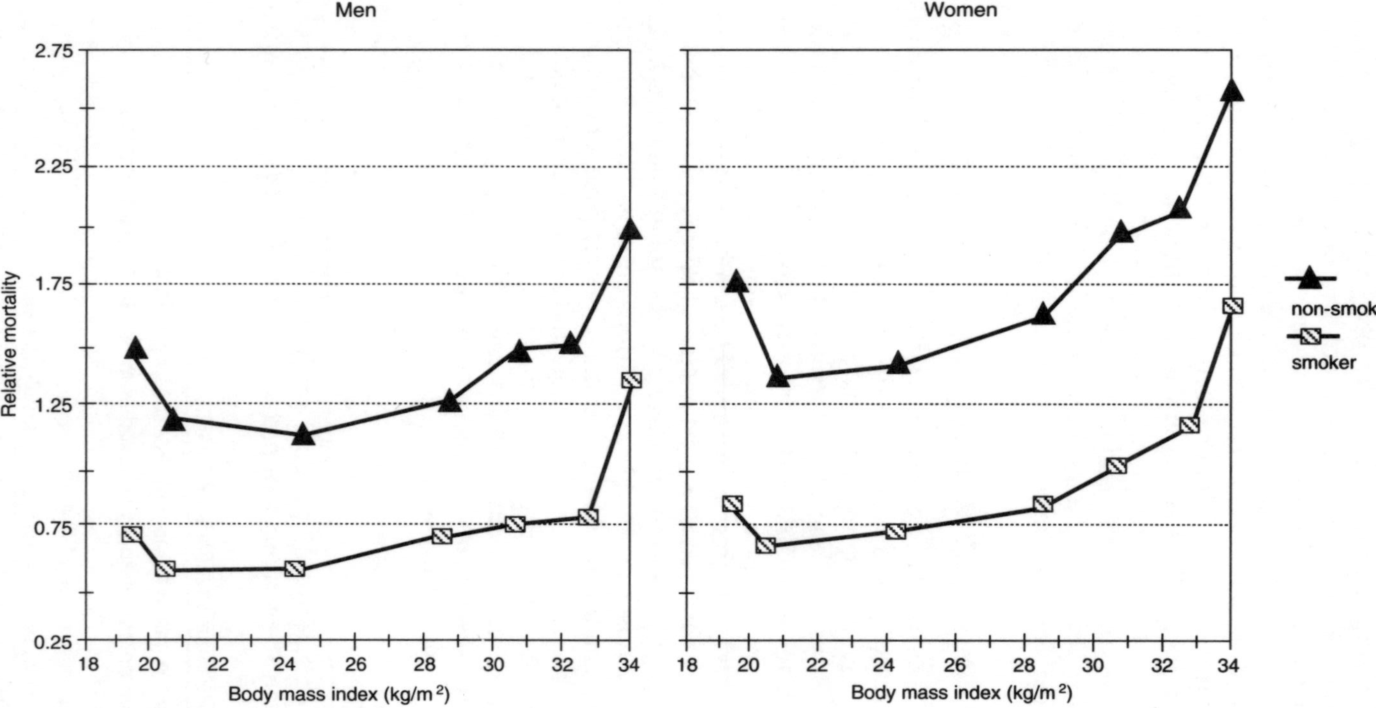

Figure 3.2 Relative mortality and body mass index
The figure shows relative mortality in smokers and non-smokers for men and women. The average mortality is 1, so a relative mortality of 2 indicates a risk of death two times the average. Body mass is a measure of fatness (weight in kilograms / height in metres squared). Note that mortality in smokers is always higher than mortality in non-smokers. Note also that mortality is lowest around the range 20–25 kg/m^2 and is higher in those with very high and very low body mass index.
Source Adapted from Expert Committeee (1983), *Journal of Royal College of Physicians* **17**, 6–65.

Table 3.4 Tobacco-related disease

heart disease
peripheral vascular disease
chronic bronchitis and emphysema
asthma
lung cancer
upper respiratory tract infections
gastritis
peptic ulcer
bladder cancer
osteoporosis
hypertension
low birth weight babies

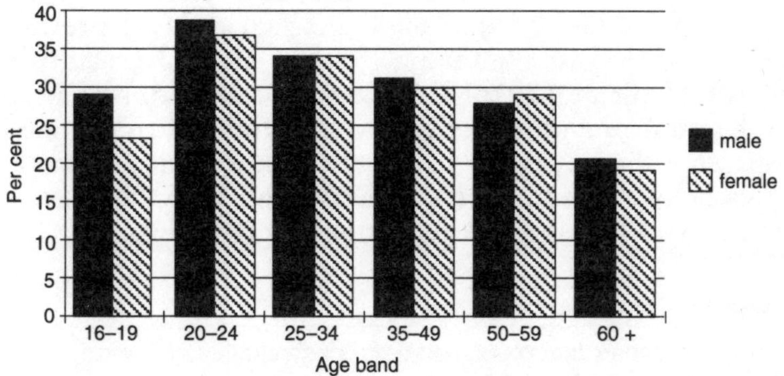

Figure 3.3 Prevalence of smoking, 1992
This figure shows the percentage of men and women who smoke in different age groups. Note that in the youngest age group women smoke more than men.
Source Data from OPCS (1993), *General household survey 1992.*

people still smoke (see Figure 3.3). It affects virtually every organ in the body and contributes to a host of diseases (some of which are listed in Table 3.4). Once they have taken up smoking, people find it difficult to stop because they have become habituated to nicotine and for a while feel uncomfortable without smoking.

PASSIVE SMOKING

Non-smokers who live or work with smokers have to breath in their smoke (this is called passive smoking). There is now strong evidence that those exposed to other people's smoke in this way have a small but measurable increase in risk of lung cancer (Jarvis 1992; Heath 1993). Children exposed to passive smoking have an increased risk of upper respiratory tract and ear infections. Very many fires are caused by the careless discarding of cigarettes. In addition to this, non-smokers are inconvenienced by the smell of smoke. There is thus a need to balance the rights of smokers to smoke against the rights of non-smokers not to have their environment degraded and their health put at risk by others smoking.

ALCOHOL

Alcohol is the second biggest lifestyle cause of ill health after smoking (see Figure 3.4). Like smoking, alcohol affects just about every organ of the body and can cause a wide range of diseases (see Table 3.5).

Alcohol is however a more complicated problem than smoking because it is accepted that individuals and society derive several real benefits from the use of alcohol, and the need is to prevent harmful use of alcohol rather than all use of alcohol (Faculty of Public Health Medicine 1991; HEA 1993). Alcohol drinking is unlikely to be harmful provided it is kept within the low risk range (for men not more than 21 units in a week, for women not more than 14 units per week) and is kept separate from activities such as driving or any work requiring skill, alertness or co-ordination.

Table 3.5 Alcohol-related disease

acute intoxication, blackouts, cerebellar degeneration, dementia
peripheral neuropathy
strokes
hepatitis, cirrhosis
oesophagitis
gastritis
diarrhoea and malabsorption
pancreatitis
cardiomyopathy
high blood pressure
pneumonia due to inhaled vomit
cancer oesophagus, larynx, pharynx
head injuries
suicide
endocrine disturbance
obesity
reactions with medication
men: loss of libido, impotency, infertility
women: sexual difficulties, menstrual irregularities
psychological disorders
Other alcohol-related problems
criminal and public disorder
problems at work
social and family problems
road and other accidents
fire and drowning

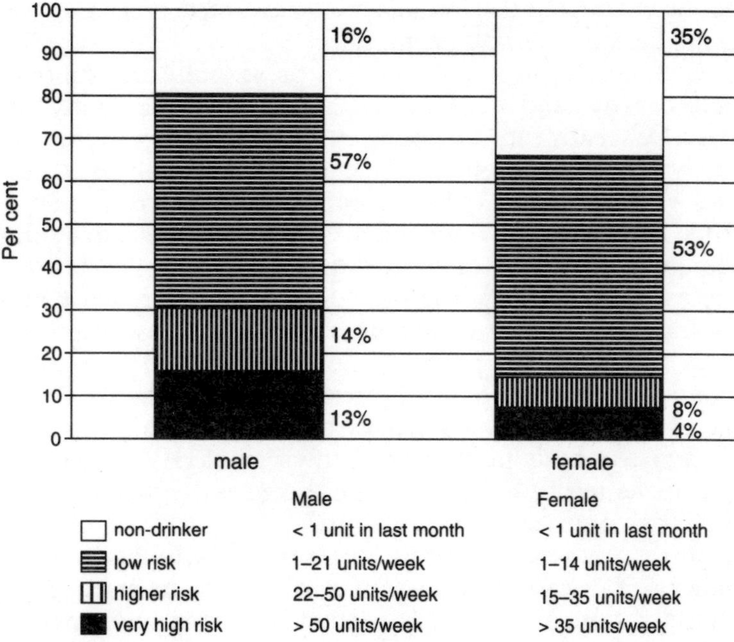

Figure 3.4 Drinking patterns in men and women, 1992
Definitions of drinking pattern are given in the key. Note that 27% of men and 11% of women are drinking above the low risk level (21 units/week men 14 units/week women).
Source Data from OPCS (1993), *General household survey 1992.*

SAFE SEXUAL PRACTICES

Sexual activity is another aspect of lifestyle which can either add greatly to happiness or be the cause of much unhappiness and ill health. Health damage can arise in three ways:

1. unwanted pregnancy
2. sexually transmitted disease (including AIDS)
3. violation of principles of self-esteem and concern for others.

The birth of a child is usually a source of great joy but when it follows an unwanted pregnancy this is not so, and the child may face increased risk of being unloved and possibly abused. If the pregnancy is terminated then the mother's health may be damaged by the physical and psychological stress of an induced abortion. Improved methods of contraception should allow women to take control of their own fertility, but lack of real understanding means that many unintended pregnancies still occur, particularly in the young. Reducing the frequency of unwanted pregnancy is clearly a contribution to health promotion.

Several infectious diseases can be sexually transmitted in both heterosexual and homosexual activity. Until recently there were effective treatments for many of these and they were often incorrectly viewed as unimportant mishaps that medicine could quickly and easily sort out. The advent of HIV infection and AIDS has forced everyone to attach a new seriousness to sexually transmitted disease. Until an effective treatment for HIV is developed, preventing its transmission is the only defence we have. Behaviours which increase the risk of acquiring a sexually transmitted disease are large numbers of partners and frequent changes of partner. Condoms create a physical barrier and offer a useful (but not complete) degree of protection. Sex practices which do not involve the exchange of body fluids carry a low risk of HIV transmission. 'Safe sex' is the term used to describe these sexual practices which minimise risk of disease transmission.

To discuss sexual activity in terms of avoiding unwanted pregnancy and disease transmission is to miss the most important health consideration. Outside the context of caring relationships, sexual activity all too easily involves the exploitation of one partner. A health promotion view of sexual activity seeks to ensure that it enhances the well-being of both partners.

PHYSICAL EXERCISE

Physical activity both promotes positive health and decreases the risk of disease (Fentem, Bassey and Turnbull 1988). People who exercise regularly increase all aspects of fitness (strength, stamina, suppleness) and most also claim that it increases their sense of well-being. A sedentary lifestyle increases risk of heart disease and other conditions such as osteoporosis.

Discussion/Activity 3.2 How healthy is your lifestyle?

Think about your lifestyle. What things about it are health-enhancing? What things about it are health-damaging? Why do you do the health-enhancing and the health-damaging things? Are the lifestyles of your patients likely to be influenced by similar considerations?

ENVIRONMENTAL INFLUENCES ON LIFESTYLE

The previous section discussed lifestyles rather as though people made up their minds about these behaviours unaffected by the situation in which they find themselves. In reality they are influenced in all sorts of ways by the society and environment in which they live and we always have to ask to what extent people really can make choices about their own lifestyle. Graham (1993) has analysed the pressures which can make it so difficult for women to choose not to smoke in some circumstances.

One set of constraints on lifestyle comes from the physical environment. A person cannot choose to swim unless they have some suitable water nearby. A woman cannot choose to go out jogging if the neighbourhood around her is not safe. Someone cannot choose to eat wholemeal bread or fresh vegetables if the shops to which they have access do not stock these things.

Money imposes another set of constraints which limit lifestyle and environment (Blackburn 1991). Those with a generous income can usually buy the things they need to exercise healthy choice. On the other hand, those on a very tight budget are barred from many games because they cannot buy the equipment needed or pay the other costs of participation. Someone may know all about health risks in the home and the need for safety equipment but if they cannot afford to replace dangerous items they have little choice but to remain at risk. If the food budget is tight and the electricity cut off because the bill has not been paid, eating choices may be restricted to the cheapest food which does not need preparation.

The culture in which a person lives also limits their choice of lifestyle in all sorts of ways. A young man who lives in an environment where heavy drinking is considered an expression of machoism and manliness is under very strong pressure to do likewise. A child whose peer group are smokers will find it difficult to resist the pressure to join them in smoking. These cultural pressures may well be augmented by advertising which subtly suggests that smoking or drinking is smart and glamorous.

INEQUALITIES OF HEALTH

One of the most striking features of health in all countries is the inequality between different groups. These inequalities will be illustrated by reference to social class and ethnicity. If we had a better understanding of why these differences existed, we could probably use that knowledge for more effective health promotion.

SOCIAL-CLASS GRADIENTS IN HEALTH

Social class can be defined in several ways but the most commonly used system in the UK is based on people's occupation. There is a

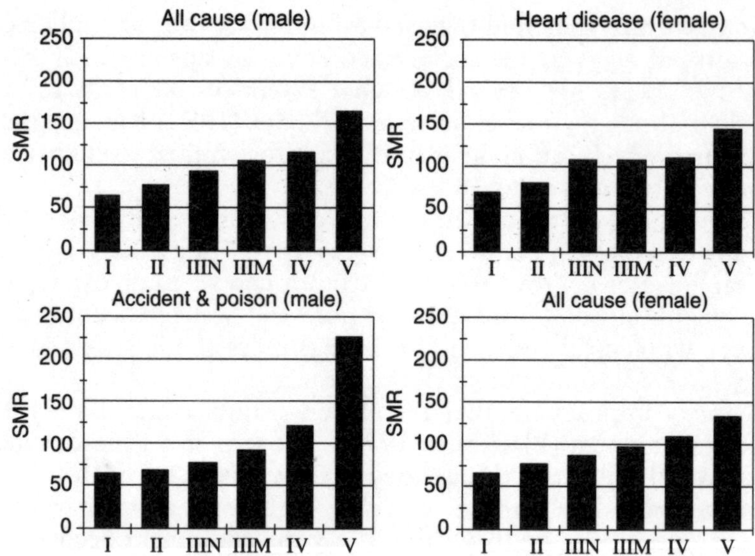

Figure 3.5 Class gradients in mortality
The figure shows Standard Mortality Ratios (SMRs) for men (all causes, heart disease, and accidents and poisoning) and for women (all causes). People are usually classified into the five classes I to V. Social class III is further subdivided into IIIN (skilled non-manual occupations) and IIIM (skilled manual occupations). Note that in every case there is a gradient of SMR from lowest in social class I to highest in social class V. (SMRs are explained in Chapter 4, pages 70 and 71.)
Source Data from OPCS (Office of Population Censuses and Surveys) (1986), *Occupational mortality: decennial supplement 1979–1980*; London: HMSO.

striking gradient in health with social class (see Figure 3.5). Social class V has higher death rates from a wide variety of causes than social class I. Those in social class V are more likely to suffer illness and disease. Children from social class V are more likely to die as babies and they grow more slowly than those from social class I.

What is it about social class that has such a strong influence on health? Lifestyle explains some of the differences. Social class V has higher smoking rates, and lower consumption of fruit and vegetables, but this is not nearly enough to explain the gradient. Poor housing, less congenial living environment, more difficulty in obtaining and using medical care, and less financial resources also explain some of the gradient but such factors are unlikely to explain it all.

ETHNIC DIFFERENCES

The UK is now a multiracial community but when we examine the health of different ethnic groups we find significant differences in health experience (Balarajan and Raleigh 1993). Among the communities with ethnic origins in the Indian subcontinent, death rates for heart disease, tuberculosis and diabetes are much higher than in the indigenous community, while death rates for most cancers are lower. Sickle cell anaemia occurs in Afro-Caribbeans but not in other groups. Strokes and hypertension are more common in Afro-Caribbeans than in the indigenous community, while heart disease is less common (see Figure 3.6).

Why do these differences exist? Genetic differences explain the occurrence of sickle cell anaemia but probably do not explain the

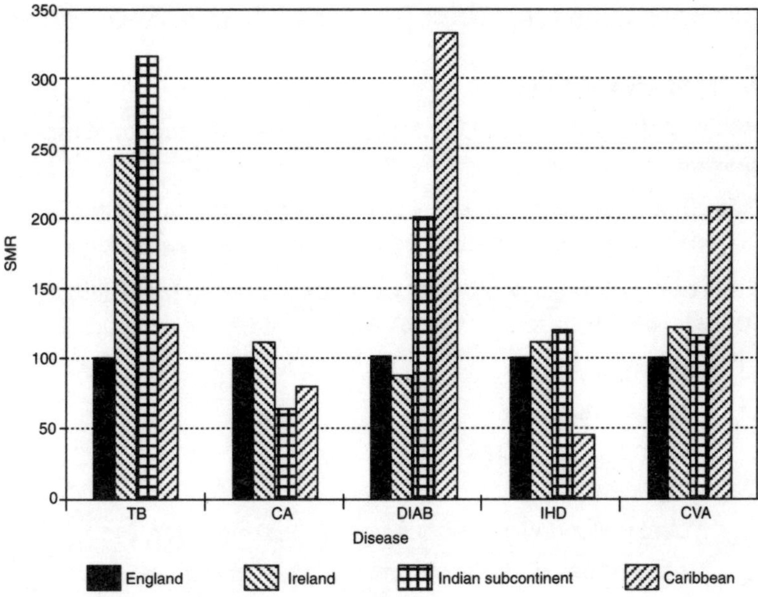

Figure 3.6 Ethnic differences in mortality
The figure shows Standard Mortality Ratios for tuberculosis (TB), cancer (CA), diabetes (DIAB), ischaemic heart disease (IHD) and strokes (CVA) for people born in different parts of the world. There are considerable differences between the various ethnic groups. Note that while the Indian subcontinent and Caribbean groups have higher SMRs for TB, diabetes and stroke, they have lower SMRs for cancer. (SMRs are explained in Chapter 4, pages 70 and 71.)
Source Data from Marmot M. Adelstein A.M. and Bulusu L. (1984), *Immigrant Mortality in England & Wales 1970–1978*. Studies on Population and Medical Subjects no. 47; OPCS/HMSO.

differences in the other diseases. Lifestyle may explain some of the other differences between ethnic groups though existing explanations are very incomplete.

UNEMPLOYMENT

Unemployed people have worse health than those in employment (Smith 1987; Office of Health Economics 1993). They have higher death rates, are more likely to commit suicide, are more likely to suffer from chronic ill health and have more psychiatric illness. In part this can be explained by people being unable to get or keep a job because they are already ill. In part it may be explained by unemployed people being deprived in other ways in addition to having no job. A job gives someone not only an income, but also status, social contact, a structure for their days, and self-esteem. It is therefore not surprising to find that being without a job harms people's health.

SUMMARY POINTS

Health is the result of the interaction of genetics, environment and lifestyle.

Genetics determines an individual's health potential but the expression of genetic potential is influenced by environment and lifestyle.

Environment describes things over which people have little or no control, such as:

- ☐ drinking water
- ☐ recreational water
- ☐ housing
- ☐ air quality
- ☐ global pollution (greenhouse gases, ozone layer, etc.)
- ☐ pleasantness of the environment (litter, graffiti, etc.)
- ☐ transport systems
- ☐ workplace

Lifestyle describes those aspect of living over which people have considerable control, such as:

- ☐ choosing a balanced diet
- ☐ maintaining body weight
- ☐ not smoking (and not exposed to passive smoking)
- ☐ following safe sex practices
- ☐ taking physical exercise

People's ability to make lifestyle choices is constrained by the physical and social environment in which they live.

There are striking inequalities in health:

- ☐ between social classes
- ☐ between ethnic groups
- ☐ between unemployed and employed

REFERENCES

Anon (1991). Ozone too much in the wrong place. *Lancet* **338**, 221–222.

Balarajan R. and Raleigh V.S. (1993). *Ethnicity and health: a guide for the NHS.* London: Department of Health.

Blackburn C. (1991). *Poverty and health: working with families.* Milton Keynes: Open University Press.

BMA (British Medical Association) (1992). *Cycling towards health and safety.* Oxford: Oxford University Press.

Central Statistical Office (1994). Transport. Chapter 13 in *Social Trends* **24**. London: HMSO.

Coleman A. (1985). *Utopia on trial: Vision and reality in planned housing.* London: Shipman.

DHSS (Department of Health and Social Security) (1984). *Diet and cardiovascular disease. Report of the panel on diet in relation to cardiovascular disease.* Committee on Medical Aspects of Food Policy. London: HMSO.

Diamant B.Z. (1992). Assessment and evaluation of the International Water Decade. *Journal of Royal Society of Health* **112**, 183–188.

DoH (Department of Health) (1990). *Group of experts. Report on cryptosporidium in water supples* (Badenoch Report). London: HMSO.

Emery A.E.H. and Mueller R.F. (1992). Genetic factors in some common diseases. Chapter 10 in *Elements of medical genetics* (6th edition). Edinburgh; Churchill Livingstone.

Faculty of Public Health Medicine (1991). *Alcohol and the public health.* Basingstoke: Macmillan Education Ltd.

Fentem P., Bassey J. and Turnbull N.B. (1988). *The new case for exercise.* London Sports Council and Health Education Authority.

Friends of the Earth (1990). *Cycling and the healthy city.* London: Friends of the Earth.

Graham H. (1993). *When life's a drag: women smoking and disadvantage.* London: HMSO.

HEA (Health Education Authority) (1991). *Health Update No. 2: Smoking.* London: Health Education Authority.

HEA (Health Education Authority) (1993). *Health Update No. 3: Alcohol.* London: Health Education Authority.

Heath C.W. (1993). Passive smoking: environmental tobacco smoke and lung cancer. *Lancet* **341**, 526.

Ineichen B. (1993). *Homes and health.* London: Spon.

James W.P.T. (1988). *Healthy nutrition: preventing nutrition related disease in Europe.* WHO European Regional Publication No. 24.

Jarvis M. (1992). Passive smoking. In Heller T., Bailey L. and Pattison S. (eds.), *Preventing cancers.* Buckingham: Open University Press.

Lowry S. (1991). *Housing and health.* London: British Medical Journal.

McMichael A. (1993) Global environmental change and human population: a conceptual and scientific challenge for epidemiology. *International Journal of Epidemiology* **22**, 1–8.

Monkley-Poole S. (1992). Nursing responses to environmental issues. *Nursing Standards* **6** (No. 28), 32–33.

National Advisory Committee on Nutrition Education (NACNE) (1983). *A discussion paper on proposals for nutritional guidelines for health education in Britain*. London: Health Education Council.

Office of Health Economics (1993). *Briefing Number 29: Impact of unemployment on health.*

OPCS (Office of Population Censuses and Surveys) (1993). *General household survey 1992*. London: HMSO.

Read C. (1991). *Air pollution and child health*. London: Greenpeace.

Royal College of Physicians (1983). Obesity. A report of the Royal College of Physicians. *Journal of the Royal College of Physicians London* **17**, 3–58.

Smith A. (1992). Setting a strategy for health. *British Medical Journal* **304**, 376–378.

Smith R. (1987). *Unemployment and health*. Oxford: Oxford University Press.

Strauss W. and Mainwaring S.J. (1984). *Air pollution*. London: Edward Arnold.

Truswell A.S. (1992). *A.B.C. of nutrition* (2nd edition). London: British Medical Journal.

Walker A. (1992). Swimming – the hazards of taking a dip. *British Medical Journal* **304**, 242–246.

WHO (World Health Organisation)(1992). *Our planet, our health*. Geneva: WHO.

Wolff S.P. and Gilham C.J. (1991). Public health versus public policy: An appraisal of British urban transport policy. *Public Health* **105**, 217–225.

CHAPTER 4

Uncovering cause

GOAL

To examine theories about causes of ill health and health and to distinguish well-founded from ill-founded theories.

OBJECTIVES

- to identify the types of evidence supporting causal theories
- to explore the strengths and limitations of epidemiological evidence in revealing cause
- to discuss the nature of evidence supporting a link between dietary fat and heart disease
- to describe what a Standardised Mortality Ratio (SMR) is and the reasons for using it
- to explore the advantages and disadvantages of high risk and population strategies in health promotion

HOW DO WE KNOW WHAT AFFECTS HEALTH?

All health promotion is built on theories that by influencing people's environment or lifestyle in particular ways their chances of enjoying health can be improved (Campbell 1993). If these theories are incorrect, the health promotion activity becomes at best useless and probably positively harmful (Skrabenek 1991). The previous chapter gave a list of environmental and lifestyle factors (Table 3.1) which influenced health and ways in which they could be modified so as to improve health. How sure can you be that the changes suggested really will make people healthier?

In general we believe these theories because they have been told to us by other people whom we trust (such as our teachers) or because we have read them in a book or journal that we believe to be reliable. Most of the time there really is no alternative to relying on others but when we do this the theories we believe are no sounder than our judgment as to whom we can trust on each particular issue.

DISAGREEMENT AND UNCERTAINTY

For any theory one can almost always find someone who is prepared to put forward a conflicting theory. Certainly every one of the theories about factors influencing health listed in the previous chapter will be disputed by someone. Sometimes very well-informed people will disagree about things (for example, the links between dietary fat and heart disease (Ahrens 1985) or between fibre and bowel cancer (Modan 1992) are denied by some very eminent medical scientists). How then do we decide which view to accept?

It is salutary to remember that much health promotion activity in the past has been based on what now seems to be incorrect theory. You do not have to look very far back to find health educators advising people to cut back on starchy foods because they were 'fattening'. Now we are advising people to eat more of those foods and suggesting that they try and use them to replace some fatty foods in their diet. At one time there used to be great emphasis on the need to cut down dietary cholesterol in order to reduce heart disease but now dietary cholesterol is regarded as relatively unimportant and the emphasis is on saturated fats. Obviously we have to scrutinise the evidence for any particular bit of advice very carefully (Kemm 1991).

SORTING SENSE FROM NONSENSE

A counsel of perfection would be to examine the evidence for each theory for ourselves. The next part of this chapter will discuss some of the ways of doing that. However, in reality there is often not enough time to check everything in this way and even if we had the time we frequently do not have the necessary skills. There are a few rough and ready rules for sorting out sense from nonsense:

- How reputable is the source?
- Is the source disinterested?
- What is the consensus view?
- Are there confirmatory studies?
- Is it biologically plausible?
- Is it statistically respectable?

In general we will attach more weight to the views of someone who has a long track record of working in the field than to the views of someone who apparently has no training or skills. The scientist who has studied the field for years (provided they stick to the topics in which they are competent) is more likely to be reliable than the campaigning journalist.

Similarly we will be suspicious of those who have an interest in the view they express. We should treat with caution the employee of the tobacco industry who claims smoking does you no harm, or the 'organic' food producer who claims that all goods produced in other ways are harmful to health. A consensus view may be some help. We may be less inclined to believe someone if all their colleagues hold a different view. When an observation is correct it is usually rapidly repeated in confirmatory studies by different workers in different populations. The observation that can only be made by one group of workers and cannot be repeated by others is unlikely to be sound.

Theories which fit in with our general understanding of how things usually work (i.e. are biologically plausible) are more likely to be correct than ones which completely overturn our usual view of the world. Thus the theory that tuberculosis is caused by infection with a particular bacterium is more plausible than the theory that is caused by a particular alignment of planets.

It is also helpful to see if there has been any attempt to apply statistical tests to the observations on which the theory is based.

None of these quick tests is absolutely reliable. There are many examples of the outsider and the revolutionary idea being correct and of the consensus being wrong. None the less, in the absence of other guidance these rules of thumb will be of some help to you in deciding which theories are a sensible base for health promotion and which are not.

Discussion/Activity 4.1 How do we decide which theories to believe?

Here are two theories about influences on health:

1. Fluoridation of water protects teeth against dental caries.
2. Eating refined sugar causes criminal or delinquent behaviour.

Think of some other theories. Apply the tests suggested in the previous section to the theories mentioned and to any others you have thought of. Think why you believe each theory to be true or untrue and how sure you are about the correctness of each judgment.

THE STANDARD OF PROOF

How sure do you have to be before acting on a particular theory linking some aspect of the environment or lifestyle to health? If before acting you require 'absolute proof' or 'proof beyond all reasonable doubt', you will probably do nothing. It is debatable whether such a level of proof is philosophically possible. Very few if any of the theories which are the current base for health promotion could be said to be proven beyond all reasonable doubt.

The question that should be asked about each theory is 'Is there sufficient evidence for it to justify action?' (Orlan 1979). There is no shortage of theories linking environmental factors or lifestyle and health for which the answer to this question is a resounding yes.

LINES OF EVIDENCE

This next section will look at some of the sorts of evidence that can be used to show whether exposure to a particular factor is likely to influence health. The word 'factor' is used as shorthand for some characteristic of the environment or lifestyle. 'Exposure' is the word used to indicate whether an individual has come into contact with that factor. For example in a study of how eating fish affected health, those who regularly ate fish would be called 'exposed' and those who never ate fish 'non-exposed'. The different lines of evidence which might be collected to investigate how a particular factor affects health are listed in Table 4.1.

CLINICAL AND ANECDOTAL EVIDENCE

The first suspicion that a particular environmental or lifestyle factor is a cause of health or disease frequently comes from chance observation. A nurse notices that the last three patients with an unusual type of cancer worked in the local sawmill and wonders if the place of work and the disease might be connected. A new factory opens in the village and the next year two of the babies born in the village

Table 4.1 Lines of evidence that a particular factor influences health

Clinical/Anecdotal
Epidemiological (showing that the factor and disease are associated)

- comparing populations (countries, regions, groups in population)
- secular trends
- case control studies
- cohort studies
- intervention studies

Animal models
Demonstration of possible mechanisms in animals and in man

have congenital malformations. Your old granny drank a glass of carrot juice every day and lived to be 101 in the best of health. Of course these things could be coincidental but they just might be the first clue that leads to the discovery of another factor influencing health.

SHOWING ASSOCIATION

Often the first step in showing that a factor such as smoking or air pollution causes disease is to show that they are associated (i.e. people exposed to the factor are more likely to get the disease). The main method of showing associations of this type is an epidemiological study. Association merely means that these two things tend to occur together. Epidemiology is further explained later in this chapter.

INTER-COUNTRY COMPARISONS

Comparison of different countries or parts of countries may show the frequency of some disease to vary with some environmental or lifestyle factors. For example we can show that cirrhosis tends to be common in countries with a high consumption of alcohol and rare in countries with a low consumption of alcohol (see Figure 4.1). This suggest that high alcohol consumption and cirrhosis are associated.

SECULAR TRENDS

If we look at secular trends in the frequency of a disease (i.e. how it has changed over time), we may find that some environmental or lifestyle factor has also changed. Figure 4.2 shows what happened in a Norwegian community when the food supply was disrupted during the Second World War. When the consumption of sugar decreased the frequency of dental caries in children's teeth decreased and when sugar consumption increased so did dental disease.

National comparisons and secular trends are the weakest sort of epidemiological evidence and the risk of confounding (see page 70) is high. Note that there is nothing in these studies to say that the people who are exposed (drinking the alcohol, eating the sugar) are the people who are getting the disease (cirrhosis, caries).

CASE CONTROL STUDIES

Case control studies are a better way of testing whether a particular factor is associated with a disease. They involve taking a group of

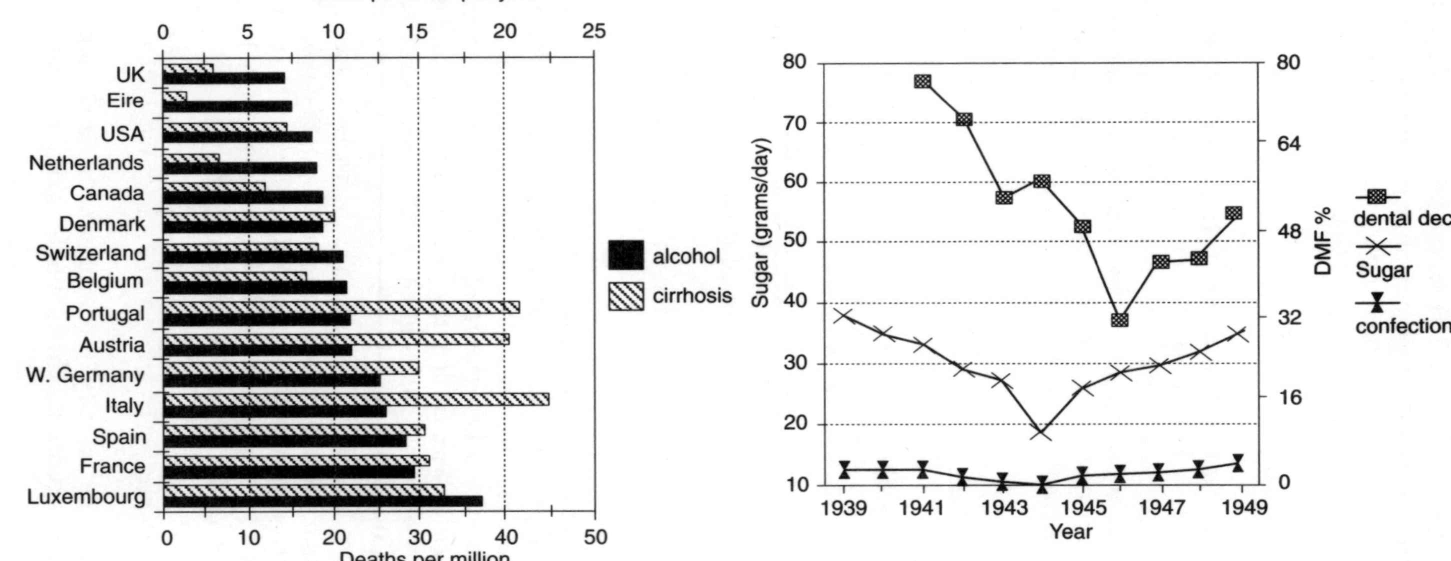

Figure 4.1 National comparisons of cirrhosis and of alcohol consumption
Note that countries with a high per capita consumption of alcohol tend to have a high cirrhosis rate and countries with low consumption tend to have a low cirrhosis rate. Also note that the relationship is not perfect (for example Portugal and Austria have higher rates of cirrhosis than their consumption would suggest). Data are for around the year 1988.
Source Consumption data from *Brewers' Society Statistical Handbook 1987*; London Brewing Publications Ltd. Cirrhosis data from *WHO statistics annual.*

Figure 4.2 Secular trends in sugar consumption and dental caries in Norway during the war
During the Second World War sugar was difficult to obtain and its consumption fell. The frequency of dental caries measured as a percentage of children's teeth that were decayed, missing or filled (DMF%) also fell. After the war these changes were reversed.
Source Data from Toverud G. (1964), *British Dental Journal* **116**, 229.

people with the disease (cases) and a group of people without the disease (controls). We then look to see how many of each group have been exposed to the factor we suspect of causing the disease. If when we compare the groups we find that a higher proportion of cases than of controls have been exposed this suggests that the factor is associated with the disease. Table 4.2 gives an example of data from a case control study showing an association between smoking and cancer of the larynx.

COHORT STUDIES

Cohort studies involve taking a group of people exposed to the factor and a group of people not so exposed. We then follow both sets of people for a period of time to see how many in each group subsequently develop the disease. If we find that more of the people exposed to the factor develop the disease, that shows that the factor

Table 4.2 Smoking and cancer of larynx: an example of a case control study

	Cases: patients with cancer larynx	**Controls**: patients without cancer or lung disease	Relative risk
Non-smokers	9	1436	1
1–20 cigarettes per day	51	780	10.4
21–40 cigarettes per day	74	575	20.5
>40 cigarettes per day	27	155	27.8
	161	2946	

This study looked at the smoking habits of 161 patients with cancer of larynx and 2946 patients admitted to the same hospital who did not have cancer or chronic lung disease. Note how very few of the patients with cancer larynx are non-smokers (9/161), while nearly half the controls are non-smokers. On the other hand, nearly two thirds of the cancer cases (101/161) but less than one quarter of the controls (730/2946) smoke more than 20 per day. This strongly suggests that smoking is associated with cancer of larynx.

This information can be used to calculate how many times greater the risk of cancer of larynx is in smokers than non-smokers (the relative risk). It can be seen that those smoking more than 40 cigarettes per day are 27 times more likely to have cancer of larynx than non-smokers. The observation that relative risk increases with the number of cigarettes smoked shows a **dose response** effect and suggests that the association is causal.

Source Wynder E.L., *Smoking and health*. USDHHS, pp. 5–35.

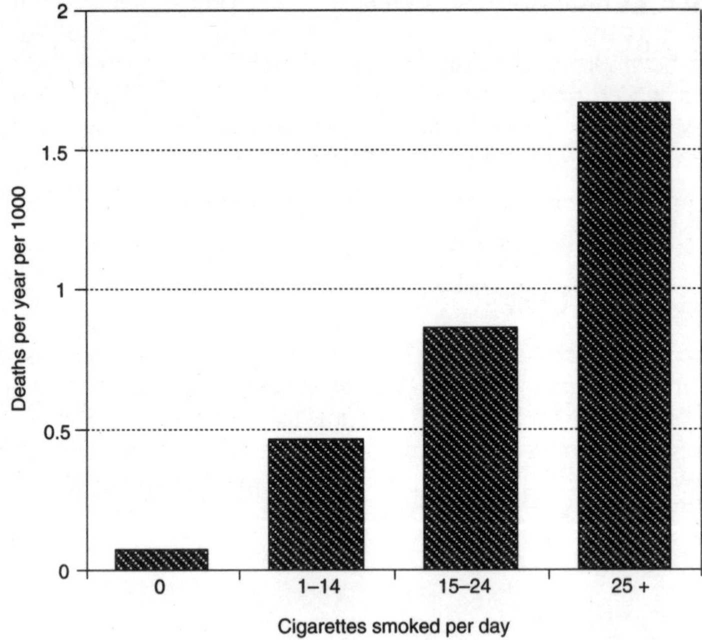

Figure 4.3 Lung cancer in British doctors: comparison of smokers and non-smokers
The risk of lung cancer (age-adjusted death rate) is far higher in smokers than in non-smokers and higher in heavy smokers than in light smokers. The study completed in the 1950s was very influential in persuading the medical profession that smoking really did cause cancer.
Source Data from Doll R. and Hill A.B. (1956), *British Medical Journal* **ii**, 1071–1081.

and the disease are associated. A study of this type on British doctors was very influential in convincing people of the dangers of smoking. Some of the data from that study are shown in Figure 4.3.

BIAS

In case control studies it is all too easy to look harder for exposure in the cases than in the controls. In cohort studies it is also easy to follow the exposed group more carefully than the non-exposed and so find more disease. If we do treat the two groups differently in this way, there is a danger that we may find an association where none really exists. Studies have to be designed in such a way as to minimise the risk of bias like this occurring.

ASSOCIATION AND CAUSE

You will note that the preceding sections have always talked about a disease associated with a factor, not about being caused by it. When we find an association between a disease and exposure to a factor there are several possible explanations:

- exposure causes (increases the risk of) the disease
- the disease causes (increases the likelihood of) exposure
- something else increases the likelihood of both disease and exposure
- coincidence

Before we accept that exposure causes the disease we have to try and rule out all other possible explanations for any association that has been found (Glynn 1993). Animal models of the disease and studies of possible mechanisms by which the disease is caused are two ways of doing this. They add strength to the argument that exposure causes the disease.

INTERVENTION STUDY

By far the most powerful proof of cause is an intervention study (Buyse, Autier and Piedbois 1992). Suppose we intervene to alter a particular factor which we suspect of causing a disease (for example, help some people to stop smoking) and that thereafter the frequency of disease in these people decreases. Suppose also that in another group of similar people we do not intervene and there is no change in the frequency of disease in them. We then have very strong grounds for claiming both that the factor was a cause of the disease and that our intervention prevented the disease.

ANIMAL MODELS OF DISEASE

Experiments in animals are another way of investigating the cause of disease. Often it is possible to induce a disease similar to that seen in humans by exposing animals to the factor under suspicion. The trouble with all animal evidence is that animals are not humans. Because one species of animal becomes ill under certain conditions it does not mean that humans will also become ill under similar conditions. Different animal species react in very different ways. For example, some strains of rat get high blood pressure when fed a high-salt diet but other strains of rat under the right conditions get high blood pressure when fed a low-salt diet. This type of study also raises ethical problems about the use of animals.

One has to decide to what extent animal experimentation can be justified on the grounds that it increases knowledge which might benefit human health.

DEMONSTRATION OF POSSIBLE MECHANISMS

Laboratory studies in animals and in humans can help by showing that there is a possible mechanism by which a particular environmental or lifestyle factor could cause disease. For example, it can be shown that feeding particular high-fibre diets to human subjects increases the speed at which residue passes through the colon, alters the way in which bile pigments are metabolised and alters the type of bacteria growing in the colon. Each of these effects might be part of a mechanism whereby high-fibre diets protect against colon cancer.

THE EXAMPLE OF DIETARY FAT AND ISCHAEMIC HEART DISEASE

It can be seen that no line of evidence is entirely convincing by itself. The case for a theory is strongest when several lines of evidence converge. The example of dietary fat and heart disease will be used to illustrate this (Ashwell 1993; HEA 1993).

International comparisons show that countries with a high intake of fat tend to have a high mortality from heart disease (see Figure 4.4). There are examples where heart disease and fat consumption have shown similar secular trends (see Figure 4.5). A few cohort studies have shown higher risk of heart disease in those on a high-fat diet (but others have not). Animal models exist and changes similar to those seen in man can be induced in animals (rabbits and primates) by feeding them high-fat diets. There are several mechanisms by which high-fat diets could cause heart disease. High-fat diets can be shown to raise blood cholesterol and fibrinogen levels and to alter blood platelet stickiness – all changes which could increase the risk of heart disease. Taken alone, no single piece of this evidence is very impressive. Taken together they add up to a powerful case that eating a high-fat diet increases a person's risk of heart disease.

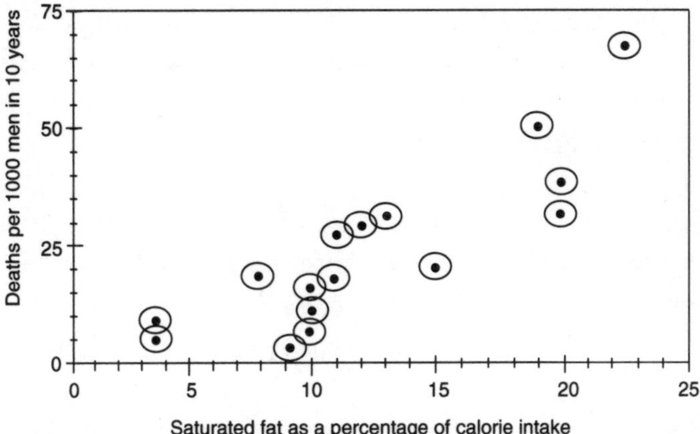

Figure 4.4 Dietary fat and heart disease: international comparisons
Heart disease tends to be most frequent in countries with the highest consumption of fat. Each point represents one population group from the 'Seven countries' study.
Source Adapted from Keys A. (1980), *Seven countries: a multivariate analysis of death and coronary heart disease*; Cambridge MA: Harvard University Press.

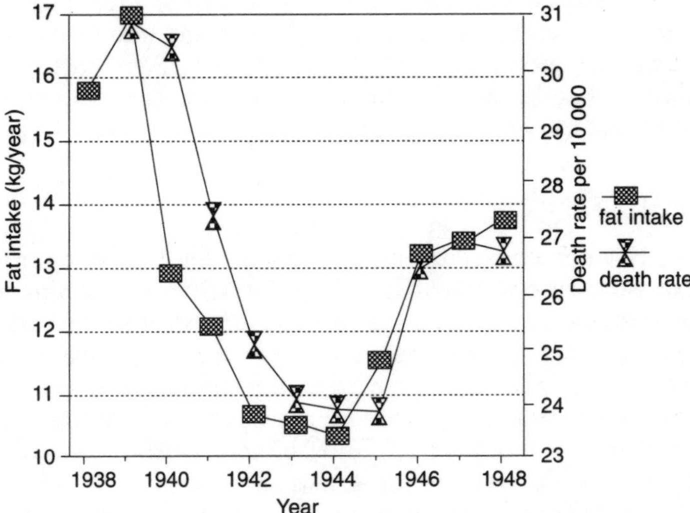

Figure 4.5 Dietary fat and heart disease: secular trends in wartime Norway
There is a striking correspondence between deaths from circulatory disease (mostly heart disease) and consumption of fat. (But what else was changing at the same time?)
Source Adapted from Strom A. and Jensen R.A. (1951), *Lancet* **i**, 126–129.

MULTIPLE CAUSATION

Very many diseases are caused by a combination of different factors. The many factors which affect one's risk of getting heart disease are listed below.

- increasing age
- male sex
- high blood cholesterol
- high blood pressure
- smoking
- high-fat diet (especially saturated fat)
- sedentary lifestyle
- stress
- type A personality (have high stress levels)

Those on the left are more important than those in the right, and the first two (age and sex) cannot be changed.

A study on the cause of oesophageal cancer illustrates the problem of investigating multiple cause. It was found that:

- people who drink a lot of alcohol are more likely to get oesophageal cancer
- smokers are more likely to get oesophageal cancer
- people who drink a lot of alcohol are more likely to be smokers

So is the association with drinking due to the fact that drinkers smoke more or is the association with smoking due to the fact that smokers drink more? Figure 4.6 shows some data on this subject and shows that both smoking and drinking are associated with increased risk of oesophageal cancer.

CONFOUNDING

Frequently when we are trying to compare the frequency of disease and exposure to one particular factor in different groups we find that the groups also differ in their exposure to other factors. These other factors are called confounding factors. For example, it is common to find that groups with a high intake of fat also have a high intake of sugar and a low intake of starch. We have to make allowance for these other confounding factors before we can be sure of the relationship between fat intake and disease.

Age is a common confounding factor. When we are trying to compare the frequency of a disease in two groups which differ in age, we have to allow for that difference in age before trying to show whether other factors are associated with the disease under study. Allowance for difference in age is made either by using age-adjusted rates (see for example Figures 1.1 and 1.2) or by using Standardised Mortality Ratios (SMRs) (see for example Figures 3.5 and 3.6).

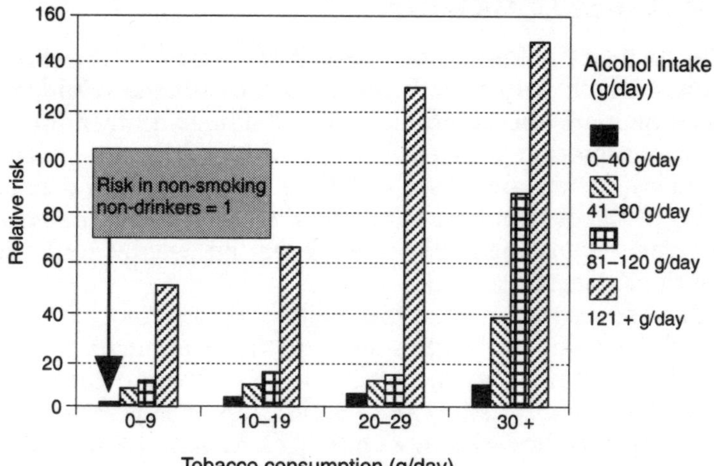

Figure 4.6 Interaction of two risk factors – smoking, drinking and oesophageal cancer
Risk of oesophageal cancer is increased by both smoking and drinking. For any level of tobacco consumption (0–9, 10–19, 20–29 or 30+ grams per day) the risk increases with amount drunk. For any level of alcohol consumption (0–40, 41–80, 81–120 or 121+ grams per day) the risk increases with amount smoked. The risk of smoking and drinking combined is much greater than the effect of either on its own.
Source Adapted from Doll R. and Peto R. (1981), *The causes of cancer*; Oxford: Oxford University Press. Data from Tuyns *et al.* (1977), *Bulletin of Cancer* **64**, 65–70.

STANDARDISED MORTALITY RATIOS

Many of the figures in this book refer to Standardised Mortality Ratios (SMRs) and they are widely used to describe disease frequency. We use SMRs to get round the problem of confounding by differences in age. Suppose we compare two districts A and B and find that the crude mortality rate (total number of deaths in a year divided by the total population) is higher in A than in B. However, the population of district A is also older than that of district B, so of course we would expect it to have more deaths. We want to know which district has the higher death rate after the difference in age has been allowed for. SMRs allow us to do this by comparing the number of deaths which actually occurred with the number of deaths we would expect in a district with that age population.

- An SMR of 100 indicates a death rate as expected.
- An SMR above 100 indicates a death rate worse than expected.
- An SMR below 100 indicates a death rate better than expected.

WHAT IS EPIDEMIOLOGY?

The previous sections have described some epidemiological techniques which help clarify the causes of disease. Epidemiological techniques are also helpful first for planning and then for evaluating health promotion activity. A useful introduction to epidemiology is given by Barker and Rose (1990). Epidemiology is defined as 'the study of the distribution of health, disease and their determinants in populations and the application of that knowledge to the control of health problems'.

The one restriction on applicability of epidemiology is that we must be able to define the health states and the determinant factors that we wish to study and we must be able to estimate them in some way. Thus if we wish to study the relationship of hyperactivity and food additives in children we must have clear criteria for deciding whether a child is hyperactive and a clear definition of what a food additive is.

You will notice that all of the examples of the use of epidemiological techniques given have been concerned with disease. This is because epidemiology was first developed to study disease and so far there are very few examples of it being used to study determinants of positive health. However, there is no basic reason why it cannot be applied to positive health. The chief difficulty to be overcome is developing clear criteria for recognising positive health together with methods for measuring it.

Epidemiology is regarded with suspicion by some health promoters but it is a very powerful and useful tool.

HIGH-RISK AND POPULATION STRATEGIES – THE PARADOX OF PREVENTION

In all health education activity we have to ask the question, 'Who are we trying to influence?' Is it everyone (population strategy) or is it just the few people at highest risk (high-risk strategy)? We will illustrate the problem by thinking about risk of harm from alcohol use but we could just as well have used risk of harm from high serum cholesterol or risk of harm from high blood pressure (Rose 1981) or several other examples.

Should the nurse working on a medical ward aim to give education on sensible drinking to all patients or just to the few who have been recognised as very heavy drinkers? It might seem sensible to concentrate on the few patients at high risk (very heavy drinkers) but most of the people who are going to suffer alcohol-related harm will not be very heavy drinkers (Kreitman 1986). This is an example of the 'paradox of prevention' and it may seem surprising. The paradox arises because a large number of people with a slightly

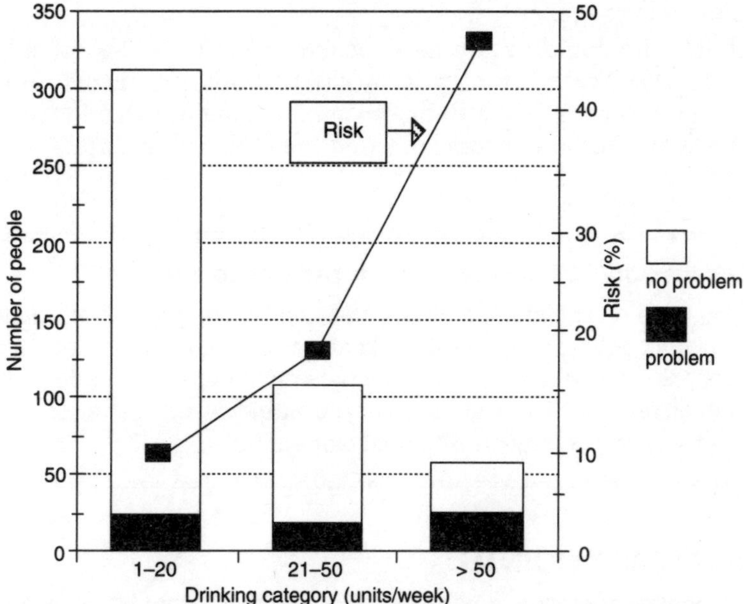

Figure 4.7 The paradox of prevention – the example of alcohol
This study of a Scottish community shows how many men had experienced any drink-related problem. Risk increased with amount drunk. Nearly half the men in the highest drinking category (more than 50 units per week) had had problems while only one in 20 of those in the lowest category (< 21 units per week) had had problems. On the other hand, because there were far more people in the lower drinking categories the number of people with problems (shown in black) was very similar in each drinking category.
Source Adapted from Kreitman N. (1986), *British Journal of Addiction* **81**, 353–363.

increased risk (e.g. 1000 people with a risk of 1 in 10) will produce more problems than a small number of people with a greatly increased risk (e.g. 100 people with a risk of 1 in 2). Figure 4.7 shows an example.

There are other problems with the high-risk strategy. Frequently we do not know who the people at high risk are. If some patients are selected to receive health education and others not, those selected may feel 'got at' or stigmatised. Sometimes the patients at highest risk may be very set in their ways and therefore derive less benefit from health education than patients at lower risk. All these reasons suggest that often we should not be trying to select high-risk groups but trying to influence all (i.e. choose the population strategy)(Rose 1992).

On the other hand, your time and resources are limited. It may not be possible to give health education to everyone. In these circumstances it is sensible to concentrate health education efforts on those who could obtain most benefit from it (i.e. choose a high-risk strategy). There are clearly merits in both arguments and usually the best approach is a judicious mix – some health education for all but with special concentration on the high-risk group.

Discussion/Activity 4.2 Which patients to educate?

You have a special interest and skill in promoting healthier eating. Think of a work setting (a general medical ward, an antenatal clinic, a general practice). There are far too many patients for you to spend much time with all of them. Think about how you would select which patients to do work with in connection with healthier eating.

SUMMARY POINTS

All health promotion is based on theories as to what influences people's health. Health promoters need to be able to distinguish true theories (sense) from untrue theories (nonsense).

There is not enough time for practical health promoters to study the evidence for every new theory but a number of 'rules of thumb' will help sort sense from nonsense.

Evidence that some factor causes disease may come from clinical, epidemiological or laboratory studies.

Epidemiology can show association between a particular factor and disease by:

- ☐ inter-country comparisons
- ☐ secular trends
- ☐ case control studies
- ☐ cohort studies

Most diseases are caused by a combination of several different factors. Care must be taken to avoid confounding (when there is variation in more than one possible causative factor).

Health promotion can be based on 'high-risk strategies', which concentrate effort on the few people at highest risk, or on the population strategy, which tries to influence everyone's behaviour. The 'paradox of prevention' is that most people who suffer harm from exposure to a risk factor will not be in the highest-risk group.

REFERENCES

Ahrens E.H. (1985). The diet heart question in 1985: has it really been settled?. *Lancet* i, 1085–1087.

Ashwell M. (1993). *Diet and heart disease: a round table of factors*. London: British Nutrition Foundation.

Barker D.J.P. and Rose G. (1990). *Epidemiology in medical practice* (4th edition). Edinburgh: Churchill Livingstone.

Buyse M., Autier P. and Piedbois P. (1992). Clinical trials in cancer prevention. In Heller T., Bailey L. and Pattison S. (eds.), *Preventing cancers*. Buckingham: Open University Press.

Campbell A.V. (1993). The ethics of health promotion. Chapter 3 in Wilson-Barnett J. and Macleod Clark J. (eds.), *Research in health promotion and nursing*. Basingstoke: Macmillan.

Glynn J.R. (1993). A question of attribution. *Lancet* **342**, 530–532.

HEA (Health Education Authority) (1993). *Health Update No. 1: Heart disease* (revised edition). London: Health Education Authority.

Kemm J.R (1991). Health education and the problem of knowledge. *Health Promotion International* **6**, 291–295.

Kreitman N. (1986). Alcohol consumption and the preventive paradox. *British Journal of Addiction* **81**, 353–363.

Modan B. (1992). Diet and cancer: causal relationship or just wishful thinking? *Lancet* **340**, 162–163.

Orlans H. (1979). On knowledge policy and practice. *Federation Proceedings* **38**, 2553–2556.

Rose G. (1981). Strategy of prevention: lessons from cardiovascular disease. *British Medical Journal* **282**, 1847–1851.

Rose G. (1992). *The strategy of preventive medicine*. Oxford: Oxford Medical Publications.

Skrabenek P. (1991). Why is preventive medicine exempt from ethical constraints?. *Journal of Medical Ethics* **16**, 187–190.

FURTHER READING

Doll R. and Peto R. (1981). *The causes of cancer*. Oxford: Oxford University Press.

CHAPTER 5

What governments can do

GOAL

To understand the things that governments and only governments can do to influence the health of populations.

OBJECTIVES

- to identify the range of government activities that affect people's environment and lifestyle and thus their health
- to discuss the role of exhortation, taxation, subsidy, prohibition and compulsion in influencing lifestyle
- to understand the need for consent if legislation is to be effective
- to describe the competing non-health interests which influence government decision making

HOW GOVERNMENTS CAN ACT

Chapter 3 explored how health is determined by the interplay of genetics, environment and lifestyle. Most of this book is about things that the individual can do to look after their own health but the discussion of health promotion is always shot through with the debate as to what is the individual's responsibility and what is society's. Decisions are made on behalf of society by its government, either national or local. This chapter considers how decisions that only governments can make affect health. Governments can act by making laws to regulate the affairs of society, by utilising the resources collectively owned by society (chiefly the general taxation fund) or by using its influence to persuade people or companies to act as it wishes.

National legislation may be divided into primary or secondary. Primary legislation is laws that are enacted in parliament, cannot be varied without the consent of parliament and are generally concerned with the broad principles. Primary legislation often contains clauses which empower the minister to make regulations on specified matters. In order to make or change these regulations, the minister only has to notify parliament of the changes. These regulations are referred to as secondary legislation and are generally concerned with details. Table 5.1 shows how primary and secondary legislation gives powers to enforce food hygiene (Ryder 1990).

Table 5.1 Food safety legislation: examples of primary and secondary legislation

Primary legislation – Food Safety Act 1990

Section 7 makes it an offence to render food injurious to health by whatever means with the intention that it should be sold for human consumption.
Section 8 makes it an offence to sell food (or supply food in the course of business) that does not comply with food safety requirements – in particular, food that has been made injurious to health or is unfit for human consumption or is so contaminated that it would be unreasonable to expect it to be used for human consumption.
Section 14 makes it an offence to sell food which is not of the nature, substance or quality demanded by the purchaser.
Section 15 makes it an offence to falsely or misleadingly label, advertise or present food.
Section 17 implements European Union obligations.
Section 19 allows registration of premises used for food businesses and licensing of food businesses.
Section 20 strengthens power of local authorities to enforce food safety regulations.
Section 40 gives the Minister power to issue statutory codes of practice to guide enforcement authorities.
Section 16 allows the Minister to make regulations on food safety (e.g. composition of food, contamination of food and food sources, microbiological standards, food processes or treatments, hygienic conditions, labelling, etc.).

Secondary legislation – made under Food Safety Act and earlier Acts)

Food Hygiene (general) regulations 1970 covers construction and cleaniness of food premises, hygienic handling of food, personal cleanliness of food handlers, washing facilities in food premises and temperatures at which certain food should be kept.
Food hygiene (amendment) regulations 1990 introduce more stringent requirements on storage temperatures for a wide range of foods.
Meat inspection (amendment) regulations 1990 require that all animals shall be inspected before slaughter for fitness to be consumed. Also set out detailed structural and hygiene standards for slaughterhouses.
Milk and dairies (general) regulations 1959 require registration of all dairy farms and all premises used as dairies. Prescribe structural standards, safe water supplies and maintenance of hygienic equipment and milking routines.
Milk and dairies (special designation) regulations 1989 lay down treatment processes for milk pasteurisation, sterilisation and ultra-heat treatment. Specify microbiological standards for raw and treated milk.

There are three broad areas in which government decisions can promote health:

1. improving the environment in which people live
2. directly influencing people's behaviour
3. indirectly influencing people's behaviour by making healthy choices easy choices.

The distinction between direct and indirect influence is not clear cut but the former concentrates on the behaviour of the individual while the latter concentrates on the behaviour of commercial groups.

IMPROVING THE ENVIRONMENT

Many aspects of the environment, such as housing, sewers, water supply and roads, cannot be materially influenced by the individual. Only governments can improve these things. They may do so either by using their own resources to make the improvements or by requiring others to do so through legislation. Where the state or local government is directly responsible for the work (e.g. roads, local authority housing), improvement may be achieved by allocating extra resources. Private individuals or companies may be required by legislation to make environmental improvements or they may be persuaded to do so without legislation. (Local authorities often make environmental enhancement a condition of giving planning consent.) There is a wide range of government agencies which are responsible for enforcing environmental legislation (HM Inspectorate of Pollution, the Rivers' Authorities, the Water Authority, etc.). At local authority level, much enforcement is done by environmental health officers.

DIRECTLY INFLUENCING PEOPLE'S BEHAVIOUR

To a limited extent it is within the power of the individual to choose what they will eat, whether they will smoke and other aspects of their lifestyle. There is a limited number of ways by which governments can directly influence people's behaviour, ranging from exhortation through gentle pressure to compulsion. The following sections give examples of all approaches but there is considerable disagreement as to how far it is proper for governments to go in their attempts to encourage citizens to adopt healthier ways of living.

EXHORTATIONS AND MASS HEALTH EDUCATION CAMPAIGNS

Exhortation through mass-media campaigns is often suggested by politicians as the solution to health-damaging habits. Only governments have the resources needed to mount big national campaigns. In this country they are often organised by the Health Education Authority on behalf of the government. The utility of this approach is discussed in Chapter 19. At this point we may merely note that such campaigns rarely offend any powerful interest groups and rarely produce any widespread change in behaviour.

TAXATION

If exhortation fails, governments can attempt to modify the individual's behaviour by making unhealthy choices slightly less attractive and healthy choices slightly more attractive. Taxation is primarily used to generate revenue for the government but it can also be used to influence price of certain goods, and therefore purchasing behaviour. When things become more expensive people may be discouraged from buying them (DoH 1989; Faculty of Public Health Medicine 1991). Figure 5.1 shows how alcohol consumption increased as alcohol became more affordable. Health benefit has been given as one of the reasons for raising taxation on cigarettes and it is likely that taxation of alcohol may be used in the

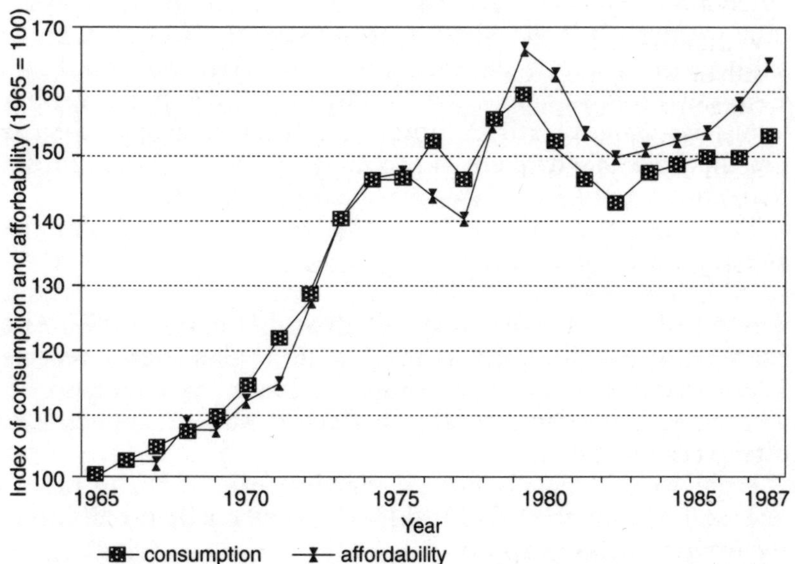

Figure 5.1 Alcohol consumption and affordability
Over the past twenty years in the UK, consumption and affordability of alcohol have varied together. The affordability index is calculated from average earnings divided by cost of alcohol.
Source Adapted from Chief Medical Officer (1989), *On the state of the public health for the year 1988*; London: HMSO.

same way. Taxation of health-damaging products is attractive not only because it discourages use of such products but also because it means that those who benefit from the product make some contribution to the costs of minimising the harmful consequences to society resulting from that product.

SUBSIDIES

Just as people can be discouraged from buying health-damaging products by taxes, they can be encouraged to buy health-favouring products by making them cheaper (or even free) with subsidies. Extensive use of subsidies was made during the Second World War, when certain essential foods were kept cheap (Hollingsworth 1957). Nowadays children obtain free vitamin drops from child health clinics, and the post-war generation benefited from free cod liver oil and orange juice (rich in vitamin C).

PROHIBITION

As an extreme measure, governments can forbid certain behaviours which damage health. This is one of the ways in which government currently attempts to prevent harm from the use of opiates and other 'drugs'. It is illegal to be in possession of or to supply such substances. There is debate about how effective prohibition is. Certainly prohibition has some undesirable side-effects, such as isolating users and creating a criminal subculture around their trade. On the other hand, there is probably less use of these substances than there would be if they could be freely traded.

The experience of the United States with the prohibition of alcohol is well known. Prohibition reduced alcohol-related disease such as cirrhosis but it had so many other effects on society that it was ended after a short time (Walsh and Hingson 1987). Another example of prohibition was the law in England (only repealed in 1950) that made suicide a criminal offence. As a method of preventing suicide it was totally ineffective and its application was often very unkind.

Prohibition is usually not an effective form of health promotion and health promoters find it difficult to reconcile prohibition with the informed-choice approach.

COMPULSION

Just as governments can forbid citizens to do some things, they can compel them to do others. Examples of states compelling people to adopt healthy behaviour are the seat-belt laws. People travelling in the front seats of cars are required by law to wear seat belts. More recently, the use of rear seat belts in cars that have them has also been made compulsory. People riding motor cycles are required to wear crash helmets. In several countries, mothers were required to have their children immunised against infectious diseases and could be fined if they did not do so.

POPULAR CONSENT TO LEGISLATION

A law that does not have the broad support of the majority of the population is very unlikely to be effective in changing people's behaviour. On the other hand, a law which is widely recognised as being just and sensible may bring about a very great change in behaviour. The most striking example of this is the seat-belt legislation. Before it became compulsory to wear seat belts, there had been numerous campaigns (clunk-click every trip) to encourage people to use seat belts but still less than half the drivers or front seat pasengers did so. After the law was introduced the percentage of drivers or front-seat passengers who used seat belts immediately increased to well above 90 per cent (see Figure 5.2). However this result was probably only achieved because the preceding campaigns had persuaded the population that it was a good idea to use belts and that the new law was therefore reasonable (Avery 1984).

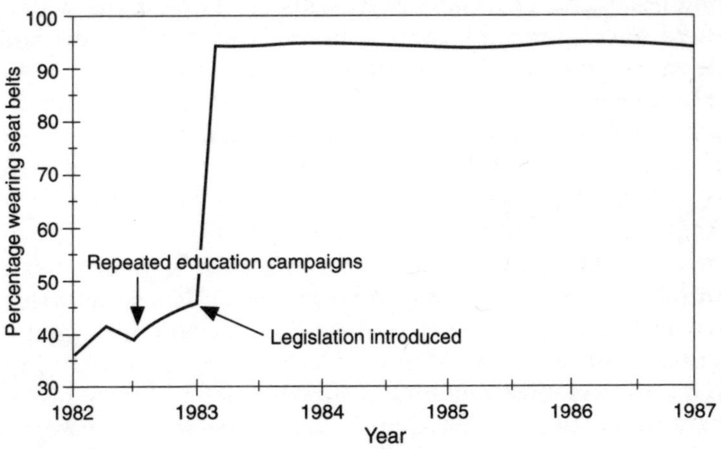

Figure 5.2 Seat-belt use before and after legislation
Despite repeated health education campaigns, seat-belt use remained low until legislation made it compulsory. Thereafter nearly all drivers and front-seat passengers used seat belts.
Source Adapted from Smith A. and Jacobson B. (1988), *The nation's health: a strategy for the 1990s*; London: Kings Fund, Figure 20.

Discussion /Activity 5.1 Legislation about individual behaviour

In France mothers have to produce evidence that their child has been immunised before they can claim child allowance. Is this a good idea?

Are there any things that you think people should be compelled to do for their health? How do you justify these?

INDIRECTLY INFLUENCING PEOPLE'S BEHAVIOUR

While the individual has some power of choice over their health-related behaviour, society sets the context in which that choice is made. Governments are likely to have a much greater impact on the individual's behaviour by influencing the availability of choices rather than by attempting to directly influence the individual's behaviour.

REGULATION OF TRADE

Instead of prohibiting individuals from using a health-damaging product, governments may set strict conditions on its trade. Regulation of alcohol sales is a good example of how consumption can be influenced. Trade in alcohol is closely regulated. Anyone wishing to sell alcohol has to obtain a licence and a special group of magistrates (the licensing bench) control the number and distribution of licences. There are limitations on the hours at which alcohol can be sold. There are limitations on who can buy alcohol, and its sale to children under 18 is forbidden. One can debate how effective licensing law is in regulating alcohol consumption but it is obviously one of the actions that governments can take.

CONTROL OF PRODUCTS

Another way in which governments can influence health is by banning the sale of health-endangering or health-damaging products. Electrical goods have to meet certain minimum safety requirements. Children's nightclothes have to be flame retardant, while children's toys must not contain sharp parts and must be safe. Child safety regulations are listed in the book *Children and their accidents* by Avery and Jackson (1993). Foods sold in the UK must not be 'injurious to the health of the purchaser' and have to meet certain compositional standards. The widespread use of British Standards (Kitemarks) further encourages the manufacture and sale of products that are safe to use.

CONTROL OF LABELLING

A number of regulations define how food shall be labelled. This all helps the consumer make informed choices about how and what they will eat. For products which raise particular health problems, special labelling may be required. In this country cigarette packages must carry a warning about the health effects of smoking and in the United States alcohol has to carry a similar warning (Blume 1987).

CONTROL OF ADVERTISING

Control of advertising is one more way in which governments can influence behaviour. Cigarette advertising is not permitted on television and alcohol advertising on television is covered by a voluntary code of conduct. Some people have argued that advertising health-damaging products should be forbidden. They are particularly concerned that advertising encourages children to take up health-damaging habits and that it makes harmful products socially acceptable (Chapman 1986). The advertisers usually argue that they should be allowed to continue on the grounds that:

- If it's legal to sell a product, it should be legal to advertise it.
- Advertising does not encourage non-users to start using the product but only brand switching by existing users.

It is hard to take this second argument seriously. Several studies have attempted to explore the effect of advertising on cigarette (Smee *et al.* 1992) or alcohol (Smart 1988) use but the subject is complex and both parties cite such studies to support their case for or against the desirability of an advertising ban.

The topic of advertising has to be extended to include not only direct advertising but also activities such as sponsorship. Companies can use sponsorship to remind people of their name or the name of their product so effectively that formal advertising becomes almost irrelevant. Motor racing cars, football shirts and other devices constantly remind viewers of the product. Some forms of sponsorship may be particularly worrying for health promoters because they associate health-benefiting activities with health-harming products. Recent examples include sailing with beer (Whitbread round the world race), rowing with gin (the Oxford and Cambridge boat race) and tennis with smoking (Kim logos on tennis shirts).

Sponsorship is attractive to the companies because it gives them allies. It is also difficult to complain about sponsorship because an attack on sponsorship may be represented as an attack on the worthwhile activities that obtain money from it.

Discussion/Activity 5.2 Limitations on tobacco sales

At the time this was written the UK was one of the few countries in the EU which was arguing against a ban on advertising of tobacco products. Do you think that opposing the advertising ban was a good thing? What are the arguments to support its case? Is this position compatible with the stated intention in *Health of the Nation* to reduce the number of people who are smokers?

Generally do you think current legislation on the sales of tobacco products is too severe, about right or not severe enough? How can you justify limiting the freedom of someone to trade in a product that is perfectly legal to use?

VOLUNTARY CODES OF PRACTICE

Frequently commercial activities are bound by voluntary codes of practice rather than legislation. The warning labels on cigarette packets and the restrictions on television advertising of alcohol are two examples. The trade and the government argue that voluntary codes are preferable because they preserve a good working relationship. Table 5.2 shows the voluntary agreement on television advertising of alcohol. However, many people are concerned that such codes are unenforceable and all too easily broken (Pendleton, Smith and Roberts 1988).

Voluntary codes are an interesting example of government using influence rather than legislation. The companies agree voluntarily to something which they probably see as against their immediate commercial interest because they suspect that if they do not agree they will be the subject of legislation that they like even less.

ENFORCEMENT

Laws will not change anything unless they are observed. Some laws are very poorly enforced. Laws on the sale of cigarettes and alcohol to young people are frequently broken but people are very rarely prosecuted for this offence. In these circumstances it is not surprising that the law is ineffective. Governments have not only to pass the necessary legislation but then also to take measures to ensure that it is enforced.

Drink-driving legislation is another example of a law where enforcement is a problem. Campaigners have demanded harsher penalties for those who drink and drive but this is unlikely to have much effect on driver behaviour. The problem is not that drink drivers do not fear the penalties but that they think they are very

Table 5.2 The IBA code of advertising standards and practice for alcohol advertisements on television

1. Liquor advertising may not be addressed particularly to the young and no one associated with drinking in an advertisement should seem to be younger than about 25. Children may not be seen or heard in an advertisement for an alcoholic drink.
2. No liquor advertisement may feature any personality whose example people are likely to follow.
3. Advertisements may not imply that drinking is essential to social success or that refusal to drink is a sign of weakness.
4. Advertisements must not feature or foster immoderate drinking. This applies to the quantity of drink being consumed in the advertisement and to the act of drinking portrayed. References to buying rounds of drinks are not acceptable.
5. Advertisements must not claim that alcohol has therapeutic qualities nor offer it expressly as a stimulant, sedative or tranquilliser. While advertisements may refer to refreshment after physical performance, they must not give any impression that performance can be improved by drink.
6. Advertisements should not place undue emphasis on alcoholic strength of drinks.
7. Nothing in an advertisement may link drinking with driving or with use of potentially dangerous machinery.
8. No liquor advertisement may publicise a competition.
9. Advertisements must neither claim nor suggest that any drink can contribute towards sexual success.
10. Advertisements must not suggest that solitary drinking is acceptable.
11. Treatments featuring special daring or toughness must not be used in a way which is likely to associate the act of drinking with masculinity.

unlikely to be caught if they drive with blood alcohol levels above the legal limit. (They are right: the chances of being stopped and tested are between 1 in 200 and 1 in 1200.) There has been a lot of discussion as to whether the police should be allowed or encouraged to perform random breath tests (i.e. to stop and test drivers when they have no particular reason to believe that they have been drinking). Some people object to this on the grounds of civil liberties. A few police dislike the idea because they think it will not lead to the detection of many more offences and thus be a poor use of their time. The great argument for 'random' breath testing is that it will change drivers' perceptions of the risk of being caught (BMA 1988). Random breath testing has been used in this way in Australia and is generally thought to have been very successful (Howell 1983).

CONTROL OF DISTRIBUTION

In some circumstances governments may influence behaviour by directly controlling distribution. The obvious example of this is food rationing in this country during the Second World War (Hollingsworth 1957). This was a deliberate attempt by government to ensure that the health of the population was not damaged by malnutrition at a time when food supplies were very limited. By ensuring a much fairer distribution than the market could have achieved, they were remarkably successful in this endeavour. Clearly wartime conditions were exceptional and such an intervention would not be acceptable today.

Discussion/Activity 5.3 Why are 'drugs' and alcohol treated differently?

Alcohol and 'drugs' such as cannabis and opiates are all taken because they have psychotropic properties, that is to say they alter a person's mood in a way that they find pleasurable. People can become addicted to any of them. They can all damage the user's health but not all people who use them have their health damaged. Why are these substances treated differently by the law? To what extent has law making been influenced by health considerations?

PROVISION OF RESOURCES

Few governmental decisions have more effect on health than decisions as to how resources will be allocated. The importance of environmental improvement has been identified but this is largely dependent on making money available. Improving houses, cleaning up dirty industry, laying decent sewers, rebuilding dangerous roads and providing proper public transport all require expenditure.

The health services are an obvious second area where what can be achieved is influenced by the resources available. How much can be achieved by health education services in the Health Education Authority, the district health promotion departments, the schools or other agencies will also depend in part on what resources they have available to them.

NON-HEALTH INTERESTS OF GOVERNMENT

It is all too easy for health professionals and others working for health to forget that health is only one of the many concerns of government. We may argue forcibly for increased taxation on cigarettes and alcohol and more spending on health services and environmental improvement. Government on the other hand will be concerned how these things will effect cost of living, employment, balance of payments, regional economies and finances available for other projects (education, police, defence, social security, and so on). At intervals governments have to get themselves re-elected, and they are unlikely to adopt measures which they think will make them unpopular.

It is proper that a democratic government should be sensitive to the views of its electorate, even if those views may sometimes be viewed as antagonistic to health. Less proper is the effect that powerful lobbyists may have on government decisions. Companies or trade unions may exercise influence to dissuade governments from bringing in health-promoting legislation which the company or union perceives as harmful to their interests. Devices by which companies may influence government include contributions to party funds, consultancies or prospects of future directorships for Members or Ministers, and suggestions that manufacture, investment and jobs could be moved to a country less concerned with health. The history of the dealings between government and the cigarette industry furnishes many examples of how powerful lobbyists can sway government decisions (Taylor 1985).

THE EUROPEAN UNION AND OTHER INTERNATIONAL OBLIGATIONS

The freedom of parliament to legislate on many health subjects is restricted by international obligations. Increasingly UK law is determined by EU legislation (Joffe 1993). While health arguments for increased taxation of alcohol may be strong, the move towards harmonisation of tariffs across the EU and the removal of import restrictions will make it very difficult to achieve this. There are very strong health arguments for labelling alcohol containers with the number of alcohol units they contain, but EU regulations make it illegal to put this information on the label of a wine bottle.

FREEDOM VERSUS 'NANNY STATE'

At the core of this discussion of what governments can do lies the issue of to what extent it is right for the state to limit the freedom of its citizens 'to be foolish' (Leichter 1991).

One extreme view is that if people want to kill themselves that is their business and the state should not interfere. The argument against this is that one citizen's choices may be limited by the actions of another. The freedom of the factory owner to pollute the air limits my freedom to breath clean air. The freedom of the local dealer to sell heroin in the school playground may limit the freedom of my children to grow up safely. The freedom of my neighbour to drive his car at 70 mph down the road in which I live may limit my freedom to cross it in safety. Secondly, if we expect society to care for us when we are ill, does not that place some obligation on us to take reasonable care to protect our health?

The other extreme view is that a beneficent state knows what is best for its citizens and will ensure that they live in a way that protects their health. This seems little more attractive than the opposite extreme and the sensible position must lie somewhere in between.

INFLUENCING GOVERNMENT

This chapter has been all about things that governments can do and, by implication, that health care workers or other individuals cannot. However, government is meant to be the servant of its citizens, so part of the health promotion task must be influencing government to play its part in health promotion. A good description of how to run a campaign has been written by Duncan (1986). MADD (Mothers Against Drink Drivers) proved highly effective in persuading governments to legislate against drink driving in the USA (Leichter 1991). CADD (Campaign Against Drink Drivers) has been similarly effective in the UK. MOPUP (Movement Opposed to the Promotion of Unhealthy Products) and BUGAUP (Billboard Using Graffitists Against Unhealthy Promotion) have used more direct methods to influence the Australian government to act against promotion of tobacco products (Raw, White and McNeill 1990).

Health professionals can act as advocates for their patients on health promotion issues by writing letters to MPs or local councillors, writing to the press and lobbying through their professional associations. The Royal College of Nursing and the Health Visitors' Association have a long and honourable history of campaigning for health promotion.

SUMMARY POINTS

Governments can improve the health of their population by:

- ☐ improving the environment in which people live
- ☐ directly influencing people's behaviour
- ☐ indirectly influencing people's behaviour by making healthy choices easier choices

Governments can improve environment through their own activities and also by planning laws and other regulations controlling how industrial and commercial firms change the environment.

Governments can in certain limited circumstances pass laws forbidding unhealthy behaviours (using drugs, driving with high blood alcohol levels) or requiring healthy behaviours (wearing crash helmets on motor cycles, seat belts in cars, etc.). This legislative approach only succeeds when it has popular support.

Governments can also attempt to modify behaviours by health education or by manipulating prices to make healthy behaviour cheaper (subsidy) or unhealthy behaviour more expensive (taxes).

Governments can also influence the availability of goods that affect health through regulation of trade (for example alcohol licensing and banning sales of dangerous goods). They can also legislate to control labelling and advertising.

The health of the population is only one of the many considerations of government. UK legislation is being increasingly influenced by European Union legislation and by other international obligations.

There is a balance to be struck in deciding how far the state should interfere – even for beneficent reasons – with the ways its citizens choose to behave (Nanny state).

Health promoters need to think how they can influence government on health issues.

REFERENCES

Avery J.G. (1984). Seat belt success: where next?. *British Medical Journal* **288**, 622–623.

Avery J.G. and Jackson R.H. (1993). *Children and their accidents*. London: Edward Arnold.

Blume S. (1987). Warning labels and warning signs: a battle continues across the Atlantic. *British Journal of Addiction* **82**, 5–6.

BMA (British Medical Association) (1988). *The drinking driver*. London: BMA.

Chapman S. (1986). Cigarette advertising and smoking: a review of the evidence. In British Medical Association, *Smoking out the barons: the campaign against the tobacco industry*. Chichester: John Wiley and Sons.

DoH (Department of Health) (1989). *On the state of the public health for the year 1988*. Annual Report of the Chief Medical Officer. London: HMSO.

Duncan N. (1986). The BMA's campaign against the tobacco industry. In British Medical Association, *Smoking out the barons: the campaign against the tobacco industry*. Chichester: John Wiley and Sons.

Faculty of Public Health Medicine (1991). Does taxation affect alcohol consumption?. Chapter 6 in *Alcohol and the public health*. London: Macmillan.

Hollingsworth D. (1957). The application of newer knowledge of nutrition. Chapter 24 in Drummond J.C. and Wilbrahim A., *The Englishman's food: a history of 5 centuries of English diet* (2nd edition). London: Cape.

Howell R. (1983) The impact of random breath testing in New South Wales. *Medical Journal of Australia* **1**, 616–621.

Joffe M. (1993). Future of European Community (EC) activities in the area of public health: European Public Health Alliance. *Health Promotion International* **8**, 53–61.

Leichter H.M. (1991). *Free to be foolish*. Princeton NJ: Princeton University Press.

Pendleton L., Smith C. and Roberts J.L. (1988). Monitoring alcohol advertisements on television: developing a consensus approach. *Health Education Journal* **47**, 71–73.

Raw M., White P. and McNeill A. (1990). MOPUP and BUGAUP. Case study 6 in *Clearing the air: a guide to action on tobacco.* London: BMA on behalf of WHO, European Regional Office.

Ryder C.J. (1990) UK food legislation. *Lancet* **336**, 1559–1562.

Smart R.G. (1988). Does alcohol advertising affect overall consumption? A review of empirical studies. *Journal of Studies on Alcohol* **49**, 314–322.

Smee C., Parsonage M., Anderson R. and Duckworth S. (1992). The effect of tobacco advertising on tobacco consumption. *Health Trends* **24**, 111–112.

Taylor P. (1985). *The smoke ring: tobacco, money and multinational politics.* London: Sphere.

Walsh D.C. and Hingson R.W. (1987). *Epidemiology and alcohol policy.* Chapter 9 in Levine S. and Lilienfeld A. (eds.), *Epidemiology and health policy.* New York: Tavistock.

CHAPTER 6

Principles of education

You cannot teach a man anything; you can only help him find it within himself.

GALILEO GALILEI

GOAL

To understand a set of theories of learning which provide a basis for educational activities.

OBJECTIVES

- to identify the steps in the education process
- to explain how educational theories can assist teaching and learning activities
- to discuss the different approaches to learning used by children, adults and elderly people

EDUCATION – WHAT IS IT?

Education is a familiar word which we read and hear frequently in the media and in general conversation. However, attempting to explain its meaning is not easy. Many people equate education with giving information and with teaching and learning. Although these activities are an important part of education they are not the whole story.

Education is a planned, systematic process used with the intention of influencing the behaviours of others by producing changes in their knowledge, attitudes and skills. It involves a cycle of actions. First, an assessment of an individual's learning needs and the learning situation must be made. Second, relevant learning opportunities are planned and implemented. Finally, an evaluation of the individual's learning and of the process completes the cycle. This doesn't necessarily end the process, however, and the cycle may be recommenced as a result of the findings of the evaluation (see Figure 6.1)

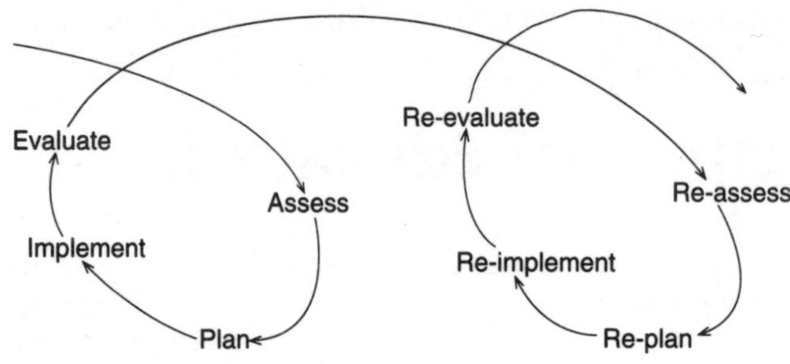

Figure 6.1 The teaching–learning process – a repeating cycle.

In health promotion the major goal of education is to help people develop the knowledge, skills and attitudes necessary to maintain and improve their health.

LEARNING

Learning is an essential part of education. It is an activity we have done throughout our lives. We learn incidentally from every day experiences or intentionally because of changes in our work and home situations. We also choose to learn as a leisure pursuit. Learning involves the acquisition of new knowledge, skills and attitudes which need to be applied in specific situations to be of value.

Learning may be said to have occurred when an individual is able to carry out specific actions or has increased their knowledge. However, the real test is whether the individual actually uses the acquired knowledge or skill appropriately. It can be argued that they are more likely to do this if they know why they should act in this way.

Learning involves many activities such as listening, observing, problem-solving, practising, watching, discussing, writing, drawing and reflecting on experiences. It results in the development of a wide range of new behaviours or learning outcomes, including the ability to demonstrate, describe, explain, analyse and synthesise information.

CASE STUDY: COMPLIANCE WITH MEDICATION

Janice had recently started as an undergraduate at university but after only a couple of weeks she developed a nasty sore throat. Her GP prescribed an antibiotic and told Janice to have one four times a day for seven days. After four days Janice was feeling much better and went back to her studies. Because she felt better she decided she didn't need the antibiotic any longer and stopped taking it.

Although Janice knew she should take the antibiotic four times a day and remembered being told to take it until the course was complete she didn't do this. Although it could be argued that learning had occurred, it is only really worthwhile if it results in the medication being correctly taken. Perhaps if Janice had also understood that the reasons for taking the antibiotic as instructed were to eradicate the infection and reduce the organism's resistance to the antibiotic she would have been more likely to comply with the instructions.

TEACHING

Although learning can and often does take place without teaching, it would be naive to think that teaching has no effect on learning.

Teaching is a process of helping others to learn and incorporate new behaviours into everyday life. This implies that teaching is part of a two-way interaction involving the teacher in activities such as informing, instructing, challenging and coaching so that the learner is able to use knowledge, skills and attitudes in appropriate situations.

The teacher's goal is to create situations and opportunities in which the individual is willingly and actively engaged in learning and does not become a passive recipient in the interaction. The teacher attempts to motivate the learner to move from dependence to independence in learning and to take more responsibility and control of their actions.

EDUCATIONAL THEORY

In line with many other disciplines, education follows specific theories which guide the teaching–learning process. There are many ideas of what constitutes a theory. A commonly held view is that a theory is a set of laws that provide a means of describing, predicting and explaining behaviours but the term is also used to describe situations where ideas have not been sufficiently tested to constitute laws. Chapman (1985) defines a theory as: 'a proposed explanation of an event or series of happenings, often demonstrating the relationship of one to another and may or may not be proven'.

Education has traditionally adopted psychological theories to assist teachers in their understanding of educational problems and help them develop ways of overcoming them. There is no single psychological theory relevant to all education but rather a number of theories which can be used to complement each other.

The aims of using educational theory in health promotion are:

- to provide a realistic view of the behaviours of the people involved in the teaching and learning process
- to enable the educator to analyse their own teaching experience
- to help the educator predict and influence future events

BEHAVIOURIST APPROACH TO LEARNING

According to behaviourists, most behaviour is learned by making a link or connection between a stimulus and a response. The process by which a link is made is called conditioning. There are two types of conditioning:

1. classical conditioning or signal learning
2. operant conditioning

Classical conditioning

This is the simplest type of learning and was originally described by Pavlov (1849–1936), a Russian scientist. In his experiments with dogs he found that a stimulus (food) elicited an involuntary, reflex response (salivation) in the dog. He described this as a natural or unconditioned situation. He then gave a second stimulus (bell) just before the original stimulus (food) which produced the response of salivation. He repeated the paired stimuli (bell followed by food) many times. Eventually he found that the bell alone produced salivation. The bell then becomes the conditioned stimulus while salivation is the conditioned response.

Generally, classical conditioning plays little part in education. In the context of health education its main relevance is to situations in which emotional responses can become conditioned. A child experiencing pain and discomfort from injections, procedures and other events may associate this with nurses, doctors, health clinics or hospitals. These stimuli may then elicit fear reactions which interfere with learning when the child comes into contact with them again later in life. Similarly, an adult may appear to be indifferent or unduly apprehensive in new learning if as a child their experience of learning provoked anxiety or was otherwise unpleasant.

The principles of classical conditioning can also be used in health promotion by making connections between cause and effects of disease. For example, linking lung cancer with smoking or HIV infections with intravenous drug abuse will help to produce avoidance behaviour.

Operant conditioning

Operant conditioning or trial-and-error learning works on the principle that humans behave in such a way as to receive gratification. The behaviour (response) occurs first and is followed by a consequence that gives satisfaction and so becomes the stimulus. For example, a child completes a mathematical problem correctly and then the teacher gives praise.

The theory of operant conditioning was developed independently by Skinner (1904–) and Thorndike (1874–1949). From his experiments with cats, dogs and chickens, Thorndike proposed that behaviour which results in success is more likely to be repeated than behaviour which does not. He also suggested that repetition of successful actions results in considerable learning, and this achievement is enjoyable for the learner.

From this perspective, operant conditioning has a useful application in health promotion. A client is more likely to learn successfully if the learning is planned to be relevant to their needs, interesting and within their capabilities.

Opportunities to practise the learned behaviour increase the likelihood that it will be repeated. Skinner emphasised the use of reinforcement as the key to learning. Reinforcement may be primary or secondary. Primary reinforcers such as food and comfort are innate and act without previous training. Secondary reinforcers, such as praise, awards and money, are more likely to influence human behaviour.

Reinforcement can also be used positively or negatively. Positive reinforcement (reward) increases the probability of the desired behaviour being repeated. Negative reinforcement (punishment) decreases the probability of the behaviour occurring. Absence of positive reinforcement usually leads to the extinction of the response. The health educator can use these principles in many ways, for example to encourage obese people to lose weight or smokers to give up smoking. The educator should reinforce the behaviour of not eating between meals rather than reprimand or criticise the individual for eating snacks between meals. Similarly, non-smoking behaviour should be reinforced and smoking behaviour ignored. Family and friends can be encouraged to use these principles too.

COGNITIVE THEORIES

Cognitive theorists are concerned with how knowledge is acquired. They view learning as a complex cognitive activity which involves the processing of information in order to solve problems. This approach was first introduced by Gestalt psychologists who believe that an individual learns best when they have an appreciation of the whole situation. An individual encountering a new problem identifies the significant elements involved in the situation. Influenced by previous experiences, the individual's perception of the problem then undergoes restructuring as they organise the elements into patterns that make sense to them. Having reflected on the problem, they can then decide on a plan of action and move towards a solution.

Gestalt psychologists derived laws that direct this process:

- laws of similarity and proximity
- laws of closure

The laws of similarity and proximity maintain that an individual groups elements together on the basis that they are similar in size, colour, shape and so on or because they are physically close or because they occur at the same time.

The law of closure requires completion of the solution for satisfaction to occur. As the individual experiences more and more problem situations he becomes adept at observing, investigating and analysing situations and arranging them into logical patterns to produce solutions. An example of this could be someone who completes crosswords. The more crosswords they complete the more competent and skilled at solving the clues they become.

In health education the educator can apply Gestalt theory by making sure the client can see each element of learning as a part of the whole. At the same time each element should be complete in itself. For example, teaching parents about artificial infant feeding can be divided into three elements: sterilisation of equipment, preparation of the feed and feeding the child. Each element is complete in itself but is also part of the larger whole process.

The educator should also try to structure learning so that the client experiences insightful learning or 'the penny dropping' phenomenon.

More recently other theories of learning have been proposed. Ausubel (1968) suggests that learning takes place as a result of interaction between new information and existing cognitive structures. Each successive learning task therefore should be related to what has gone on before. He describes this linking of new to old as 'meaningful learning'.

Ausubel also claims that learning is more effective if educators use 'advance organisers'. The use of patient teaching flow sheets, which provide an overview of the information to be learned, is an example of using 'advance organisers' in patient education. These help the educator and client assess what the client already knows and needs to learn. They also provide an aid to documenting and evaluating the teaching–learning process so that learners and teachers can see the progress that has been made. Patient teaching flow sheets are particularly useful when a multi-disciplinary team is involved in teaching (see Chapter 14).

HUMANISTIC THEORY

Humanistic theory is derived from a belief that self-fulfilment is the ultimate goal in a person's life. Their values, beliefs and attitudes guide and motivate them to become self-directed learners. They are capable of choosing appropriate actions that will help them pursue their goals. Self-awareness, life experiences and personal involvement are fundamental to humanistic learning.

Humanistic psychologists maintain that when learning activities are being planned, each individual's needs, interests and concerns must be considered so that learning becomes relevant. They believe that individuals like to participate in assessing their learning needs, planning goals and evaluating activities as well as being actively involved in learning activities. In addition, they contend that learning is best achieved in an informal, comfortable and non-threatening environment where the teacher works in an equal partnership with the learner, encouraging them to become independent, self-reliant, imaginative and innovative.

Carl Roger's (1969) work in developing humanistic theories is well known. He claims that in order to use this approach the traditional role of the teacher must change to become that of a facilitator of learning. An effective facilitator is someone who questions, challenges, fosters curiosity, guides others towards relevant learning resources and encourages their active participation in all aspects of the learning process. The facilitator becomes a confidante who shares not only their knowledge but also their feelings with the learner.

Knowles (1978) captures the essences of humanistic principles in his theory of adult education, which he terms androgogy. He identifies four important assumptions about adult learners:

Self concept The individual moves from being a dependent learner towards being an independent, self-directed learner who is responsible for their own actions.

The individual's experience Adults have occupied many roles and had a wide range of experiences. They use these experiences to help them learn.

Readiness to learn Adults become ready to learn when they see the significance of learning or experience a need to know something or how to do something.

Orientation to learning Adults usually prefer a life-centred and task-centred approach to learning.

The psychological and learning theories outlined above offer guidance to the health promoter and help them be more realistic in developing aims and goals for teaching and learning. Humanistic approaches are particularly helpful for health education with adults because they promote a partnership for learning. The individual learner is provided with necessary support and retains control over the learning situation.

Discussion/Activity 6.1 Turning theory into practice

Bill is a widower aged 86. He comes into the medical ward confused and in very poor shape. He is noted to have several cuts that won't heal up, bleeding around the gums, a petechial rash on his skin and he is anaemic. It rapidly becomes clear that he is vitamin C deficient, and when he is given vitamin C and some good food he makes a rapid recovery.

It turns out that for the past year Bill has been mostly living on ginger-nuts and cups of tea. Until his wife died a year ago Bill had always had someone to cook for him and look after him. When his wife died he had no idea how to plan meals, buy food or cook.

Use the various theories of learning to plan an educational approach that will help Bill look after himself in the future.

AIMS, GOALS AND OBJECTIVES

Aims, goals and objectives direct the learning experience.

Aims describe the longer term direction and the broad reasons why particular activities are being organised or done.

Goals describe the desired outcomes or results of learning and answer the question, 'What is the purpose of learning?' A goal summarises the learning objectives that follow.

Learning objectives are more specific and may be:

1. behavioural objectives, which describe precisely what knowledge or skills the client intends to gain, or
2. experiential objectives, which describe what are worthwhile experiences.

Behavioural objectives are highly specific statements and according to Mager (1962) have three parts:

1. a verb or action word which will describe the behaviour to be achieved, e.g. choose, demonstrate, describe, explain, organise, perform, plan, select, use
2. the conditions or special circumstances that are required, e.g. 'before going home' or 'using specific equipment'
3. the standard or level of performance – how well something must be done, e.g. speed, accuracy, frequency.

CASE STUDY: AN EXAMPLE OF SETTING AIMS, GOALS AND OBJECTIVES

Simon is 14 and has been diagnosed as having diabetes mellitus. He requires insulin.

Aim To assist Simon develop the knowledge and skills required to self-administer insulin so that he can manage his treatment effectively.

Goal Simon will administer his own insulin safely before he goes home from hospital.

Objectives Simon will be able to:

1. monitor his blood glucose accurately before giving his insulin
   will monitor his blood glucose – action
   accurately – conditions
   before giving insulin – special circumstances
2. draw up and inject safely the prescribed units of insulin before breakfast
   draw up and administer the prescribed units of insulin – action
   safely – conditions
   before breakfast – special circumstances

The use of objectives has been criticised on several grounds, not least of which is the time needed to develop them. However, if client and health educator work together to develop objectives they begin to create an effective working partnership. The objectives then provide a direction to work towards and a scale against which progress can be monitored.

BLOOM'S TAXONOMY OF OBJECTIVES

Learning requires changes in a range of behaviours relating to skills, knowledge and attitudes. Bloom *et al.* (1956) developed a system of classification of objectives for the three types of learning:

1. **cognitive,** which is related to knowledge and intellectual ability
2. **affective**, which is related to attitudes, values and interests
3. **psychomotor,** which is concerned with motor skills.

Bloom subdivided these categories into hierarchies, and learning advances through the different levels (see Figure 6.2).

Health promoters using Bloom's hierarchy to set objectives should be able to examine their goals carefully and work with clients to provide a clear direction of what must be learned. Such objectives also provide a basis for evaluating learning. This approach, however, does have a number of critics. Lawton (1973), Quinn (1980) and others believe that this type of classification places too much emphasis on measurable behaviour and trivial outcomes, which narrows the learning field.

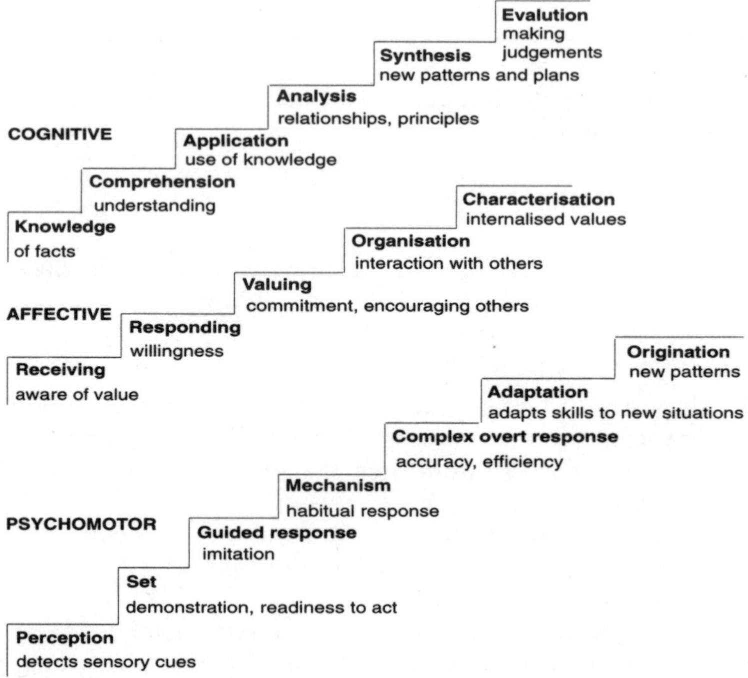

Figure 6.2 Taxonomy of educational objectives
There is a hierarchy of objectives in cognitive, affective and psychomotor domains.

EXPERIENTIAL TAXONOMY

Steinaker and Bell (1979) use an approach to teaching and learning called 'experiential learning' which sees human behaviour as an holistic process. People are deliberately exposed to certain situations and experiences in order that learning may occur. The steps in this process are described by an 'experiential taxonomy' (see Figure 6.3).

APPLICATION OF THE EXPERIENTIAL TAXONOMY IN HEALTH PROMOTION

When clients first encounter a particular experience they receive information and consider whether to accept or reject it. The health promoter's role at this stage is that of motivator, encouraging the clients to explore the subject in more detail so that they recognise that there is more to be learned. Asking questions, presenting information and drawing examples from things they have done or experienced will help to introduce the subject and make them want to explore further.

Clients may then be willing to progress to the second level – participation – where they begin to become involved in learning through discussions, role play and supervised practice. The health promoter acts as a catalyst, creating situations which promote exploration of the experience.

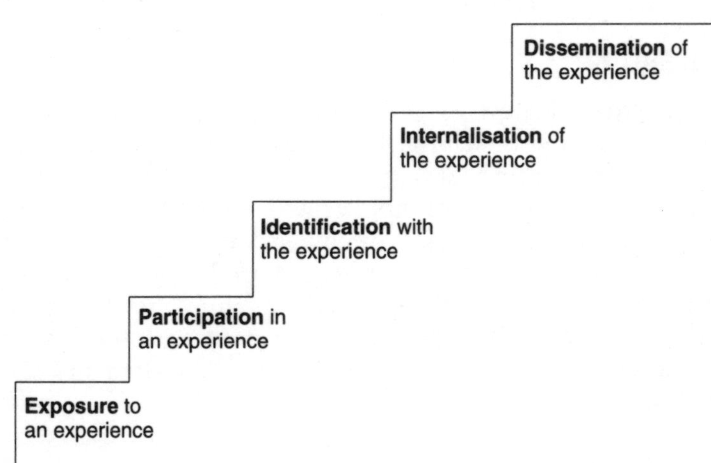

Figure 6.3 Experiential taxonomy of learning.
The progressive stages through which the learner passes are represented by a series of steps.
Source Steinaker and Bell (1979).

Successful participation results in satisfaction and leads to the third level – identification. Clients become familiar with the subject and are able to express opinions about it and share these with others such as partners or family members. The health promoter can support clients by providing additional reading or initiating group discussions and debates.

At the next level – internalisation – clients have taken on board the new ideas or behaviours which become part of their lifestyle. They are able to apply the new behaviours in different situations. The health promoter's role is to sustain and reinforce the new behaviours.

Dissemination is the highest level of knowledge and skills in the experiential taxonomy. At this level clients want to talk about their new learning and to pass it on to others. The health promoter will find that clients who have reached this level adopt the role of health promoter and introduce new clients to the health topic.

LEARNING APPROACHES AND PREFERENCES OF DIFFERENT GROUPS OF PEOPLE

Until recently education and teaching styles have focused on the needs of children. During the 1970s important differences in the learning needs of children and adults were recognised and specific strategies and approaches for adults were identified. Thus the concepts of pedagogy (education of children) and androgogy (education of adults) were developed. Some health professionals also believe that there are techniques which are best suited to the elderly, and Bille (1980) describes this as 'geragogy'.

CHILDREN

The traditional view of child learning concentrates on a formal classroom setting in school. However, experiences from pre-school years form the basic foundation for future learning.

Childhood is a period of rapid growth – physical, mental, emotional and social. It is essential that the child's developmental stage is considered when teaching–learning strategies are being devised. It will also be necessary to consider the parents and family members as a unit.

Although each child is unique there are certain characteristics (see Table 6.1) which are common to all children in the learning situation.

ADULTS

The needs of adults are different from children though there are some similarities. The wealth of personal and occupational

Table 6.1 Educating children

Characteristics	Guidelines for educators
• Learns through parents	• Orientate teaching to parents
• Learns through environment	• Provide stimulating environment with different shapes, colours and textured objects
• Learns through imitation	• Use to advantage to develop a healthy lifestyle
• Learns out of interest and curiosity	• Involve child in deciding what to learn and how • Make learning enjoyable • Use play and imagination • Encourage risk taking in a controlled way • Teach safety rules
• Learns best through active involvement and play	• Encourage storytelling and 'acting out' procedures on dolls; use colouring books
• Thinks literally and only relates to actual things and events	• Use simple, straightforward words • Be honest – if it's going to hurt, say so
• Needs great support when learning	• Consistently offer praise • Be consistent in teaching • Acknowledge child's wishes
• Has short attention span	• Make learning experiences of short duration
• Likes examples from everyday life experiences	• Involve fictional heroes • Use drawings and models to explain things
• Capable of abstract thought	• Use verbal or pictorial illustrations for explanations
• Strives to develop own identity	• Encourage child to control own learning • Encourage to assume responsibility for learning

experience adults have should be acknowledged and used to the best advantage in the learning situation (see Table 6.2).

ELDERLY

As people get older they experience many physical and psychological changes. Often these occur so commonly that even when they are a result of one of more pathological processes they are accepted as a 'normal' part of ageing. It is extremely difficult, therefore, to determine whether or not learning ability is directly affected by ageing because of the complexity of factors evident in the learning process (see Table 6.3).

Discussion/Activity 6.2 Educational approaches for different age groups

You are asked to plan a learning programme about healthy eating for an overweight patient. How would your approach differ if they were 10, 30 or 70 years old? How would the patient's gender affect your educational approach?

Table 6.2 Educating adults

Characteristics	Guidelines for educators
• Usually learns best in familiar, non-threatening environment	• Never put individuals on the defensive • Use conversational style and simple terminology • Be patient and flexible • Develop good rapport
• Learns best in response to a perceived need	• Focus first on areas the individual recognises as learning needs • Raise interest in other important areas before attempting to teach
• Learns when new material is related to old	• Build on what is already known
• Learns best when material is meaningful	• Relate new material to life experiences • Introduce only relevant information
• Likes to be actively involved	• Use problem-solving approaches • Encourage discussion and questions • Give direction only when needed
• Retains learning if it can be put to immediate use	• Provide opportunity for practice with feedback • Present information in a logical sequence • Encourage to summarise
• Likes to be responsible for learning	• Encourage individual to control learning situation • Do not expect individual to do what the teacher is not able to do • Never do anything for individuals that they can do for themselves • Remember that ultimately change in behaviour rests with individual

Table 6.3 Educating older people

Factors in the elderly which affect learning	Guidelines for educators
Visual deterioration	
• Decreased ability to: focus discriminate colour see fine detail adapt to light • cataracts	• Use large print in written materials • Use strong contrasting colours • Yellow, orange and red appear more visible • Have minimum detail in pictures • Use bright but diffused lighting • Figures should be clearly outlined • Clean spectacles
Hearing loss	
• Progressive loss of hearing and sound discrimination	• Speak slowly • Enunciate clearly without exaggerated lip movement • Speak in normal voice • Educator's face clearly visible • Exclude background noise • Use body language • Hearing aids switched on and working
Reduced sense of touch and ability to co-ordinate movement	
• Difficulty in: handling small objects writing • Increased response time	• Leave plenty of time to practise • Give encouragement
Changes in memory	
• Memory to past events is superior • Difficulty transferring information from short- to long-term memory	• Slow the pace of new learning • Repeat demonstrations • Explain procedures carefully and slowly • Link new material to old

SUMMARY POINTS

- ☐ Education involves a planned systematic process which includes assessment, planning and implementation phases.
- ☐ Psychological theories are used to promote understanding of educational problems and ways of overcoming them.
- ☐ Previous experiences of learning influence future experiences.
- ☐ Different people like to learn in different ways.
- ☐ Behaviour that results in success is more likely to be repeated than behaviour which does not.
- ☐ Reinforcement is a key to learning. Newly learned behaviours are more likely to be repeated if positive reinforcement is used.
- ☐ Organising and structuring activities will help learning occur.
- ☐ Learning is more effective when new information is linked to existing information (meaningful learning).
- ☐ Individuals' needs, interests and concerns should be considered when planning learning activities to ensure learning is relevant.
- ☐ Aims, goals and objectives help to direct learning experiences and facilitate evaluation of learning.

REFERENCES

Ausubel D.F. (1968). *Educational psychology: a cognitive view.* New York: Rinehart Winston

Bille D.A. (1980). Educational strategies for teaching the elderly patient. *Nursing and Health Care* 1, 256–263.

Bloom B.S., Krathwohl D.R. *et al.* (1956). *Taxonomy of educational objectives. Handbook 1.* London: Longman.

Chapman M.C. (1985). *Theory of nursing, practical application.* Lippincott Nursing Series. London: Harper & Row.

Knowles M. (1978). *The adult learner: a neglected species* (2nd edition). Houston TX: Gulf Publishing.

Lawton D. (1973). *Social change, educational theory and curriculum planning.* London: Hodder and Stoughton.

Mager R. (1962). *Preparing instructional objectives.* California: Fearon.

Quinn F. (1980). *The principles and practice of nurse education.* London: Croom Helm.

Rogers C. (1969). *Freedom to learn.* Ohio: Merril.

Steinaker N. and Bell R. (1979). *The experiential taxonomy: a new approach to teaching and learning.* London: Academic Press.

CHAPTER 7

Health behaviours and behavioural change

GOAL

To understand the factors which motivate people to engage in health-related behaviours.

OBJECTIVES

- to identify the factors which influence health beliefs and health-related behaviour
- to explain how theories of motivation and models of health belief can assist health promotion and education activities
- to discuss the role of the health educator in motivating clients towards changing health-related behaviour

INTRODUCTION

The previous chapter highlighted the importance of the education process in helping people develop new behaviours aimed at maintaining and improving their health and lifestyle. However, even the best education strategies and techniques cannot guarantee that learned behaviours will be internalised by the individual and incorporated into everyday life. Whether newly acquired attitudes, skills and knowledge will be utilised or not depends on the characteristics and situation of the individual.

Mass-media advertising in newspapers and magazines, TV programmes, and government health warnings must have made most people in this country aware of the harmful consequences of tobacco smoking. The numbers of smokers are dropping but almost a third of the population still continues to smoke cigarettes (Figure 3.3) (DoH 1991). Similarly, a great deal of health information focuses on the potential hazards of being overweight but obesity is increasing in both women and men. In 1980, 8% of women and 6% of men were obese but by 1986 this had risen to 12% and 8% respectively (DoH 1993).

Providing people with information is obviously not enough by itself to help them incorporate new health behaviours in their lifestyles. Therefore we must consider what factors will influence them to adopt health-promoting behaviours. What will motivate them to sustain these new activities in their lifestyle and what can the health care professional do to assist them?

THEORIES AND MODELS OF MOTIVATION

As with educational theories, no single theory entirely explains motivation. However, a number of theories and models have been put forward in an attempt to explain the relationships between health beliefs and health-related behaviour. These theories help health care professionals to understand what makes individuals behave as they do. Thinking about the theory should enable you become more effective in helping clients make changes towards a healthier lifestyle (Bunton, Murphy and Bennett 1991).

The following theories are particularly relevant to health promotion work.

MASLOW'S HIERARCHY OF HUMAN NEEDS

Maslow (1954) developed a theoretical model which is useful in health care and educational settings. Maslow's theory is based on the assumption that all human beings have needs which must be satisfied and that these needs tend to direct an individual's behaviour until they are satisfied. Maslow identified five categories of need (see Figure 7.1) as being basic to human motivation – physiological needs, safety and security needs, love and belonging needs, self-esteem needs and self-actualisation needs. He organised these into a hierarchy, with the physiological and safety needs being the most basic and self-actualisation the highest level of need. Progress through the hierarchy to higher-level needs only occurs when lower-level and more important needs have been satisfied.

When a particular need emerges it produces a state of tension in an individual. For example, a child admitted to hospital is likely to be anxious and unsettled in a new and strange environment and therefore the need to feel safe and secure will emerge. The child will be motivated toward behaviours which reduce the tension and feelings of anxiety, such as clinging to its mother or cuddling a blanket or favourite toy. The health educator has to gain insight into the

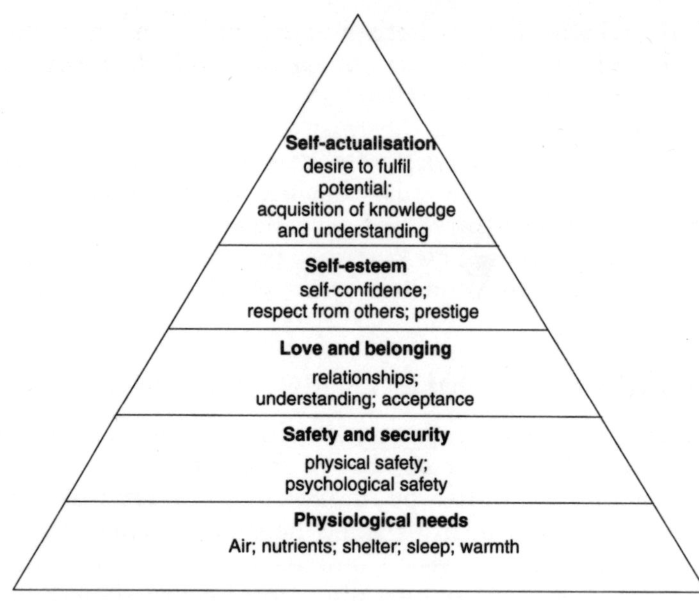

Figure 7.1 Maslow's hierarchy of needs
The individual is considered to have a hierarchy of needs. Higher-level needs only motivate behaviour when lower-level needs have been satisfied.

individual's unsatisfied needs in order to understand why they are motivated towards a particular behaviour.

As well as helping health care professionals understand what motivates behaviours, Maslow's hierarchy of needs is also useful for prioritising health promotion activities. Health behaviours which relate to basic physiological needs, and life-saving activities in particular, should be addressed first.

SOCIO-COGNITIVE THEORY – INCENTIVES AND EXPECTANCIES

Socio-cognitive theory is also important in understanding human motivation. It helps to explain human behaviour by considering the relationship and interaction between an individual and their social environment.

A considerable contribution to our understanding of motivation and behaviour has been made by Bandura. Bandura (1986) suggests that behaviour can be predicted and explained by three concepts:

1. incentives
2. outcome expectancy
3. efficacy expectancy

Incentives refers to the value the individual places on the outcome or consequence of a behaviour, such as health status, appearance, financial gain, etc.

Outcome expectancy refers to how much the individual believes that a certain action will result in the desired outcome.

Efficacy expectancy refers to the degree to which the individual feels confident they can perform the activity that will result in the desired outcome.

For example, an overweight 20 year old will be more likely to change their lifestyle to include a reducing diet and an exercise regime if they believe that:

- loss of weight will increase their attractiveness (incentive)
- changing their lifestyle will produce the loss of weight they want (outcome expectancy)
- they are capable of continuing with the diet and exercise plan (efficacy expectancy)

Bandura (1977) has also contributed to our understanding of learning as a consequence of social interaction. He highlights the importance of observing and imitating others, whom he calls models, in producing behaviour change. He suggests that this occurs in three ways. The individual:

1. copies a new behaviour not previously in their repertoire
2. modifies established behaviour by strengthening or inhibiting their responses to previous cues
3. responds to new cues offered by a model (the 'response facilitation effect')

The models an individual uses changes throughout life and in different circumstances. They include family, peers, teachers and health care professionals, and each can have a significant influence on health behaviour.

HEALTH LOCUS OF CONTROL

The health locus of control has its origins in socio-cognitive theory (Rotter 1954; Wallston and Wallston 1981) and is concerned with how an individual perceives their ability to influence and control their life. It is based on the premise that people who feel they control their lives are more likely to embark on health-promoting behaviours than those who feel powerless to act or who abdicate this responsibility.

Locus of control varies along an internal to external continuum (see Figure 7.2). Wallston and Wallston (1981) suggest that beliefs about health control fall into three categories:

1. **Internal or self-control**: the extent to which the individual believes that they themselves are responsible for their health.
2. **Powerful others**: the extent to which the individual believes that other people such as health professionals are responsible for their health.
3. **Chance**: the extent to which the individual believes that things happen to them by fate or luck rather than because of what they choose to do.

In a study of over four thousand adults aged 18 years and over, Calnan (1988) found that people who reported having good health tended to have higher scores on the internal dimension than those who reported poorer health. The people who described their health as poor were more likely to believe that health was a matter of chance than those reporting good health.

A number of social and demographic factors – such as socio-economic status, age, sex, education, family background and occupation – are said to affect locus of control. Hussey and Gilliland (1989) claim that individuals of a low socio-economic status typically exhibit external locus of control characteristics. Calnan (1988) found that older people, women, people with little formal education and those with manual occupations tended to score higher on the 'chance' and 'powerful other' dimension.

An understanding of locus of control will help the health educator to understand the relationship between health beliefs and health-related behaviour, and so to plan health education activities.

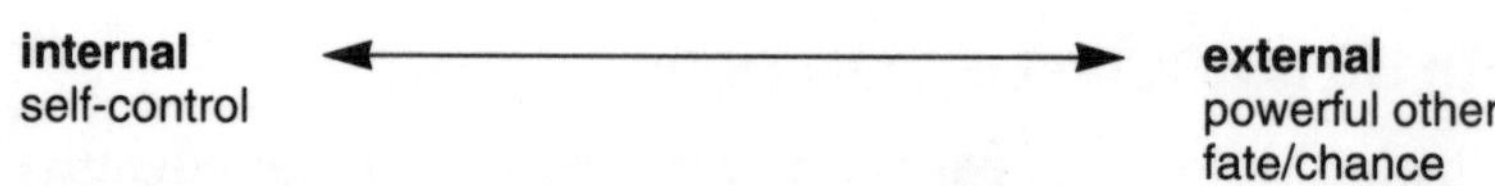

Figure 7.2 Locus of control continuum
People vary in the degree to which they believe their life and health to be under their own control (internal), or under the control of fate/chance or other people (external control).

SELF-EFFICACY

From an early age children copy their parents in many activities, including problem-solving. The degree of success they achieve, together with the feedback on their performance that they receive from others, give them a view of their competence which will influence their confidence and ability to perform in future. Bandura (1986) describes this as self-efficacy, which he defines as 'a judgment of one's ability to accomplish a certain level of performance'.

According to Bandura (1986), an individual's self-judgment arises from:

1. the degree of personal mastery or performance attainment
2. vicarious experience – the opportunity to see others perform successfully
3. verbal persuasion – having others persuade the individual about their ability
4. physiological feedback – feelings of anxiety or elation

An understanding of how an individual's self-efficacy influences their learning can help the health educator plan health education activities. When low self-efficacy hinders learning there are techniques which can be used to enhance it. Poor self-efficacy often results from failure to achieve and perform throughout life and from rejection by people who are important to the individual. Health educators should aim to correct this situation and create success instead. This will require working together with individuals to:

- identify achievable, short-term (rather than long-term) goals with which the individual feels comfortable
- structure learning to provide logical progress and increasing levels of difficulty, at the individual's rate
- use methods suited to the individual, including demonstrations
- provide frequent, positive feedback, reward and reinforcement
- provide a non-threatening environment

HEALTH BELIEF MODEL

The health belief model (see Figure 7.3) was developed in the 1950s and 1960s by social psychologists in the USA. It attempts to explain what motivates people to engage in activities aimed at preventing and avoiding diseases. The model described by Rosenstock (1966) suggests that an individual's motivation to take preventive action is dependent on:

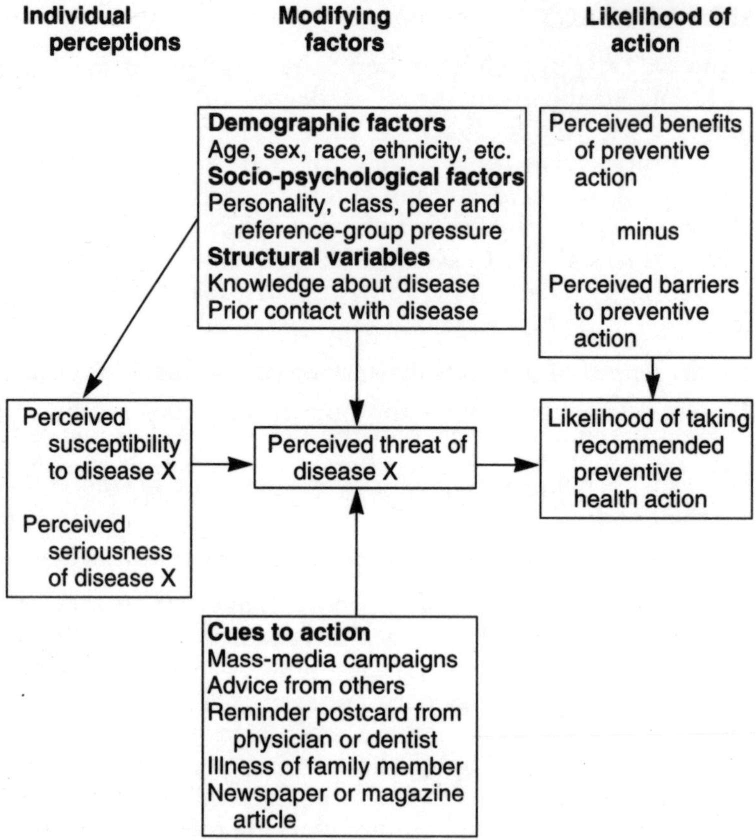

Figure 7.3 Health belief model
Source Adapted from Rosenstock I. (1974), *The health belief model and personal health behaviour* (ed. Becker M.); Thorofare NJ: Charles Slack.

- **perceived level of susceptibility**: how vulnerable or at risk to the disease or condition the individual feels
- **perceived severity**: how serious the physical, emotional and social consequences of having the disease or condition are believed to be
- **perceived benefits**: how beneficial or effective the actions are believed to be in preventing the condition or reducing its severity
- **perceived barriers**: the physical, psychological, financial and other barriers the individual would need to overcome

The model suggests that a stimulus or cue is required to trigger the process so that the individual becomes aware of a potential health risk and initiates the appropriate behaviour. Cues may be provided by things such as a TV programme, a health care professional, an advertisement or an article in a newspaper or magazine. The model also suggests a number of demographic, psychological and cultural factors that modify the individual's perceptions of the benefits of and barriers to preventive actions.

Rosenstock (1974) acknowledged that the health belief model needed further development, and he later (Rosenstock *et al.* 1988) incorporated both socio-cognitive theory and self-efficacy into the model. He recognised the importance of observational learning in which peope model (imitate) the behaviour of others. He also recognised the importance of self-efficacy (see page 113) in explaining health-related behaviour.

Health educators may find the health belief model helps them understand which people perceive themselves to be susceptible to a particular health problem and so to target their educational activity better. It will also help the educator alleviate each client's particular anxieties and plan activities with the client that will meet their specific needs.

WHY DO WE MAKE THE HEALTH CHOICES WE DO?

People take decisions about their health behaviours by weighing up the risks and benefits of a behaviour. This is often done subconsciously. Damrosch (1991) describes this as clients undertaking a 'kind of cost–benefit analysis', in which the perceived benefits of doing something are weighed against the perceived cost (see Figure 7.4).

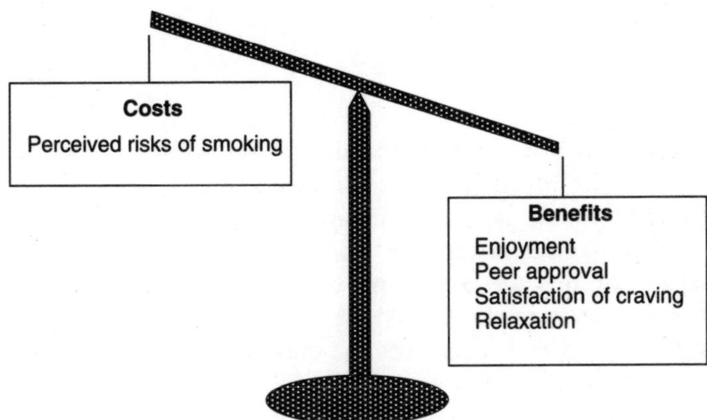

Figure 7.4 Making decisions about smoking – weighing up costs and benefits
In making a decision about an issue such as whether to start or give up smoking, the individual weighs up the costs and benefits of the change.

CASE STUDY: AT-RISK AND BENEFICIAL BEHAVIOURS

Jane, aged 24, is a language graduate who works as a travel consultant. As part of her job she is given discount travel vouchers which she uses to visit hot countries to relax in the sun. In her spare time Jane likes to be active and is a member of a local health club. She exercises and swims three times a week and uses the club's facilities to top up her tan.

In an effort to keep her trim figure, Jane also has a high-fibre, low-fat diet and rarely eats red meat. She began smoking about four years ago while still at university and despite several attempts to give up, continues to smoke 15 cigarettes a day.

The brief case study highlights the following:

- 'at risk' behaviours: smoking and frequent sun-tanning
- 'beneficial' behaviours: regular exercise, high-fibre, low-fat diet, trim figure

There are many factors which may have influenced Jane to start and continue these behaviours, such as:

- knowledge or lack of knowledge of the consequences of a behaviour
- enjoyment from activities
- stress reduction / relaxation
- habit
- peer / family / social pressure
- rewards
- age
- gender
- advertising
- occupation
- self-concept

It is unlikely that Jane is ignorant of the consequences of smoking yet she continues to smoke 15 cigarettes a day. Factors such as social / peer pressure, age and the need for stress reduction while studying at university may have influenced Jane to start smoking. Even though Jane appreciates the consequences of smoking, her perception of the risks is outweighed by the other influences of habit, peer pressure and the need to reduce stress. In Jane's case the perceived risk of smoking is low in comparison with perceived benefits. To have more chance of success at changing Jane's smoking behaviour the balance of perceptions must be shifted so that the perceived costs of smoking come to outweigh the perceived benefits.

One single factor seldom operates on its own to influence a change in behaviour and many of the following influencing factors are interrelated.

KNOWLEDGE OR IGNORANCE OF THE CONSEQUENCES OF A BEHAVIOUR

Knowledge about the consequences of a behaviour is important in making decisions and choices about health behaviour. If people are unaware of the possible consequences of excessive alcohol consumption, smoking, unprotected sex or frequent exposure to the sun, then they are unable to make informed decisions about whether to undertake a behaviour. On the other hand, even if they do have an understanding this does not guarantee that healthy behaviours will occur. In a study of almost 650 children aged between 14 and 17, 98 per cent knew that smoking harmed their health and 89 per cent knew that passive smoking was also harmful yet 1 in 5 were or had been smokers (MacFarlane *et al.* 1987).

ENJOYMENT FROM ACTIVITIES

It is extremely difficult to give up activities if these are enjoyable. Enjoyment acts as a reinforcer to a behaviour. Similarly, people are attracted to take part in activities which appear interesting, fun and challenging. Sometimes activities are taken up for health reasons and then become hobbies. For example, an individual may start keep-fit classes in an effort to get fit and lose weight but find over time that the enjoyment and company gained from attending the class become the motivation for continued attendance.

REWARDS

Rewards are important in influencing behaviour (see operant conditioning, page 94). People will be motivated by different rewards. Wiles (1992) found that notions of attractiveness were important in encouraging people to adopt and maintain health behaviour. In women the desire to be slim was commonly equated with attractiveness and in men physical fitness. As a result, weight-reducing diets and exercise regimes were adopted. Wiles concluded that attractiveness rather than health enhancement appeared to be the chief motivator.

STRESS REDUCTION AND RELAXATION

Many aspects of our working and social lives can be stressful, putting our mental health at risk. An attempt to relax and to reduce stress may be the reason for adopting both 'high-risk' behaviours and 'beneficial' behaviours. Smoking and drinking are examples of the former, and exercise, yoga, music and massage are examples of the latter. Activities may be chosen because they are readily available, easy to do or enjoyable, or may be ignored because they require too much effort or do not coincide with the individual's self-image.

AGE AND GENDER

Age may influence health behaviours. Physical education is now a compulsory part of the curriculum for all children and the percentage of adults participating in sport and physical activities is slowly increasing (DoH 1991). Generally, participation decreases with age.

Gender is also an important influence on behaviour. Women are less likely to be physically active than men. There are also gender differences with alcohol consumption. One in four men is drinking more than the levels advised by the medical Royal Colleges but only 1 in 12 women is exceeding these recommended levels (see Figure 3.4) (DoH 1991).

OCCUPATION

Occupation may be linked with age and gender in influencing health behaviours. Several studies have been conducted on the subject of smoking and health service professionals. In the nursing professions, for example, Hawkins, White and Morris (1982) report differences in smoking prevalence in nurses from different specialities. They found psychiatric nurses smoked most heavily and those in the community least.

In another study, comparing two age groups (20–50 and 51–79 years) of middle-class private patients, Wiles (1992) found differences in the factors that motivated and constrained health-enhancing behaviours. In the younger age group, employment was identified as a major constraint, causing lack of time or opportunity to take some form of exercise. Employment also constrained ability to change and improve their diet either because they only took time to eat a quick snack or because they travelled away from home and found they ate rich diets with a high fat content. Wiles found that in the older age group two constraints were reported: firstly, that confusing media messages discouraged health-enhancing behaviours; and secondly, that some felt they were 'too old' to worry about changing their behaviour, taking the view that health-enchancing behaviour was for younger people.

PEER/SOCIAL/FAMILY PRESSURE

Family members, peers and other members of society play an important role in establishing and modifying an individual's behaviour patterns. Peer pressure is often seen to be a barrier to change in health behaviour (Currie, Amos and Hunt 1991). The amount of influence peers have will change over time. Family members play an important part – often throughout life. Children learn much of their early behaviour, such as eating habits, general health maintenance, dental care, and attitudes towards smoking and alcohol, from parents and grandparents. Patterns of child rearing are also passed on from generation to generation, as well as beliefs about how much responsibility individuals should take for keeping themselves healthy. Smoke-buster clubs are a good example of using peer pressure in health promotion (Raw, White and McNeill 1990).

Peers become important models for imitation from school age onwards, and are especially influential around the age of puberty. However, young people are more likely to be influenced by their peers in matters such as dress, pop music and hobbies than in health matters. Teachers and health care professionals will also have varying degrees of influence on shaping an individual's behaviour.

ADVERTISING

Advertising can be very influential, particularly on children and young people. This is especially the case when pop stars and other idols are used to put over the message. From a health promotion point of view the image that athletes and sports personalities portray has gone some way to encouraging people to take up sports and other activities. TV personalities and programmes have also influenced many women to start fitness and dietary plans. This is discussed further in Chapter 19.

Popular magazines for both men and women frequently contain articles relating to health, particularly to sexual health and personal relationships. This makes such information much more accessible than previously. Although advertising and TV programmes can contribute positively to health promotion, they may also be instrumental in encouraging less healthy behaviours. Examples of this occur when drugs, alcohol and smoking are linked with rich, glamorous and attractive people.

SELF-CONCEPT

Self-concept refers to the beliefs that individuals holds about themselves and the importance they attach to those beliefs, though these beliefs may not necessarily reflect reality. If people see themselves as successful, they are more likely to be successful. On the other hand, people who see themselves in a negative or inferior way are more likely to engage in counter-productive behaviour. For example, people who see themselves as overweight and unattractive may over-eat, starve or binge to compensate for feeling unhappy about their appearance. Alternatively, people who feel alive and energetic are likely to be active and busy to confirm these positive beliefs about themselves.

Self-concept is a learned attribute which can be influenced, manipulated and changed. It develops from the first few months of life and continues to affect every aspect of behaviour throughout life. It is moulded by personality, past experiences, upbringing, relationships, family and social circumstances. How people feel about themselves will therefore influence their health behaviours and their readiness to develop new health behaviours.

SOCIAL CLASS

There is evidence to suggest that different patterns of health-related behaviours are practised by different social classes. Calnan (1985), in a study of a large sample of middle-aged women, showed that women from social classes I and II were more likely than those from social classes IV and V to wear seat belts, to brush their teeth regularly, to change their diet for health reasons, to take regular exercise and be non-smokers. Figure 7.5 shows differences in smoking and drinking behaviour between different occupational classes.

In a later study, of women between the ages of 21 and 55, Calnan (1986) found that health education has had more impact on middle-class groups than on working-class groups. On the whole, women from classes IV and V were more sceptical about the possibilities of disease prevention than professional women. He provided three possible explanations for this:

1. Women in the social classes IV and V feel less able to influence their lives.
2. They need to rationalise their own behaviour, particularly their smoking behaviour.
3. Different modes of reasoning were used by the two groups: women from social classes IV and V seemed to use a mode of reasoning based on their own experience, whereas women from classes I and II tended to use a mode of reasoning based on statistical theories of probability found in epidemiology.

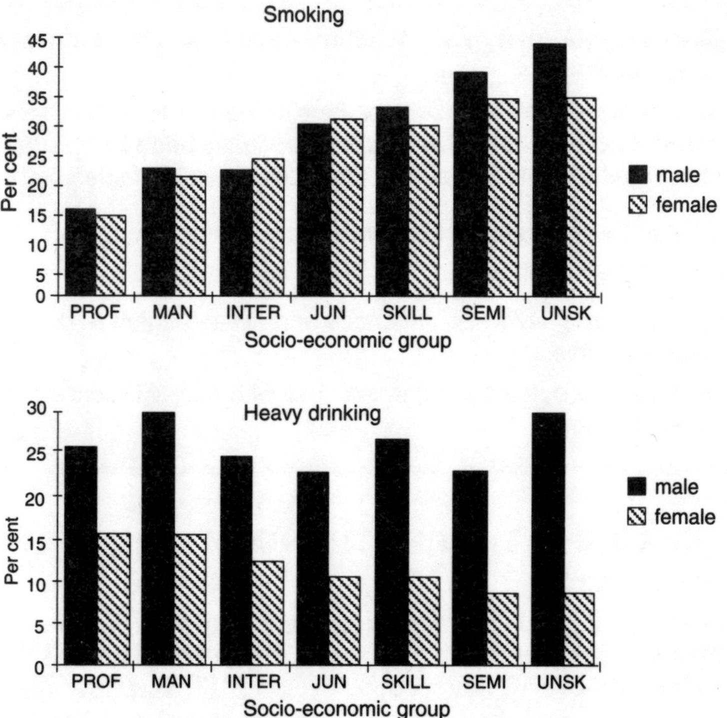

Figure 7.5 Social-class differences in smoking and drinking behaviour
The information is taken from the General Household Survey for England and Wales 1992. The groupings used are Professional (PROF), Managerial (MAN), Intermediate Skilled Non-manual (INTER), Junior Skilled Non-manual (JUN), Skilled Manual (SKILL), Semi-skilled (SEMI) and Unskilled (UNSK). These groupings are very similiar to social classes I to V used elsewhere in this book. Heavy drinkers are defined as men drinking more than 21 units per week or women drinking more than 14 units per week. Note the large differences for smoking in men and women and for heavy drinking in women.
Source Data from OPCS (Office of Population Censuses and Surveys) (1993), *General household survey 1992*; London: HMSO.

Health educators should be able to use approaches that will best influence the individual or group. For people from social classes IV and V, the use of examples from within the individual's own experiences will be more effective than quoting statistical evidence on mortality and morbidity rates.

Discussion/Activity 7.1 What influences a patient's health behaviour?

Look again at the case study of Jane on page 116. Now choose a patient or client with whom you have recently been involved and think about their lifestyle in a similar way. List the behaviours you believe:

1. are beneficial to that patient's or client's health
2. put their health at risk

Consider carefully what influences or motivates them to do each of these activities.

Compare the outcome of this exercise with that of Discussion/Activity 3.2 in Chapter 3.

THE ROLE OF THE HEALTH EDUCATOR IN MOTIVATING CLIENTS

People will often put off adopting a health-promoting behaviour. Frequently we hear smokers say, 'I'll give up when I've finished this packet' or overweight people declare, 'I'll start the diet after the weekend'. These delaying tactics may be employed because the individual does not know what to do or how to go about overcoming the barriers to change. They may lack confidence in their ability to take up a new behaviour, or fear failure and the risk of being ridiculed by others.

Because people have a natural tendency to delay, the health educator must try to motivate them sufficiently to act. Although the final decision for engaging in health-promoting behaviours rests with the individual, the health care professional has a responsibility to advise and guide clients towards making an informed choice. Some key tasks for motivating clients are listed in Table 7.1.

Individuals are motivated to different degrees by different factors depending on the situation. The health educator has the opportunity to promote or diminish an individual's motivation to learn and incorporate new health behaviours. Initially an individual's motivation may be weak. They may even be unaware of their own motivation or unwilling to share it with others.

The health educator's key task, therefore, is to create a situation in which the individual's attention is focused on the subject in question. The individual may then experience involvement and develop interest which will motivate them to learn. Health care professionals should be confident and caring in their approach and put over a positive message which shows they genuinely believe

Table 7.1 Key tasks of the health educator in motivating clients

The health educator...	**...helps the individual to:**
• with knowledge of the individual uses strategies and techniques to raise awareness and understanding of the importance of health issues to the individual	• focus attention on the subject, activity, idea in question
• creates situations where the individual is tempted to do things, such as comment, accept, reject, choose, handle, operate	• become involved and want to continue to be involved
• continues to stimulate, challenge and support the individual	• develop interest and be motivated to act

that the activity will help the client. Health educators should therefore:

- **Project the right image**: the old adage 'first impressions are lasting impressions' is often true. A smart, confident, caring professional who appears healthy will help to set the scene and give a positive message to clients.
- **Consider being a role model**: although no one expects every health professional to be perfect in their own health behaviours, it is important to bear in mind the effect they may have on others.
- **Prepare** what they are going to do and say and have sufficient knowledge and skills to cope with the unexpected.

Discussion/Activity 7.2 Motivating a family to adopt healthier dental behaviours

Susan has three children aged two, four and seven. Her partner has recently left them so Susan has to care for the children by herself. The two older children have extensive dental caries. No member of the family owns a toothbrush and all the children have sweets in their mouths most of the time. Susan says that she cannot afford a toothbrush and anyway she is too busy looking after the family to have time to help the children brush their teeth. She also says that 'the children like sweets, poor darlings, and why shouldn't they have them'. And if she does not give the children sweets they will make her life impossible until she does. Discuss how you might motivate the family to adopt a more tooth-friendly lifestyle.

BEING A ROLE MODEL

Role modelling is a technique often used by health promoters. A role model is someone who demonstrates certain behaviours in a real-life setting. Role modelling is based on social learning theory and involves imitation and identification. For example, a nurse interacting with an elderly person provides the carer with a model of effective care by specific behaviours.

According to Narrow (1979), three conditions favour role modelling:

1. The behaviour to be learned must be seen as desirable by the learner. If the behaviour results in enjoyment, satisfaction or reward for the role model the learner is more likely to attempt the behaviour.
2. Learners must be capable (intellectually, physically or emotionally) of copying the behaviour they see.
3. The learner must know what to observe – the role model must point out the essential cues to the learner.

The health promoter also has to beware of the risk of being a negative role model. For instance it will be very difficult for a client to believe in the importance of stopping smoking when they know that the health care professional smokes. If the health promoter cannot be a role model for the completed behaviour, they may be able to be a role model for making the behavioural change.

There will also be occasions when the health care professional cannot offer any sort of role model. 'Do as I advise, not as I do' is a difficult message to sell but in such as situation all the health care worker can offer is honesty. A frank discussion of the difficulties and barriers to change may help the client to adopt the healthier behaviours that the health promoter cannot.

CASE STUDY: GETTING FITTER TOGETHER

Frank is a man of 35 who is unemployed. He lives with his mother for whom he is caring. He weighs 18 stone and wants to lose weight. He has tried following several reducing diets but not lost any weight. Frank mentioned his weight problem to the community nurse who was visiting his mother. In the discussion that followed, the community nurse revealed that he too was overweight and wanted to lose about 2 stone because he felt uncomfortable and his clothes were too tight.

Frank and the nurse agreed to have a competition to see who could lose half a stone in the following month. They discussed diet and exercise and the effects this should have. The community nurse was able to borrow an exercise bike for Frank to use and they agreed to weigh themselves weekly and discuss progress when the community nurse visited. Gradually both the community nurse and Frank lost some weight. The community nurse acted as a role model. Both he and Frank experienced the benefits together.

THE CHANGE PROCESS

Adoption of a new behaviour does not happen instantly. Prochaska and DiClemente (1983) have described the states through which an individual passes before adopting a new behaviour (see Figure 7.6):

- **Pre-contemplation**: the individual is content with their existing behaviour and sees no reason to change.
- **Contemplation**: a change of behaviour is considered.
- **Action**: a change in behaviour is attempted.
- **Maintenance**: the new behaviour is continued.

Maintenance may be followed by:

- **Relapse**: the individual reverts to the old behaviour and returns to the contemplation stage.
- **Termination**: the new behaviour becomes entrenched and all temptation to return to the old behaviour is lost.

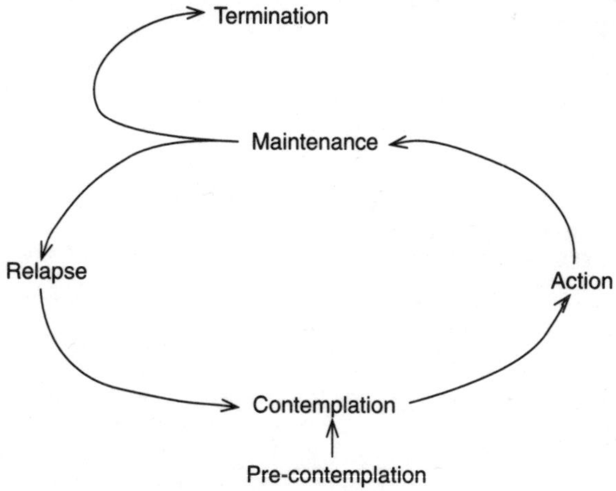

Figure 7.6 Cycles of behavioural change
The process of behavioural change involves progression from a state of pre-contemplation into a cycle of contemplation, action, maintenance and relapse. The cycles continues until the new behaviour becomes established (termination).

Most people have to make several attempts before achieving a stable new behaviour (e.g. not smoking), passing through the contemplation → action → maintenance → relapse cycle several time before reaching termination (see Figure 7.6). Health educators must try to assess which stage their patients are at, and choose activities appropriate to that stage. An episode of ill health may move patients from the pre-contemplation to the contemplation phase. In this state presentation of the reasons for behavioural change will reinforce contemplation. In the action phase, strategies for change will be helpful, while in the maintenance phase strategies to reduce desire for the old behaviour and boost rewards from the new will be needed.

DIFFUSION OF IDEAS

The spread of new ideas and new patterns of behaviours through communities has been studied by Rogers (1983) (see Figure 7.7). At first, take up of a new idea is slow and only a few people (innovators) try it. Then the idea starts to spread and more people in the community try it (early adopters, early majority, late majority). Finally, diffusion of the idea slows again as only resistant and 'hard to reach' groups are left (late adopters) (Rogers 1983). Different approaches to health promotion are required, depending on whether one is trying to get innovators to introduce a new idea, encourage the spread of an established idea from innovators and early adopters to the majority, or trying to reach the hard core of late adopters.

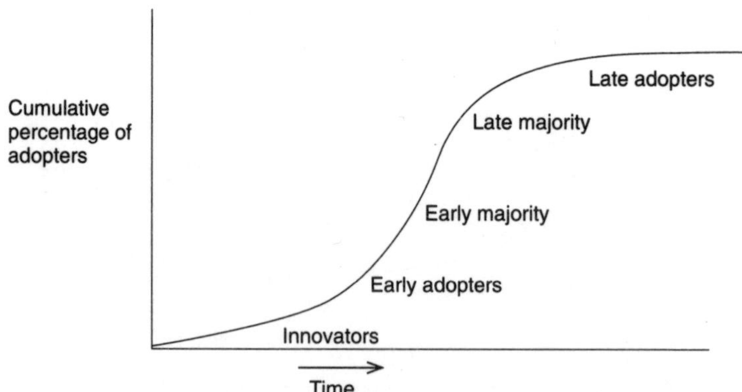

Figure 7.7 Prevalence curve of adopters
The time taken for new ideas to be adopted by different sections of the community.

SUMMARY POINTS

- ☐ Many factors are believed to influence people's health beliefs:
  - social factors
  - demographic factors
  - individual's locus of control
    - self
    - powerful others
    - chance
- ☐ People take decisions about their health by weighing up the costs and benefits of a behaviour.
- ☐ Individuals are motivated by different things in different situations.
- ☐ People are more likely to engage in health-promoting behaviours if:
  - they have an incentive for doing so
  - the health behaviour produces the outcome they want
  - they believe they are capable of performing the behaviour
- ☐ The health educator has the opportunity to promote or diminish an individual's motivation to learn health-promoting behaviours.
- ☐ The key task of the health educator is to assist the individual to:
  - focus attention on the subject
  - become involved and find the experience enjoyable
  - become interested and motivated to act
- ☐ People undertaking behavioural change pass through a cycle of pre-contemplation → contemplation → action → maintenance → relapse/termination. The health education activities must be appropriate to the individual's position in this cycle.

REFERENCES

Bandura A. (1977). *A social learning theory*. Englewood Cliffs NJ: Prentice-Hall.

Bandura A. (1986). Self efficacy. In *Social foundations of thought and action*. Englewood Cliffs NJ: Prentice-Hall, pp. 390–453.

Bunton R., Murphy S. and Bennet P. (1991). Theories of behavioural change and their use in health promotion: some neglected areas. *Health Education Research* **6**, 153–162.

Calnan M. (1985) Patterns in preventive behaviour: a study of women in middle age. *Social Science and Medicine* **20**, 263–268.

Calnan M. (1986). Maintaining health and preventing illness: a comparison of the perceptions of women from different social classes. *Health Promotion* **1**, 167–177.

Calnan M. (1988). The health locus of control: an empirical test. *Health Promotion* **2**, 323–330.

Currie C.E., Amos A. and Hunt S.M. (1991). The dynamics of behavioural change in five classes of health related behaviour – findings from qualitative research. *Health Education Research* **6**, 443–453.

Damrosch S. (1991). General strategies for motivating people to change their behaviour. *Nursing Clinics of North America* **26**, 833–843.

DoH (Department of Health) (1991). *The Health of the Nation*. London: HMSO.

DoH (Department of Health) (1993). *Health of the Nation: one year on*. London: HMSO.

Hawkins L., White M. and Morris L. (1982). Smoking, stress and nurses. *Nursing Mirror* **155**, 18–22.

Hussey L.C. and Gilliland K. (1989). Compliance, low literacy and locus of control. *Nursing Clinics of North America* **24**, 605–611.

Macfarlane A., McPherson A., McPherson K. and Ahmed L. (1987). Teenagers and their health. *Archives of Diseases in Childhood* **62**, 1125–1129.

Maslow A. (1954). *Motivation and personality*. New York: Harper & Row.

Narrow B. (1979). *Patient teaching in nursing practice. A patient and family-centred approach*. New York: John Wiley and Sons.

Prochaska J.O. and DiClemente C.C. (1983). Stages and processes of self change in smoking: toward an integrative model of change. *Journal of Consulting and Clinical Psychology* **5**, 390–395.

Raw M., White P. and McNeill A. (1990). Smoke busters. Case study 8 in *Clearing the air: a guide to action on tobacco*. London: BMA on behalf of WHO European Regional Office.

Rogers E. (1983). *Diffusion of innovations*. New York: Free Press.

Rosenstock I.M. (1966). Why people use health services. *Millbank Memorial Fund Quarterly* **44**, 94–124.

Rosenstock I.M. (1974). The health belief model and preventive health behaviour. In Becker M. (ed.) *The health belief model and personal health behaviour*. Thorofare NJ: Charles Slack.

Rosenstock I.M., Strecher V.J. and Becker M.H. (1988). Social learning theory and health belief model. *Health Education Quarterly* **15**, 175–183.

Rotter J.B. (1954). *Social learning and clinical psychology*. Englewood Cliffs NJ: Prentice-Hall.

Wallstone K.S. and Wallstone B.S. (1981). Health locus of control scales. In Lefcourt H.M (ed.), *Research with the locus of control construct*, vol. 1. New York: Academic Press.

Wiles R. (1992). Middle-class health behaviour: motivations and constraints in a sample of private patients. *Health Education Journal* **51**, 179–183.

SECTION 2

Necessary skills

CHAPTER 8

Influencing policy makers and managers

GOAL

To understand how to promote healthier environments in situations where the health worker is apparently powerless.

OBJECTIVES

- to appreciate the importance of advocacy
- to identify the key decision makers
- to clarify the issues – health and other
- to explore ways of influencing individuals and the advantages/disadvantages of each way
- to understand how to build alliances for health
- to explore ways of advocacy and lobbying using press and politicians

INTRODUCTION

Chapters 3 and 5 emphasised that individuals have little control over many of the things that determine their health. Much of this book is about making the most of the relatively few (but very worthwhile) things that they can do to improve their own health. However, one of the main themes of Health for All is empowerment, and part of that must include extending people's ability to influence decisions about things which affect their health. While health care professionals may accept that producing change should be part of their job, they may feel, especially if they are in fairly junior posts, that they have little power to do so. A great deal has been written on how people in managerial positions can motivate their teams and achieve their managerial goals. This chapter takes a slightly different viewpoint and is more concerned with how you influence people who are more senior than yourself. Some health care workers are very successful at doing this (Furley 1991). This chapter is about how to produce change in situations where you apparently have little or no control.

ADVOCACY

Health care professionals know that advocacy is often an important part of caring for individual patients or clients (Stutor 1993). The carer may have to speak up for the client to ensure that they obtain their entitlements to treatment, dignity and conditions which enable them to be healthy. Advocacy may need to be addressed to other members of the caring team (Marshall 1992) or to outside organisations such as housing departments, benefits offices, or water and gas companies. Advocacy may be needed for groups rather than individuals. At all levels, advocacy is an important tool in the health promoter's kit. Health workers have to think about how to be effective as advocates: in other words, how to influence others on behalf of their patients or clients.

WHO ARE THE KEY DECISION MAKERS?

In the health service there is an increasingly clearly defined management structure. Nursing services have well-defined lines of accountability. In the hospital or unit, staff are accountable to line managers, who are in turn accountable to more senior managers, who are in turn accountable to a chief executive or unit manager. In his or her turn the chief executive is accountable to the trust or district health authority board and its chairperson, and they are accountable eventually to the NHS management executive and the Minister of Health.

In the local authority there is a similar chain: social workers, housing staff, environmental health officers, librarians and other local authority employees will be accountable through line managers to a chief officer who will in turn be answerable to the elected local council members. The powers of the local councils are prescribed by Parliament.

In schools the classroom teacher is accountable to the head teacher, who is accountable to the board of governors and in some circumstances to the local education authority, and so on. Private firms have similar layers of management.

For each sphere of action there is usually a chain of authority with higher levels setting the framework within which lower levels make detailed decisions. At one end of the chain (the sharp end, the coal face), people are directly involved with helping individual patients or clients. At this end of the chain people make decisions about details and usually control relatively few resources (money and people). At the other end of the chain people are concerned with broad policy and control very large resources.

Table 8.1 takes the example of health promotion related to alcohol to show how different people have power to authorise different actions.

Other people can help individuals to influence these chains within organisations. Local councillors and Members of Parliament can make enquiries and if necessary representations about matters affecting their constituents. Community Health Councils were set up by the NHS Act of 1974 with the duty to act as watchdog on health authority decisions. They will assist individual patients to pursue enquiries and raise matters of general service provision (Heginbotham 1994).

Professional associations such as the Royal College of Nursing and the Health Visitors' Association are very willing to raise matters concerning either their members' interests or the general public health, at both national and local level. Trade unions such as UNISON are often involved in workplace health and safety issues and will also take up issues of members' welfare or public health.

Table 8.1 Ability to make decisions: examples related to alcohol

Action	Competent decision maker
• put up safe-drinking poster in ward	• ward sister
• encourage all nurses in hospital to include assessment of alcohol consumption in nursing plan	• director of nursing
• institute alcohol policy for all hospital employees	• personnel director / chief executive of hospital trust / health authority board
• increase regional/national priority given to care of patients with alcohol dependence	• regional chief executive / regional outpost of NHS management executive / chief executive of the NHS / NHS board
• provide better alcohol education in local school	• teacher / head teacher/ board of governors
• enforce existing drink–drive legislation more strictly	• chief constable
• increase taxation on alcohol	• Chancellor of the Exchequer
• increase penalties for drink–driving	• Home Secretary

INFORMAL INFLUENCE

The preceding section described where power lies as it appears in organisational plans and theoretical descriptions. In real life it may be rather different. It is rumoured that Mrs Wilson (the wife of Woodrow Wilson, President of the US, 1913–21) exerted enormous power towards the end of her husband's presidency but you will find nothing in the United States constitution about the powers of the President's spouse. Similarly, in any organisation you will find people with great power to influence decisions who do not appear on any organisational plan. In most committees the opinions of all members in theory carry equal weight but in practice it is very rarely true. Several managers may be of equal seniority but some are likely to be much more influential than others. Nearly always there are all sorts of informal relationships such as membership of professional organisations, shared interests outside work, friendships and so on through which influence is exercised. Doctors are notorious for using these channels of influence to great effect. In order to influence the many things which effect people's health you need to know who has the power to make changes.

Discussion/Activity 8.1 Obtaining better occupational health services

The nurses in your hospital feel they need a better occupational health service. In particular they would like more and better counselling on handling stress, and the female nurses would like to be able to have cervical smears taken at work when they are due. (If these issues are not relevant to your place of work think of some that are.)

Who has the power to make the necessary decisions? How can they be influenced to improve the service?

THE PROBLEM OF ACCESS

The first step in influencing anything is to work out to whom you have access. You and I might like to influence the Prime Minister or Minister of Health but we would probably never be able to get to their offices or speak to them on the phone. On the other hand, if we write to our MP they will very possibly raise the matter on our behalf and obtain an answer from the relevant Minister. Similarly, it is unlikely that you will be able to have lengthy chats with the chief executive or chairman of the health authority about the running of your unit. On the other hand, you can raise your concerns with your line manager or professional representative and they may either be able to make the necessary decisions or raise them with higher levels of management.

POWER TO INFLUENCE

Handy (1985) identifies five sources of power that enable people to exert influence:

- **personal power**: power that comes from being liked or admired (charisma)
- **expert power**: power that comes from knowing a great deal about the topic in hand
- **resource power**: power to control the use of resources (staff time, health promotion materials, money, and so on)
- **position power**: power from position giving access to key people or information or the right to organise things (i.e. being the boss)
- **physical power**: power to threaten force

Health promoters would not use physical power and often they have little position or resource power. This means that attempts to influence have to be based on expert power and personal power. Frequently the health care worker has the detailed knowledge by virtue of having worked closely with the people whose needs are being discussed, and therefore in that situation has expert power.

STRATEGIES OF INFLUENCE

Management texts list a number of way in which people can be influenced (Kipnis *et al.* 1984):

- reason: persuading that your suggestion is best
- bargaining: promising to give or do something in return
- friendliness: being nice to people
- coalition: giving mutual support to others
- assertiveness: being confident and self-assured
- higher authority: giving orders
- sanction: threatening penalties for non-agreement

The greater a person's position and resource power the wider the variety of influence strategies they tend to use. Health care workers who are not managers will have to rely mostly on reason to carry their case by persuasion. In some situations it may also be possible to obtain the change you want by offering to provide something that the other parties want in return for agreement (bargaining). Friendliness and coalition are particularly effective as ways of influencing colleagues of similar seniority. The nature of communication in attempts to influence has been analysed in detail (Mulholland 1991; Fisher, Ury and Paaten 1991). Skills of stating your view, active listening, supporting, clarifying and building on the contributions of others will all improve your chances of influencing others. (Note the similarity with motivation in teaching – see Chapter 7, page 122.)

ARGUING FOR RESOURCES

- Know what you want.
- Know who has the power to make it available.
- Know why you want them.
- Know what benefit will come from using them.

For some health promotion activities very few resources are needed – maybe just a little of your time, a little of someone else's, use of a room and a bit of photocopying – so there is no need to go off and ask for more. Often, however, much more extensive resources are needed for a health promotion activity – weeks of managerial effort, large numbers of helpers, use of equipment and large sums of money. If you need to get extra resources for a health promotion activity you must be clear what you want.

Having decided what you want, the next question is 'Who has the power to make them available?'. You then need to decide if you can ask for the resources directly, or if it is better to get someone to ask on your behalf. Either way the person asking will need to have a list of what is needed, what will be done with it, and why the activity is worth doing.

This process of seeking resources can have several outcomes. You may be given what you need straight away, more likely you will have to negotiate and end up with less than you wanted, but enough to do something less ambitious. You may get nothing and then you will have to start your planning again.

MAKING THINGS CHANGE – FORCE-FIELD ANALYSIS

In any situation there will be forces working in favour of change and forces working against change (Turrill 1986). If you are trying to encourage change it is helpful to think about what these forces are. How could you increase the forces favouring change and reduce the forces blocking change? Figure 8.1 gives an example of this approach. Sometimes the forces against are a reaction to the forces in favour. Maybe everyone is fed up with hearing about the issue at every meeting and the best way to make progress is to back off and be a little less enthusiastic.

MAKING THINGS CHANGE – COMMITMENT PLANNING

People can take different views of any particular change:

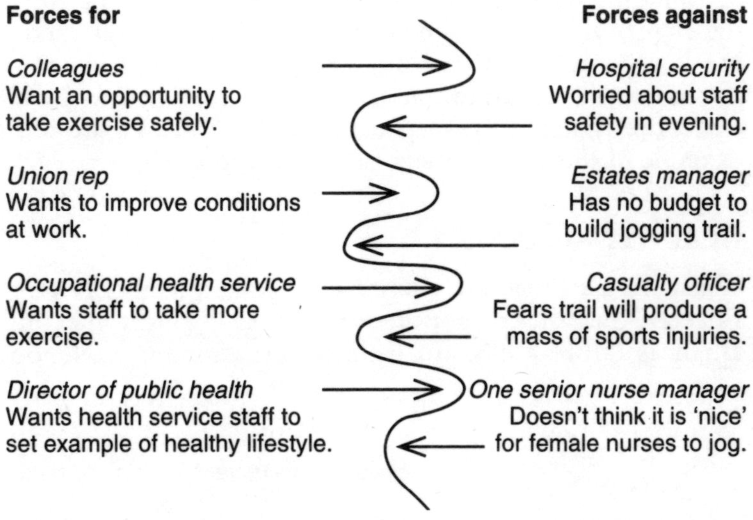

Action

To strengthen forces in favour:

- encourage colleagues to say they would like to use a jogging trail
- ask union rep to raise matter with management
- ask occupational health service to spell out the effect of more exercise on staff health and sick leave
- ask director of public health to stress the value of health staff setting example of healthy living

To weaken forces against:

- suggest to hospital security that the trail only be used during daylight hours
- point out to the estate manager that the trail can use existing paths
- get casualty officer to talk to occupational health service
- what can be done about the senior nurse manager?

Figure 8.1 Force-field analysis
Example *Getting a jogging trail for the hospital*
For any change there will be forces favouring that change and forces against. To encourage change you must strengthen the forces for and weaken the forces against.

- **oppose** – will try and block the change
- **indifferent** – will neither assist nor oppose the change
- **help** – mildly favourable to the change but will not lead
- **make** – very committed and will put all their effort into making change happen

If the change is to happen then different key people must have appropriate levels of commitment. The change will not happen if some key people oppose it. These key people must be moved at least to an indifferent position. Other people will have to positively want the change if it is to happen. It is therefore a useful exercise to list the key people who can influence the situation, work out their present level of commitment and how that has to be altered to allow the change to take place (Turrill 1986). Figure 8.2 gives an example of this commitment-planning approach.

HEALTHY ALLIANCES

When we act alone our ability to change anything is very limited. Effective health promotion very often requires the building of alliances (DoH 1993). In isolated situations it is all too easy to

	Oppose	Indifferent	Help	Make
Local councillor	O ⟶	x		
Residents		O ⟶	x	
Borough engineer		O ⟶	⟶	x
Local bus company	O ⟶	x		
Police	O ⟶	x		
Local press		O ⟶	x	
Road safety unit		O ⟶	x	

Figure 8.2 Commitment planning
Example Traffic-calming measures in a residential street
When a change is proposed, the different people and agencies involved will vary in their commitment to change: from opposition through indifference and vaguely favouring to full commitment. In order to bring about change you should identify different people's current commitment and how this needs to be altered. In the figure, O indicates people's current commitment and X the state of commitment that would allow change.

delude yourself that you are the only one who cares about people's health but a little more thought will reveal a host of potential allies:

- other health care professionals
- those who work for other caring and public service agencies (e.g. social services, education, environmental services, youth services, etc.)
- churches and voluntary organisations
- Community Health Councils
- patients' and residents' groups
- leisure and amenity groups

A single voice will not carry much weight but a coalition of voices may be able to achieve a great deal. The first step in making allies is to explain the issues that concern you and find out the issues that concern others. Some allies may have exactly the same aims as yourself. For example, if you are a school nurse concerned about child accident prevention, you will probably find that the other community staff, the local primary care teams and the other school staff all share your concern. Other allies may have rather different priorities but are still eager to make common cause over relevant issues. The prime interest of the police is law enforcement and crime prevention but they will probably be very ready to support the accident prevention activities. Commercial firms may also find they have interests in common with you. Electrical firms may see that support for accident prevention could increase their market (coiled flexes, safety kettles, safety plugs, etc.).

Successful alliances are built by getting together people who are committed to common goals. Negotiating these common goals is a vital part of alliance building and you may well have to modify your first choice of goals in the process. For example, you might not have included first aid in your initial plans for child accident prevention, but when the local Red Cross or St John's Ambulance express an interest you could make the alliance much more powerful by taking these issues on board.

Alliances are made up of people and so they have all the strengths and all the weaknesses of people. They need to be cherished and valued if they are to work well. People work harder for a cause when they are thanked and their contribution acknowledged. They need to know that their ideas are being heard and that they are participating in the decision making. This is particularly true in most health promotion settings, where people are usually in the alliance because they are enthusiastic rather than because their job description says they should be.

GETTING THE PRESS BEHIND YOU

The press is a powerful ally. When they take up a story it immediately becomes more important. Managers and politicians will not ignore an issue which is receiving press coverage. There are two main ways of getting health promotion issues into the local papers:

1. provide news stories
2. write letters to the editor

They may also run general interest features and if you build up a good relationship with the newspaper staff, you may be able to suggest topics for these – such as healthy eating, looking after yourself on holiday, and similar themes.

Local papers exist to entertain people. They have to provide interesting copy and produce a product that people want to read. They must work to very tight schedules and all their staff are busy. They may well be very willing to run stories on health promotion activities but you must make it easy for them to do so. Press releases need to be sharp and make the topic sound exciting (see Table 8.2). The press are much more likely to be interested in stories with human interest. Names and quotations help journalists make an interesting

Table 8.2 How to write a press release

1. State date of release and any embargo time.*
2. Give the source of the press release, e.g. OLDTOWN COMMUNITY HEALTH TRUST.
3. Use a short title and put it in capitals – this should make it clear WHAT THE PRESS RELEASE IS ABOUT.
4. Write in short paragraphs.
5. Put the most important item in first paragraph:
   - WHAT has happened or is going to happen
   - WHEN and WHERE did it or will it happen
   - WHO is involved
6. Supporting paragraphs should add further details. WHY it is happening.
7. Quotations from named local people are a good idea, e.g. 'I am worried that some child will be killed unless a crossing is installed', said Oldtown health visitor Jane Smith.
8. Keep it short: two sides of A4 maximum – one side is better.
9. At the end of the release, put your name, position and telephone number for further enquiries.
10. Use double-spaced typing.

Note that the structure of a press release is different from most other forms of writing. It starts with the main point without any introduction. Background information – if any – comes later in the press release.

* Embargo time: sometimes the press is asked not to release the news before a certain date and time but they are given the information earlier to make it easier for them to cover the story.

story. The editor may also be attracted by the prospect of being able to take a good photo of someone doing something. Local celebrities, children, nurses in uniform, people in fancy dress or animals may all be of interest. Remember it is the journalist's job to produce a good news article. It is your job to make it easy for them and thereby get your health promotion message across for free.

The timing of press releases is important. If they relate to a specific event, it is best to send them to arrive three or four days before the event. This gives the news editor time to get them into the reporter's diary but is not too far ahead. Many weekly papers go to press on Thursday, so the best day for them to receive a press release is Monday or Tuesday. You need to know what best suits your local press.

Similar considerations apply to getting letters to the editor published. The letter must be short, interesting, preferably linked to previous correspondence or some current news issue and preferably slightly controversial (Howe 1993).

Remember that many employers lay down rules for communications to the press in their terms of employment. You may feel that this is unreasonable but before issuing any press releases you would be well advised to check that it is being done in a way that does not infringe your own terms and conditions of service.

Discussion/Activity 8.2 Writing to the press

The staff of the accident and emergency department are very worried by the number of children who are being brought to casualty with burns and scalds. Next month will be bonfire night (5 November). Write a letter to the editor of your local newspaper stressing the need for safety in handling fireworks.

The local health visitors in conjunction with school staff are running a 'Be Safe at Home' week for children attending the local school. Many more people will be reached if the local media can be persuaded to carry a story on this subject. Which local media should be notified of this event? Write a press release to tell them about it.

LETTERS TO POLITICIANS

Politicians like to be involved and may well be able to lend powerful support (see Chapter 5, page 88). Letters to local MPs or councillors are a simple way of getting support. If you organise several people to write to their local MP about a health problem, the MP is very likely to take an interest. MPs regard any subject on which they receive letters from five to ten constituents as important. They will probably respond by writing to the people who might resolve the problem (local authority, health authority, etc.) and letters from MPs are difficult to ignore.

SUMMARY POINTS

Individual health workers even if they are not managers can change things to promote health.

Change may be obtained for individual clients or for communities by using advocacy.

To produce change you have to identify the key decision makers and influence them. Community Health Councils, professional organisations and trades unions can raise matters on the individual's behalf.

Power to influence comes from several sources but the two sources available to most health care workers are expert power (detailed knowledge of subject) and personal power. Influence will mostly be exercised by reason and bargaining, together with friendliness and coalition.

Arguments for resources must clearly state what is required and why, and must be made to someone who has the power to supply those resources.

The local press can be a powerful ally. Health workers can use both news stories and letters to get their points into the local press. Health stories should be released to the press in a way that makes it easy for the press to cover them.

Letters to MPs and councillors are also a good way of gaining support for issues.

REFERENCES

DoH (Department of Health) (1993). *Health of the Nation: working together for better health*. London: HMSO.

Fisher R., Ury W. and Patten B. (1991). *Getting to Yes: negotiating an agreement without giving in* (2nd edition). London: Century Business.

Furley A. (1991). Campaigning for change. *Health Visitor* **64**, 371–372.

Handy C.B. (1985). On power and influence. Chapter 5 in *Understanding Organisations* (3rd edition). London: Penguin.

Heginbotham C. (1994). Consumer groups. Section 3.4 in *NHS handbook* (8th edition). Tunbridge Wells: IPR for NAHAT.

Howe J. (1993). The 'Standard' guide to writing effective letters. *Nursing Standard* 7 (No. 35), 44–45.

Kipnis *et al.* (1984). Patterns of managerial influence: shotgun manager, tacticians and bystanders. *Organisational dynamics* **12** (No. 3), 58–67.

Marshall M. (1992). Advocacy within the multidisciplinary team. *Nursing Standard* **6** (No. 27) 28–31.

Mulholland J. (1991). *The language of negotiation*. London: Routledge.

Porrit L. (1990). Management: the art of getting things done. Chapter 9 in *Interaction strategies: an introduction for health professionals* (2nd edition). Edinburgh: Churchill Livingstone.

Stutor J.A. (1993). Can nurses be effective advocates? *Nursing Standard* 7 (No. 22), 30–32.

Turrill T. (1986). *Change and innovation: a challenge for the NHS*. London: Institute of Health Service Managers.

CHAPTER 9

Planning health promotion at a local level

GOAL

To understand how to plan health promotion activities at a local (district) level.

OBJECTIVES

- to understand the need for planning
- to know what information is needed to plan activities
- to be able to set aims and objectives for health promotion activities
- to identify target groups
- to clarify and select options for health promotion activity
- to plan evaluation

COMMUNITIES AND INDIVIDUALS

In this and the next chapter we will think about how to plan and evaluate health promotion activities for large groups of people. In Chapter 11 we focus on health promotion with individual patients. The general principles are the same but the ways in which they are applied differ as the focus shifts from groups to individuals.

THE NEED FOR PLANNING

Health promotion is self-evidently good and there is a huge job to be done. However, if it is to be most effective and make the best use of resources, activities must be planned. Planning involves assessing the health promotion needs, identifying the resources available for the task and the barriers to be overcome, selecting priorities, setting aims and objectives, devising methods for implementation and criteria for evaluating the results of the activity (see Figure 9.1). Proper planning ensures that important health problems or sectors of the population are not forgotten, that projects are not embarked on without sufficient resources to complete them and that everyone knows what they are doing and why.

GATHERING INFORMATION – HEALTH NEEDS ASSESSMENT

The first step in local health promotion planning is to collect information on the local scene:

- population size, age structure, ethnic mix (demography)
- frequency of disease
- health-related lifestyles
- environmental influences on health
- attitudes to health; health knowledge of population
- sources of health information
- health resources

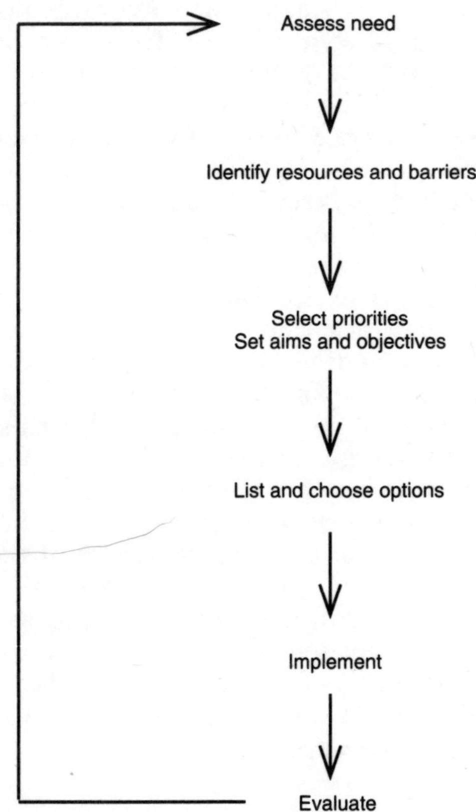

Figure 9.1 The planning cycle for health promotion

DEMOGRAPHIC INFORMATION

You will need to know the basic make-up of the population in your locality. Are there parts which are mostly populated by families with young children, or are there parts where most of the residents are elderly? Are there areas in which the residents mostly belong to one particular ethnic group? This information is needed to decide what aspects of health promotion will be most relevant to the local community. In years when the census is taken (last census taken in 1991, next census due in 2001), these questions can be answered precisely. In other years you may have to rely on general knowledge of your district. The public health department or the local authority should be able to help with this information (St Leger, Schneiden and Walsworth-Bell 1992).

INFORMATION ON FREQUENCY OF DISEASE

The next step is to identify the main local health problems. You can get information on death rates for different diseases and compare these with national averages. Information will also be available on hospital admission rates for different diseases. These sorts of information may reveal particular local problems but their interpretation is not straightforward. The public health department may both provide this information and advise on how it should be interpreted (Faculty of Public Health Medicine 1991). Death rates and hospital admission rates might show whether conditions such as heart disease, strokes, lung cancer, asthma, suicide, or road traffic accidents are more or less common in your district than elsewhere. This information will be useful first in deciding whether to concentrate efforts on one or more of these problems and second for raising local interest in the problem if you do decide to do something about it.

Note that death rates and hospital data only tell you about the more serious diseases. They tell you little about ill health such as aches and pains, lack of energy, anxiety and feeling low, and nothing about well-being and how many people are feeling fit and well. Information on these things is highly desirable but very difficult to get. Methods of measuring the frequency of this type of ill health have been devised (such as the General Health Questionnaire for mental ill-health (Goldberg and Williams 1982), and the SF36 (Jenkinson, Coulter and Wright 1993) or Nottingham Health Profile (Hunt, McEwan and McKennna 1986) for general ill-health). This type of information will only be available if someone in your district has done a special survey.

HEALTH-RELATED LIFESTYLE

One also needs to know about health-related lifestyle. How many people take exercise, eat low-fat, high-fibre diets, brush their teeth, and look after their health? How many people smoke, drink too much and are overweight? Information on these things comes from three sources:

1. extrapolation from national data
2. local surveys
3. health service sources

There is fairly good information on most aspects of lifestyle from the national surveys listed in Table 9.1. These tell us about the lifestyle of the nation as a whole and sometimes about the lifestyle of different regions. Often you will have to extrapolate from national results and assume that what is true for the whole country is also true for your district.

Sometimes a local lifestyle survey will have been done in your own district. If this is available you can check whether lifestyles in your district are different from the country-wide average. You may consider organising your own survey to collect information on health or lifestyle but be warned, this will require considerable time and resources (Luck *et al.* 1988; Kemm and Booth 1992).

Table 9.1 Some national lifestyle surveys

- General Household Survey (contains data on smoking and drinking)
- National Food Survey (in collaboration with MAFF*)
- Nutrition Survey
- Health Survey (includes data on blood pressure and body mass)
- surveys of smoking in schoolchildren
- surveys of infant feeding
- surveys of drinking

All these surveys are carried out by the Office of Population Census and Surveys (OPCS). All are published each year except the survey of smoking in schoolchildren and the General Household Survey, which are done every other year, and the infant feeding and drinking surveys, which are done at irregular intervals.

*MAFF = Ministry of Agriculture, Fisheries and Food.

Results of local surveys need to be examined carefully since they are often not done with the care and skill that is used in national surveys. One must also look carefully to see how the sample was chosen and whether it is likely to be representative. You must also consider how precise the numbers are. For example, the statement that 30% of the population smoke will not mean that exactly 30% of the population smoke, but does it mean that between 29% and 31% smoke, or does it mean that between 15% and 45% smoke? You should particularly look to see that the surveys used a representative sample with adequate numbers and that valid questions were asked.

It may be possible to obtain some information on lifestyle from health service records. In theory every patient coming into hospital should be asked about their smoking, drinking and weight. However, this information is unreliably obtained and badly recorded so that it is difficult to obtain worthwhile data from this source. Some general practices have started to collect information on risk factors for heart disease. If you are lucky, one or two of the practices in your district will be able to give you a very good picture for patients registered with them of weight, blood pressure, and smoking, drinking and exercise habits. It is to be hoped that recent changes in the way general practices are paid for doing health promotion will increase the numbers of practices who can provide this sort of information.

ENVIRONMENTAL INFLUENCES ON HEALTH

Environment is just as important as lifestyle and must be included in the planning process. What features of the local environment threaten health? What is the state of housing in different parts of the district? Where are the dangerous roads? What are the conditions like in the different workplaces? What are the local sources of pollution? Where can people go for recreation and to take leisure? Where do people go shopping and what foods are available in these shops? This sort of information can be gathered by looking around and asking other people. For example, community health staff and the housing department will know where the housing problems are, while staff in accident and emergency departments and ambulance staff will know the areas in which accidents most frequently occur.

ATTITUDES TO HEALTH

Any successful health promotion activity has to start 'where people are'. What are the things that worry people? How prominent are health worries among their other concerns? How do they feel about health-related behaviours such as smoking, drinking and exercise? The style of any health promotion activity must be guided by this sort of information. If everyone wants chips in the hospital restaurant you would probably be better advised to try and ensure that the chips are well drained and cooked in a polyunsaturated oil rather than try to persuade them not to eat chips. If, on the other hand, everyone is complaining of the smoky atmosphere in the rest room the moment is probably right to argue for a non-smoking rest area. Information on attitudes is difficult to obtain but conversations with local residents and with local health workers should give you some guidance. The local press may also be very helpful in indicating what issues are currently bothering local people. Occasionally it will be necessary to undertake a special survey to collect information to find out how people feel about a particular health issue.

KNOWLEDGE OF HEALTH

You also need to know how much people know about health in order to plan health education. People will only be irritated by health education activities designed to inform them of things they already know. For each subject we need to know whether there is a need to impart information, or to increase the salience in people's minds of information already held, or to accept that lack of knowledge is not the problem and concentrate on something else. Skills have to be considered at the same time as knowledge. Do people have the health skills they need, such as being able to shop and prepare for healthy meals, or the social skills to refuse a drink when they are driving?

SOURCES OF HEALTH INFORMATION

Different communities have different sources of information. Effective health promotion must influence the sources from which people obtain their health information (see Table 9.2). For each source we have to consider how many people notice it, how credible it is and how persuasive. Some sources such as advertising are noticed by most people but have low credibility and are not trusted. Other sources such as teachers and 'experts' have high credibility but little persuasive power. We believe what they say but do not change our lifestyle. Usually health professionals are seen to be credible sources and, more importantly, sources of advice which may influence people to change their behaviour. Health education must make full use of these sources. Similarly, one needs to know who are used as behaviour 'models' in the community (see Chapter 7, page 124).

Table 9.2 Sources of health information

- nurses, midwives, health visitors
- primary care team
- hospital staff
- teachers, youth leaders
- magazines, papers, television
- parents, children, relations
- friends
- community leaders

HEALTH RESOURCES

The information base for health promotion planning must also include the health resources available. First think what resources are available through the health services, what skills and enthusiasms there are in the district. Are there people with special interest and knowledge in stress management, fitness, heart disease, asthma, rehabilitation, diet, air pollution or other things who could be used to support health promotion? What other local resources are there? Are there people in environmental services, housing departments, schools or libraries who could play a part in health promotion? Are there any local celebrities who would support activities? Often a celebrity who has suffered a health problem in the past will be willing to play a part in helping prevent that problem in other people.

Discussion/Activity 9.1 Local health needs

Think about your town or district. Make a list of its health promotion needs. What information do you need to make a better assessment? How much of this could easily be found out? Where would you get this information?

SETTING AIMS

With all this information you are now in a position to set aims, the broad areas in which you intend to make progress. There is not enough time and resources to do everything, so one has to select what is most important. The items which feature on this priority list will be influenced by:

- professional assessment of the local health situation
- views of local residents
- national priorities

- resources available
- equity

The information on the groups in the population, the frequency of different health problems, the frequency of health-damaging lifestyles, the environmental check and knowledge of what can be changed will lead to a list of health problems which seem most important to health care professionals. However, the information gathering will also have produced a list of issues which seem most important to the local residents, and these may well be different from those on the professionals' list. There is also a third list of health issues that are national priorities, such as the health areas identified in *Health of the Nation* (see Chapter 1, page 17). Topics featured in health education campaigns chosen and run at a national level need to be considered for inclusion as local priorities. The eventual list of aims will be a negotiated compromise between the local professional, local resident and national priority list.

The final list of aims may also be influenced by consideration of local health resources. If the first set of aims leaves some major local resource untapped, it is probably sensible to revise those aims to make use of all your strengths. The first list of aims may also need to be revised in the light of equity considerations. Is there some group in the community who will not benefit, or will local health inequalities be unchanged or even increased? If so, the aims may need to be adjusted to produce a more equitable outcome.

There is a temptation to produce a very long list of aims – one which pleases everyone by including everything. You must be tough enough to cut the list down to a length that can reasonably be achieved with the time and resources available.

SETTING OBJECTIVES

The aims merely mark out the broad areas that health promotion will address. These now need to be refined into much more specific objectives that spell out what will be changed, by how much and by when (see the example in Table 9.3). The objectives are important because they will guide the activity actually undertaken and because they will be used to evaluate the activity at the end.

Discussion/Activity 9.2 Setting aims and objectives

Working from the assessment made in Discussion/Activity 9.1, produce a set of aims for local health promotion. Now pick one of these aims and develop a set of objectives based upon it.

Table 9.3 Example of health promotion aims and objectives

Aim To reduce suicides

Objectives

1. To establish a help-line and safe house for 'Asian' women in the next year.
2. To ensure that in the next year all patients admitted for attempted suicide are seen by a consultant psychiatrist and that care plans are made to help with underlying conditions.
3. To ensure that within the next two years patients with schizophrenia managed in the community are reviewed at least monthly and more frequently when their state requires it.
4. To set up a help-line and drop-in service for secondary-schoolchildren before next Christmas.

Notes

All objectives relate to clearly defined target groups (because they are high-risk groups for suicide). It will be easy to establish whether each objective has been met or not.

A time is stated within which the objective will be met.

Outcome objectives such as 'To reduce suicides by 25% in the next three years in 'Asian' women' may be appropriate for a Region (5 million population) but they are not appropriate for a District (0.5 million population). This is because the number of suicides in this category expected in any year is small so that large percentage changes from year to year are likely to occur by chance (e.g. one single suicide might represent a 25% change).

TARGET GROUPS

Just as health education activities with single clients (see Chapter 11) are tailored to meet the needs of the individual, health promotion activities for communities must be matched to the needs of the group. Therefore one has to be clear about which group's needs are to be met and target the health promotion approach accordingly. Attempts to suit the health education needs of everyone all too often end up bland and suiting the needs of no one. Of course you have to remember that health education materials are likely to be seen by individuals outside their intended target group and you have to be careful not to give unnecessary offence. When trying to target a mixed community such as a whole city it is usually better to plan a series of linked activities aimed at different groups rather than a single activity for everyone.

An example of the need for targeted activities could be an activity to increase awareness of safe sex. Literature for the gay community may need to use very explicit language if it is to be seen as relevant. Literature for youth clubs would need to be different, as would literature for ethnic minority groups, literature for schools and literature for general distribution.

Different groups of the population have different health needs. These should have been identified during the information-gathering exercise. Information on the target group will guide you in selecting what objectives to set (a stop-smoking activity is not appropriate for a community where no one smokes), the most acceptable approach (sexual health education would be differently handled in schools serving different communities) and the most effective approach (language, level of literacy, and so on).

LISTING THE OPTIONS

When the objectives have been set and the target group identified, one has to consider what activities will be undertaken to achieve the objectives. The several different ways in which the objective could be achieved need to be listed with their advantages and disadvantages. Table 9.4 gives an example of the options available to meet the objective of increasing the number of women taking up the invitation to attend for breast screening. The options considered should not be limited to health education but should also include practical help options. Similarly, the advantages and disadvantages

Table 9.4 Options to increase uptake of breast screening

Background Lower Puddlethorpe is a town with a population of 50,000 and is served by three group practices. Invitations to be screened are sent to all women on the practice registers aged 50–65. The women are expected to travel to the breast-screening unit at the local hospital 3 miles away. In the last round only 50% of those invited attended.

Objective To increase the percentage of women from Lower Puddlethorpe who attend for breast screening from 50% to 75%.

Option	Advantages	Disadvantages
1. Poster and leaflet campaign	Fairly cheap	Unlikely to be effective on its own
2. Invitation delivered personally by practice staff	Opportunity to explain individually Likely to be effective	Expensive in time Might be seen as pressurising
3. Personalised letter of invitation from practice	Easy to arrange	Leaves choice with women
4. Offer taxi to take women to screening unit	Likely to be effective Acceptable to women	Expensive
5. Seek support from local townswomen's Guild	Easy to arrange	Will not reach all women
6. Talks to groups of women at local health centre	Easy to arrange	Unlikely to reach non-attenders

The choice of options will depend on local circumstances but one possible choice might be **1**, **3** and **5**.

considered include likely effectiveness, resources needed and acceptability to target population.

RESOURCES REQUIRED

Having chosen the activities to be undertaken, the next step is to list the resources, time, people, materials and money needed for their execution. You can then check that all these are available.

GOING ROUND THE LOOP

This chapter has been written as though health promotion planning were a linear process going logically from needs assessment to choice of options. In reality it is more likely that when you get towards the end of the planning process you realise that your initial objectives and choices are for some reason unsustainable. Local politics demand that some other topic or group is given higher priority, the resources needed are not available, and so on. You will therefore revisit and adjust you initial aims and objectives and modify plans for implementation until you have a satisfactory compromise between what you first wanted to do and what you can actually do.

CONTRACTING AND HEALTH PROMOTION

The National Health Service has moved to a situation in which health authorities assess the need of their resident populations for health services including health promotion and then make contracts with provider units for the provision of such services. In this new environment health promoters therefore have to 'sell' their services to the purchasing authorities. The purchasers will increasingly specify the health promotion services that they wish to buy on behalf of their populations. Ideally, purchasers will be open to advice from health promotion providers as to what services they should purchase and the process will be one of co-operation not antagonism (Killoran 1992). None the less the nature of the relationship between health promotion staff and health authorities is changing. Well-justified plans for local health promotion will play an ever more important part in determining what health promotion is to be done.

SUMMARY POINTS

Effective health promotion relies on planning following the cycle of:

- ☐ health needs assessment
- ☐ setting aims and objectives
- ☐ list and choose options

- ☐ implement
- ☐ evaluate

Needs assessment involves gathering information on population size, frequency of disease, lifestyle, environment, attitudes and knowledge and sources of information.

The needs assessment informs setting of aims from which quantified and measurable objectives are developed.

Different ways of meeting the objectives (options) are then listed, together with the resources needed.

Finally the best options are chosen and implemented.

Planning by health promotion providers should be done in co-operation with purchasers and form the basis for contracts.

REFERENCES

Faculty of Public Health Medicine (1991). *Health measurement toolbox* (3rd edition). London: Faculty of Public Health Medicine.

Goldberg D.P. and Williams P. (1982). *A user's guide to the General Health Questionnaire*. Windsor: NFER Nelson.

Hunt S., McEwan J. and McKenna S. (1986). *Measuring health status*. London: Croom Helm.

Jenkinson C., Coulter A. and Wright L. (1993). Short form 36 (SF36) health survey questionnaire: normative data for adults of working age. *British Medical Journal* **306**, 1437–1440.

Kemm J.R. and Booth D. (1992). *Promotion of healthier eating: how to collect and use information for planning, monitoring and evaluation*. London: HMSO.

Killoran A. (1992). *Putting health into contracts*. London: Health Education Authority.

Luck M., Lawrence B., Pocock R. and Reilly K. (1988). *Consumer and market research in health care*. London: Chapman and Hall.

St Leger A.S., Schneiden H. and Walsworth-Bell J.P. (1992). Obtaining data. Appendix A in *Evaluating health services effectiveness*. Milton Keynes: Open University Press.

FURTHER READING

Chalmers J., Lockerbie L., Hepburn W. and Lutz W. (1992). *Health and community surveys*. London: Macmillan / International Epidemiological Association / WHO.

CHAPTER 10

Evaluation of health promotion

GOAL

To understand why it is important to evaluate health promotion activities and the principles used in these evaluations.

OBJECTIVES

- to understand how evaluation is used to improve health promotion activity
- to appreciate the managerial context of evaluation
- to understand the difference between outcome and process evaluation
- to choose appropriate outcomes for evaluation
- to understand the difference between monitoring and evaluation
- to describe different evaluation designs
- to recognise costs involved in evaluation
- to be willing to act on results of evaluation

INTRODUCTION

Everyone agrees that health promotion ought to be evaluated yet good evaluations are few. Evaluation tries to answer the questions:

- What difference has a particular health promotion activity made?
- What health gain has it produced?

This chapter will explain how this sort of question might be answered and in the process suggest why good evaluations are not done more often.

THE PARTIES TO AN EVALUATION

Classic descriptions of evaluation describe three parties (Fitzgibbon and Morris 1987):

- the manager
- the evaluator
- the programme worker

The manager The person who makes decisions about resources. They will use the evaluation to help them decide whether each health promotion activity should be continued, repeated or stopped.

The evaluator The person who collects information about the health promotion activity and its results and then interprets that information to find out what the health promotion activity has achieved. The evaluator has no predisposition for or against continuing the activity. They are only interested in trying to assess its effect.

The programme worker The person who is doing the health promotion activity. They have detailed knowledge of how it is working but are likely to be committed to it and therefore find it difficult to take a detached view.

For the evaluator, keeping proper detachment is difficult. In order to collect information on a health promotion project the evaluator will need to understand what it is trying to do and how it works and will therefore need to be closely involved with the project and its workers. At the same time, the evaluator must be trusted by the manager to understand the framework of managerial decisions and give an evaluation which is not simply a repetition of the project workers' views.

In reality the situation is more complex and one person has to play more than one role. Sometimes the manager also acts as the evaluator. More often the programme worker doubles as evaluator and attempts a 'self-evaluation'. In either case if they are to do the evaluation satisfactorily the evaluator must take – and be seen to be taking – a detached view of the health promotion activity.

QUALITY ASSURANCE AND AUDIT

Evaluation is an essential part of quality assurance and the main method by which effectiveness (which is one of the key components of quality) is demonstrated. Evaluation is also linked to audit but there are important differences to note. Audit is a process by which health care workers improve the quality of their work. They do this by noting their own current practice, comparing it against quality standards and then modifying their practice to match the standards. Audit works best if it is separate from management so that people are free to admit to themselves and their peers where their practice falls short of standard. Evaluation may form part of the audit process but such an evaluation must not be confused with an evaluation as part of the management process.

INPUT, PROCESS AND OUTCOME

In any health promotion activity we can distinguish:

- inputs
- process
- outcomes

Inputs are the resources used, such as people, time, materials and money. **Process** is all the activities which make up the health promotion, such as meetings, one-to-one talks and exhibitions. **Outcomes** are the desired results, such as people learning how to count their drinks in units of alcohol, people stopping smoking, obtaining a crossing on a dangerous road, and preventing suicides. **Impact** is often added as a step between process and outcome. It refers to the degree to which the processes reach and are noticed by the target group.

PROCESS EVALUATION

Process evaluations ask questions such as:

- How many people attended the meeting?
- Did they enjoy it?
- How many people requested leaflets?
- Are the leaflets well designed and suitable for their purpose?
- Were the methods used appropriate?

This detailed examination of process will show how the activities might be improved and give insight into the operations of the project. Evaluation of written materials is discussed in Chapter 12.

OUTCOME EVALUATION

Outcome evaluation asks whether the health promotion activity has influenced people's knowledge, attitudes, behaviour or health in the desired direction. It asks questions such as:

- How many mothers have a better knowledge of infant feeding?
- How many people intend to take more exercise?
- How many mothers continued breast feeding after the first week?
- How many people lost weight?
- How much has the death rate from lung cancer been reduced?

This sort of evaluation tends to be more difficult but it is needed to assess whether the health promotion has been effective. Most good evaluations contain a mixture of process and outcome evaluation.

IMPACT EVALUATION

Impact evaluation assesses how successful the health promoter was in making contact with their target group. What proportion of the target group had heard of or noticed the health promotion activities? How much notice had they taken of it? Could they remember any of the images or messages used?

SUMMATIVE AND FORMATIVE EVALUATION

Summative evaluation takes place at the end of a health promotion project and is used to decide whether the project should be continued or repeated. It will tend to concentrate on outcomes. Managers tend to be most interested in summative evaluation.

Formative evaluation takes place while the project is running and is used to find ways in which the project can be improved and made to run better. It will tend to concentrate on process and will be of greatest interest to the project workers.

QUALITATIVE OR QUANTITATIVE

Evaluation methods may concentrate on describing in qualitative terms how things have changed, how people felt about the activities, and so on. Alternatively they may concentrate on measuring quantitatively what has happened – the number of people who saw an advertisement, the percentage of the leaflet content remembered, the number of people who stopped smoking, and so on. Each of these approaches is suited to different tasks. Quantitative methods may seem more scientific but if used to answer the wrong questions they may force you into collecting the wrong information. There is a common belief that qualitative methods are easy and quantitative hard, but the reverse is usually true. There can be no fixed rule that quantitative methods are better than qualitative or vice versa. The procedure must always be to decide what questions have to be answered and then choose the method best suited to that particular question.

PARTICIPANT OBSERVATION

Most of the methods described in this chapter require the evaluator to try to stand outside the process and observe and measure what goes on without becoming involved. The participant-observer method takes exactly the opposite approach, arguing that the best way to understand a complex process is to be as closely involved in it as possible. It gives the evaluator insight into the hopes, disappointments and feelings of those involved in a way no other method can. It can identify changes of attitude and increases in group members' well-being that more formal measurement techniques will miss. The weakness of the method is that because the evaluator identifies closely with the project and its clients, they run the risk of changing roles and becoming the advocate rather than the evaluator of the project. The participant-observer approach has been widely used in the evaluation of community development health projects (Beattie 1990).

EVALUATION AND DEVELOPMENT

Different types of evaluation are appropriate to the different stages in development of a health promotion activity (Nutbeam, Smith and Catford 1990). When someone suggests a new way of health promotion, the first question is 'Does it work?' Experimental studies using predominantly outcome evaluation will be needed to answer this question. Having shown that the method works in one place with one health promoter, the next questions are 'Will it work elsewhere with other people? and 'Can it be improved?'. Demonstration studies using a mixture of process and outcome evaluations are needed to answer these. Finally one wants to know if the method can be widely implemented, and this will be shown by dissemination studies using mostly repeated process evaluations (see Figure 10.1).

CLARIFYING OBJECTIVES

The first item in any evaluation must be to clarify the objectives. If the objectives have been clearly written down in quantified and measurable terms, this is easy. Sometimes, however, the objectives are only present in someone's head or, worse still, have never been fully thought through. In this situation it may require considerable

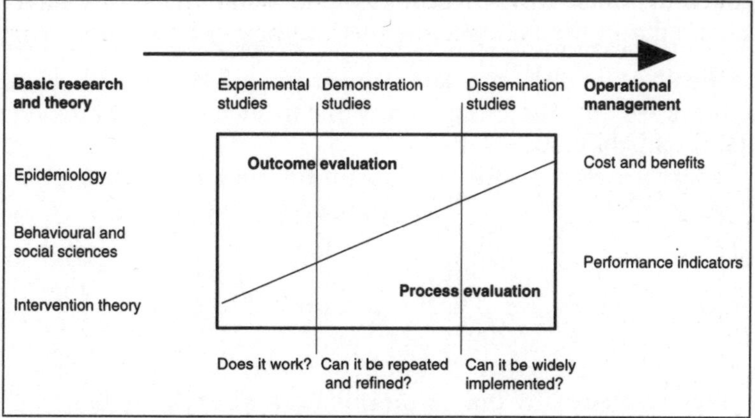

Figure 10.1 Types of evaluation at different stages in the development of a health promotion activity
The balance between outcome and process evaluation shifts as one moves from experimental study through demonstration studies to widespread dissemination of methods which have been shown to work elsewhere. (See text for further explanation.)
Source Adapted from Nutbeam, Smith and Catford (1990), *Journal of Epidemiology and Community Health* **44**, 83–89.

time and effort to work out what the implicit objectives of the health promotion activity were.

DESCRIBING INPUTS AND PROCESS

It is important to know not only the effect of a health promotion activity but also what the activity was. Evaluations should therefore include a description of the inputs:

- staff and skill mix used
- equipment and materials used
- time
- money

This should then be followed by a description of the activities, for example:

- posters: how many were displayed and where
- leaflets: which ones and how they were used
- meetings held: topics covered and who attended
- talks given: topics covered and who attended
- people visited

CHOICE OF OUTCOMES

A health promotion activity has as its long-term goal the promotion of positive health and the prevention of disease. It attempts to achieve this by changing environment, awareness, knowledge, attitudes or behaviour.

There are thus a series of short-term, medium-term and long-term outcomes (see Table 10.1). Impact can be thought of as a very short-term outcome but it is usually considered separately.

In order to do an outcome evaluation we have to decide what outcome to measure. There is a trade-off to be made between long- and short-term outcomes (see Figure 10.2). It is the long-term outcomes which are most desirable in themselves. The short-term outcomes are generally only desirable because they are believed to lead to the desirable long-term outcomes. On the other hand, the long-term outcomes tend to be very difficult to measure. These outcomes develop many years after the health promotion activity, they are linked to the intervention by a long causal chain that can be affected by other factors and any change in outcome is likely to be small. The short-term outcomes in contrast are relatively easy to measure. For most purposes it is usually appropriate to base evaluation on measures of short-term outcome.

Discussion/Activity 10.1 Choosing outcome measures

Look again at Figure 10.2. Now choose two health promotion areas (such as prevention of coronary heart disease or promotion of mental health). For each of the areas you have chosen, decide how you would measure short-term, medium-term and long-term outcomes.

Table 10.1 Short-term, medium-term and long-term outcomes

Outcome level	Explanation	Example
Impact	Awareness of activity Awareness of topic	Seen AIDS posters Read HIV pamphlets Concerned about HIV and AIDS
Short-term	Knowledge Skills Attitudes	Know about HIV and AIDS Know about safer sex Think it worth preventing
Medium-term	Behaviour	Use condoms Restrict number of partners
	Environment	Condom vending machines widely avaible
Long-term	Physiological Disease prevention	Fewer HIV positive Fewer AIDS cases

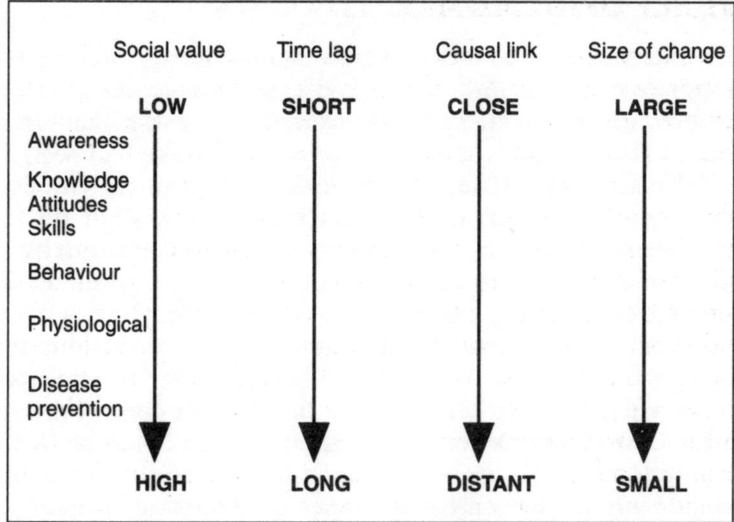

Figure 10.2 Characteristics of outcome measures
The health promotion outcomes vary in social value, how quickly they change, the closeness of the causal link to intervention and the likely size of change.

MONITORING AND EVALUATION

We must at this point distinguish between monitoring and evaluation. Monitoring asks the question 'Have things changed?' while evaluation asks the much more difficult question 'Have our health promotion activities influenced things?' In order to answer the evaluation question we have to try to compare the changes that do or do not occur with how things would have been if we had not intervened with a health promotion activity.

OUTCOME EVALUATION STUDY DESIGNS

There are a range of designs for outcome evaluations:

- randomised controlled trials
- comparison trials
- lagged intervention trials
- comparison of self-selected groups
- message tracing
- uncontrolled before and after comparisons

RANDOMISED CONTROLLED TRIALS

It is relatively easy to measure how things change after a health promotion activity. The problem is to decide whether our activity helped, hindered or had no effect on this change. To answer that question we need to know what would have happened if there had been no activity. Theoretically we need to compare two identical groups, one of which experienced the health promotion activity while the other did not. We could then tell if our activity made any difference by comparing what happened to the two groups. The randomised controlled trial is the nearest one can get to this desired study.

In a randomised controlled trial of health promotion, all people taking part would be randomly allocated either to an intervention group which had the health promotion or to a control group which had no health promotion. Random allocation could be by tossing a coin or some similar process. The importance of random allocation is that everyone has an equal chance of being put in either group so we should end up with two groups that are exactly the same in all respects. Since the two groups are exactly the same to start with, any difference between them after the health promotion activity must be due to the activity.

Randomised controlled trials have been carried out for health promotion activities such as advice on smoking and drinking in general practice, advice on reducing risk of coronary heart disease and effect of breast screening. The results of one such trial are shown in Table 10.2.

Often, however, a randomised controlled trial is impossible or too difficult to do. Frequently people cannot be randomly allocated to receive the health promotion or not. There are ethical problems in denying the health promotion to some people. Some of the people offered the health promotion activity may not take it and some of those not offered it may take it. All these things make randomised controlled trials difficult to mount.

COMPARISON TRIALS

Comparison trials are a second best when randomised controlled trials are not possible. Once again two groups are compared, one of which receives the intervention while the other does not. However, instead of creating the two groups by random allocation, pre-existing groups are used. For example, one might use two wards, or two towns, or two schools. The idea is to pick two groups which are as similar as possible so that the only difference between them will be that one receives the intervention while the other does not. This ideal can never be achieved since there will always be differ-

Table 10.2 Evaluation of a leaflet on eating and health: example of a randomised controlled trial

A sample of people living in the Southampton area was randomly allocated to one of two groups. One group (the intervention group) was sent a copy of a leaflet 'Eat well, Be well'. The other group acted as control and no leaflet was sent. After five weeks both groups were sent a questionnaire, and a nutrition knowledge score (maximum 17) was calculated from the responses.

	Intervention group	Control group
Number in group	243	243
Number of replies	146	153
Mean knowledge score	9.1	8.6
% remembering seeing healthy eating leaflet or poster	49	33

The difference in knowledge between the two groups is tiny and could easily have arisen by chance. There is no evidence that being sent the leaflet has increased the knowledge of the intervention group. We know that they probably received it since a significantly higher percentage of the intervention group remember seeing a leaflet or poster in the last three months. Note that 33% of the control group also claimed to have seen a healthy eating leaflet or poster, indicating that both groups were exposed to other sources of information.

Source Nicholas S., Waters W.E., Woolaway M. and Hamilton-Smith M.B. (1988). *Journal of Human Nutrition and Dietetics* **1**, 233–238.

ences between different wards, towns and schools but it may be possible to find pairs of groups where the differences are small. The groups to receive the intervention may have been decided before the comparison groups were identified, or the choice of groups which are to receive the intervention may be made by tossing a coin or some similar chance method.

The comparison trial still has the ethical difficulty that one group is denied the health promotion and the practical difficulty that the effect of any activity may spill over from the intervention group to the non-intervention group. Table 10.3 gives an example of a comparison trial.

LAGGED INTERVENTION TRIALS

The lagged intervention trial is similar to the comparison trial but instead of one group getting the health promotion while the other does not, the different groups receive the health promotion at different times. This study design has the advantage that no one is denied the health promotion intervention. For example, one town might receive the health promotion six months before another town. It should then be possible to tell the effect of the intervention by comparing the changes over time between the first and second towns.

Table 10.3 Evaluation of a Healthy Heart Week: example of a comparison trial

A Healthy Heart Week was organised in Halstead, a small town in Essex (the intervention town). No event was organised in the similar town of Saffron Walden which was used as the comparison town. Knowledge of coronary risk factors was measured in both towns before the Healthy Heart Week and two weeks and six months after. Knowledge was measured by interviewing a random sample of about 200 people in each town on each occasion.

Coronary risk factor	**Percentage mentioning coronary risk factors**					
	Before		**Two weeks after**		**Six months after**	
	Hal	SW	Hal	SW	Hal	SW
Diet	58	66	72*	66	71*	72
Smoking	39	38	47	42	47	44
Exercise	39	46	61*	49	56*	49
Stress	22	36	27	27	27	31

* Indicates value significantly different from the result of the survey done before the Healthy Heart Week in same town.

These results show:

- knowledge of risk factors was similar in the two towns before the Healthy Heart Week
- knowledge of diet and exercise as risk factors (but not of smoking and stress) increased significantly in Halstead after the Healthy Heart Week
- knowledge of risk factors did not increase significantly in Saffron Walden

It is reasonable to conclude that the Healthy Heart Week was effective in increasing knowledge of diet and exercise as risk factors.

Source: Watson D., Moreton W. and Jessop E.G. (1988). *Health Education Journal* **47**, 49–53.

COMPARISON OF SELF-SELECTED GROUPS

In all the previous study designs the people running the study have decided which groups get the health promotion activity and which do not. An alternative is to offer the health promotion activity to everyone and let them decide for themselves whether to take part. For example, we might invite everyone to an exhibition or invite everyone to take a leaflet. People who come to the exhibition or take a leaflet can then be compared with people who did not. We might hope to show that those who had taken part in the health promotion activity in this way had better knowledge or more favourable attitudes than those who had not.

The difficulty with this approach is that the two groups were different before our health promotion activity. At the very least they differ in their readiness to come to exhibitions or take leaflets and they almost certainly differ in other important respects such as their interest in health matters. It is therefore essential to collect information on the other ways in which the groups might differ (age, sex, ethnicity, employment, education, and so on) and try to demonstrate that none of these things could account for differences in outcome between the groups.

MESSAGE TRACING

Message tracing is a study design that tries to avoid the need for a comparison group by using each individual as their own comparison. In this technique, change in knowledge or behaviour related to the health promotion message is compared with change in knowledge or behaviour of some closely linked subject about which no message was given. For example, we might run a health education event intended to increase people's knowledge of the number of alcohol units in beer and cider but make no mention of wines and spirits. If we then find that people's knowledge of the alcohol content of beers and ciders has increased but that their knowledge of the alcohol content of wines and spirits has not, it is fairly safe to conclude that the educational activity contributed to their increased knowledge. If on the other hand we find that their knowledge of the alcohol content of drinks not mentioned in the educational activity had also increased then it is less likely that their increase of knowledge was due to the activity.

UNCONTROLLED BEFORE AND AFTER COMPARISONS

The crudest form of evaluation is simple before and after comparison without comparison groups. One may, for example, measure people's knowledge of baby care before and after they attend mothercare classes. If there is no increase in knowledge, then we know that we must look carefully at the mothercare sessions to make them more effective. Of course if there is an increase in knowledge it is dangerous to assume that it was due to the mothercare classes. The increase could have been due to magazines or information from friends or many things other than the education. Simple before and after comparison is an unreliable form of evaluation but it is better than nothing.

RESOURCE COSTS OF EVALUATION

Evaluation requires time, thought and a limited amount of resources. Costs of evaluation ought to be included in the costing of every health promotion activity. Resources invested in evaluation are well invested because they should enable us to recognise effective health promotion activities and maybe enhance them, and also to recognise ineffective health promotion activities and avoid wasting further resources by repeating them.

Discussion/Activity 10.2 Planning an evaluation

Think of some health promotion activity with which you have been involved. How could you do an outcome evaluation on this? What study design would you use? How would you do it? What resources would you need? Who would be interested in your results when the evaluation was complete? Do you think that an outcome evaluation is necessary? What process evaluation would you want to do?

COST EFFECTIVENESS AND COST BENEFIT

This chapter has been about measuring the effect of health promotion activities. Once this has been done, two further questions arise:

1. Was it cost effective? i.e. Could the same effect (outcome) have been achieved for less cost?
2. Was it cost beneficial? i.e. Could more health gain have been obtained by some other activity?

Health economists attempt to answer these questions. The measurement of costs involves assessment and valuation of all resources used and it is difficult (Tolley 1993). Valuation of benefits is even more problematic. While there is likely to be disagreement about conclusions of these health economists, the process of identifying and trying to value the different elements should give useful insights into how health promotion could be improved.

REPORTING OF EVALUATION

When someone has gone to all the time and trouble of doing an evaluation it ought to be widely reported inside and outside their organisation. This will ensure first that everyone concerned with the activity evaluated can learn from the findings and second that the lessons can be applied to other health promotion. There is an understandable tendency for people to report only positive evaluations which demonstrate that activities have been successful. This is unfortunate because some of the most helpful evaluations are the ones which demonstrate problems and therefore give insight into ways in which the effectiveness of health promotion can be improved.

THE NEED FOR MORE EVALUATION

The key to making health promotion more successful is discovering which activities are effective and how to make them even more so. Evaluation is the tool that enables us to do this. It is disappointing that there are not more examples of good evaluation. All of us working in health promotion have a duty to do more and better evaluations and to make our results much more widely available.

SUMMARY POINTS

Three roles are involved in an evaluation: programme manager, evaluator and programme worker.

Evaluation is an important aid to quality assurance in health promotion.

Evaluations may cover input, process, outcome and impact.

The choice of quantitative or qualitative methods depends on the nature of the evaluation.

Outcomes chosen for evaluation may be short term (knowledge and attitudes), medium term (behaviour) or long term (physiological and disease prevention).

Long-term outcomes have the most social value but are very difficult to use in evaluations.

Designs for outcome evaluation studies include:

- ☐ randomised controlled trials
- ☐ comparison trials
- ☐ lagged intervention trials
- ☐ message tracing
- ☐ comparison of self-selected groups
- ☐ uncontrolled before and after studies

Resources need to be allocated for evaluation.

REFERENCES

Beattie A. (1990). Evaluation of community development initiative in health promotion: a review of current strategies. In *Baseline review of community development and health education*. London: Health Education Authority.

Fitzgibbon C.T. and Morris L.L. (1987). *How to design a programme evaluation.* London: Sage.

Nutbeam D., Smith C. and Catford J. (1990). Evaluation in health education: a review of progress, possibilities and problems. *Journal of Epidemiology and Community Health* **44**, 83–89.

Tolley K. (1993). *Health promotion: how to measure cost-effectiveness*. London: Health Education Authority.

EXAMPLES OF DIFFERENT TYPES OF OUTCOME EVALUATION STUDIES

Randomised controlled trial design

Fehily A., Vaughan-Williams E., Shiels K. *et al.* (1989). The effect of dietary advice on nutrient intakes. Evidence from diet and reinfarction trial. *Journal of Human Nutrition and Dietetics* **2**, 225–235.

MRFIT Research Group (1990). Mortality rates after 10.5 years for participants in MRFIT trial – findings related to a priori hypotheses. *Journal of the American Medical Association* **263**, 393–396.

Comparison trial design

Nutbeam D. and Catford J. (1987). The Welsh Heart Programme evaluation strategy: progress plans and possibilities. *Health Promotion* **2**, 5–18.

Salonen J.T., Kottke T.E., Jacobs D.R. and Hannan P.J. (1986). Analysis of community based cardiovascular studies. Evaluation issues in the North Karelia project. *International Journal of Epidemiology* **15**, 176–182.

Walter H.J., Hofman A., Vaughan R.D. and Wynder E.L. (1988). Modification of risk factors for coronary heart disease – five year result of a school based intervention trial. *New England Journal of Medicine* **318**, 1093–1100.

Young I. (1993). Healthy eating polices in schools: an evaluation of effect on pupil knowledge and behaviour. *Health Education Journal* **52**, 3–9

Comparison of self-selected groups design

Gibbs J.O., Mulvaney D., Henes C. and Read R. (1985). Work-site health promotion. Five year trend in employee health care costs. *Journal of Occupational Medicine* **27**, 826–830.

Uncontrolled before and after design

Cameron I.H. and McGuire C. (1990). Are you dying to get a suntan – pre and post campaign survey results. *Health Education Journal* **49**, 166–170.

Hill A. and Mayon-White R.T. (1987). A telephone survey to evaluate an AIDS leaflet campaign. *Health Education Journal* **46**, 127–129.

McEwan R.T., Bhopal R. and Patten W. (1991). Drama on HIV and AIDS: an evaluation of a theatre in education programme. *Health Education Journal* **50**, 155–160.

McGovern E., MacAuley D. and Anderson V. (1992). A nurse-led stop smoking initiative. *Nursing Standard* **7** (No. 25), 26–29.

CHAPTER 11

Putting health education into practice

GOAL

To develop and deliver a health education plan using education and communication principles and the steps in the education process to help learning occur.

OBJECTIVES

- to identify the steps involved in the communication process
- to discuss the principles of effective communication
- to describe effective communication techniques in health promotion
- to explore methods of assessing health learning needs
- to describe the activities used for planning health education activities
- to discuss the techniques available for implementing the plan
- to evaluate individuals' learning and the effectiveness of the health education process

COMMUNICATION

This chapter deals with the health education process in relation to individuals. Effective communication is fundamental to the health education process and in this situation it is frequently called therapeutic communication (Kasch 1984). There is considerable evidence that communication and interaction between clients and professionals in health care settings are often limited (Parkin 1976; May 1990; Wilkinson 1992).

Communication is an extremely complex process, the detailed discussion of which is beyond the scope of this book. This chapter therefore attempts to provide a brief overview of the communication process and concentrate on the principles and techniques which are essential to the delivery of health promotion.

WHAT IS COMMUNICATION?

Communication essentially involves the exchange of information between two or more people (Porrit 1990). In health promotion this may be at different levels:

1. in one-to-one, or small-group situations with clients
2. indirectly with clients via the media, written materials, television and advertising (see Chapters 12 and 19)
3. between professionals – in relation to the organisation and management of health promotion activities (see Chapter 8)

Communication is a two-way cyclical process which requires a sender, a message and a receiver. Once a message is received, the receiver indicates their response and thus becomes the sender (see Figure 11.1).

Although the process outlined above appears simple, it is made complicated by the way each individual involved interprets the messages from their own point of view and subject to influences from their previous experiences of life.

The aim of effective communication is to send a message which is understandable to the person receiving it. This involves:

- **the sender** preparing the message and deciding on its content and format
- **the message,** which should be clear, simple and straightforward
- **the mode of transmission**, which should involve appropriate verbal and non-verbal techniques to enhance the recipient's understanding

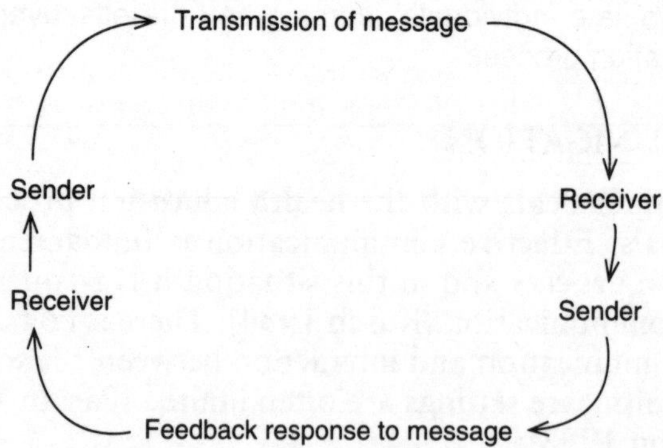

Figure 11.1 The process of communication
The role of sender and receiver alternates between health educator and client as they alternately transmit (message or response) to and then receive from the other.

- **the receiver** attending, observing, actively listening, interpreting the message and reacting and responding to it

In preparing the message the **sender** needs to consider:

- What do I want the recipient to understand?
- What is the best method of doing this, e.g. writing, face-to-face?
- What are the potential barriers and how can they be overcome?
- How will I know the message has been understood?

The **recipient**, on the other hand, needs to consider:

- What does the sender want me to do as a result?
- Am I interpreting correctly the message the sender wishes to convey?
- Are there any factors hindering my understanding?
- Are there any hidden messages being conveyed?
- What messages do I need to send back to show I have understood?

The health educator and client both act alternately as sender and receiver, providing, receiving or seeking information, reassurance and encouragement. The health educator will seek through communication to persuade and motivate the client to contemplate changes in health-related behaviour.

BARRIERS TO EFFECTIVE COMMUNICATION

There are many factors that act as barriers to effective communication. Some of these are identified in Table 11.1. There are also principles and techniques which health promoters can use to minimise or overcome these barriers (Phillips 1992).

In sending the message, use the KISS rule:

Keep
It
Simple
and Straightforward

Messages must be clear and avoid ambiguity. Using simple words and short sentences will help clarity. Avoid jargon and technical words. Ambiguity can lead to confusion and frustration for both sender and recipient. Brief, clear messages will be understood more easily and thus minimise misunderstanding.

Table 11.1 Barriers to communication

- Unclear message (leads to distortions of content and feelings being communicated).
- Inappropriate level of language (leads to lack of understanding, feelings of inadequacy or loss of confidence).
- Distractions in the message, the sender or the setting (lead to message being misheard, misread or misunderstood).
- Poor presentation, including lack of organisation of information and inappropriate methods (leads to boredom, inattention, confusion and frustration).
- Inaccurate expectations – of the purpose of the communication and the abilities of the people involved.
- Interpersonal feelings – the way in which those involved in the communication feel about each other.
- Poor communication skills.
- Lack of knowledge and information about the subject.
- Lack of self-awareness and lack of awareness of the effect their communication has on others.
- Those attempting to communicate hold conflicting values.
- Sensory impairment or deprivation such as hearing or speech loss.
- Having a judgmental approach or making belittling remarks.
- Client's lack of interest in the subject – topic of little relevance to them.
- Fear of hearing painful or unwanted information.

Allow time for communication and make sure that the client does not feel hurried. Choose a suitably quiet and private place where you will not be interrupted.

Discussion/Activity 11.1 Distortion of messages

Work with your colleagues in groups of five or six. Choose a short factual report about 300–500 words in length from a newspaper and ask your colleagues to go and wait outside the room. Then invite one colleague back into the room and read the article to them but do not let them see the written text. The person to whom the article has just been read then invites another colleague back and passes on to them as much of the article as they can remember. The new person then invites the next colleague back into the room and passes on to them what they have just been told. This continues until everyone has been invited back into the room. Each person stays in the room after they have passed the message on but keeps quiet and listens to the message being relayed to each newcomer.

Listen carefully to how the message changes and information is distorted. Observe carefully your colleagues' ways of putting the information across. Read the original report to your colleagues and discuss with them what factors acted as barriers to communication.

USING QUESTIONS

The health promoter uses questions to help the client explore particular issues or feelings. Questioning can also be used to focus on specific points if a client is wandering off the agreed subject. Open or closed questions can be used.

Open questions require more than a single-word response and often ask the question 'How?'.

- 'How do you cope with your treatment now?'
- 'Tell me what you believe is your problem?'

Closed questions can be answered in a single word, which is often 'yes' or 'no'.

- 'Have you lost any weight?'
- 'Do you normally have difficulty sleeping?'

NON-VERBAL COMMUNICATION

Non-verbal communication plays an important part in sending information and supporting the verbal message. Non-verbal communication includes:

- body language
- touch
- silence

Body language is expressed in facial expression, posture, gestures, eye contact, and in many other ways. Attitudes such as interest, sympathy and attentiveness can be shown by body language. Negative attitudes such as boredom, impatience and apathy are also all too easily conveyed through body language.

Touch can also be used to communicate feelings of empathy. Silence is a way of indicating interest and a willingness to wait for the recipient to put their thoughts in order. Alternatively, silence can be used destructively to indicate disapproval, anger or disinterest.

ACTIVE LISTENING

The health promoter must develop active listening skills since the ability to receive information is just as essential to effective communication as is the ability to send information. The health promoter must be sensitive to the client's values and beliefs. These have developed through previous experiences and will affect the way in which the message is interpreted.

When listening, the health promoter must focus attention on the client to pick up not only the verbal message but also the non-verbal cues the client is conveying. However, care should be taken not to overdo this. Excessive eye contact may interfere with communication by making the client uncomfortable because they feel they are being stared at.

Reinforcement techniques can encourage continuation of communication. Restating and reflecting are ways of indicating that you have received both the feeling and the content of a message, for example: 'You were saying you felt unhappy about the amount of weight you had put on since Christmas'. They also encourage the sender to continue and elaborate on what they were saying. Phrases such as 'go on' and 'uh huh' and nodding gestures can also do this.

Watch out for signs that your message is unclear. The recipient may look confused, disinterested, or fail to give an appropriate response. Seek clarification, by asking the recipient to restate or review the message. Rephrasing the message may be required in order to get confirmation of understanding.

Effective communication also requires a proper setting (see pages 186–188).

Discussion/Activity 11.2 Methods of communication

Consider a recent face-to-face communication you have had with a client. What information did you pick up from the other person in addition to words spoken? What influence did their appearance, dress, age, posture, gestures and expression have on your interpretation of the message?

TYPES OF COMMUNICATION

The number of people reached by a communication can vary from one to millions (Tones 1986). The degree of involvement for each individual also varies from very high, as in a one-to-one counselling situation, to very low, as when someone is half listening to a radio broadcast (see Figure 11.2).

METHODS FOR INDIVIDUALS AND SMALL GROUPS

Methods suitable for individuals or small groups (less than 10) include one-to-one counselling, discussion, questions and answers, problem-solving, providing materials for independent learning (self-instruction),

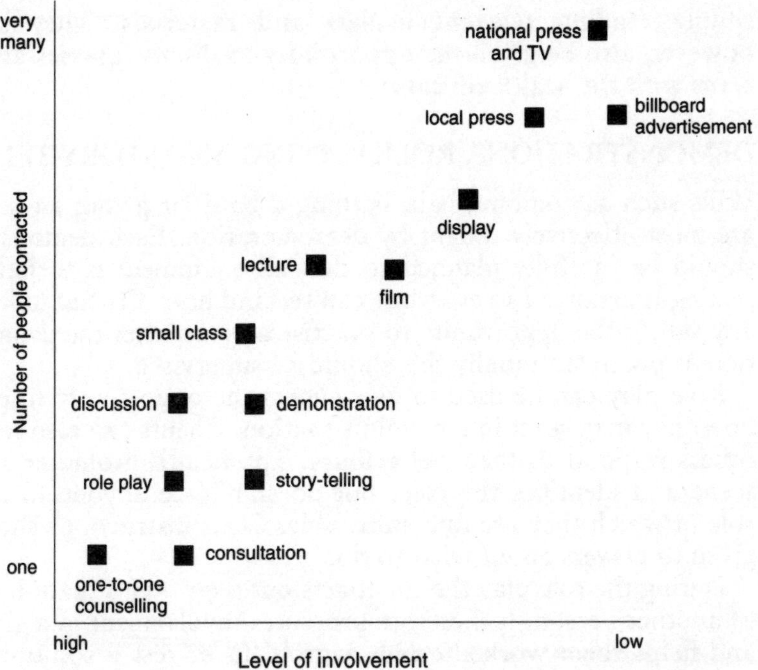

Figure 11.2 Levels of involvement in different health education methods
Health education methods vary in the number of people contacted (from one to millions) and in the degree to which each person is involved. In general, methods which contact very large numbers have a low level of involvement.

demonstration, role playing and story-telling. All encourage interpersonal interaction and actively involve individuals in learning.

INVOLVING THE CLIENT

Discussion, answering questions and problem-solving involve the participants asking questions of each other or posing problem situations which are then discussed to promote understanding, increase knowledge and, in some cases, a change in attitude. The use of these techniques with groups enables members to share experiences or perceptions of a situation and learn from each other. The health promoter facilitates group processes and dynamics to ensure all members are able to participate in and benefit from discussions. It is important to help clients decide on solutions to problems rather than advise or direct them.

Some people prefer to learn independently using prepared learning packages, interactive videos and computer programs or by simply reading relevant leaflets and materials. They should, however, also be given the opportunity to discuss queries and concerns with the health educator.

DEMONSTRATIONS, ROLE PLAYING AND STORY-TELLING

Skills such as combing hair, bathing a baby or giving an injection are most effectively taught by demonstration. Each demonstration should be carefully planned so that all equipment is to hand and seating is arranged so everyone can see and hear. Crucial to learning any skill is the opportunity to practise as soon after the demonstration as possible. Initially this should be supervised.

Role play can be used to give clients the opportunity to explore how they may react in a certain situation. Clients can also test how others respond to their behaviours. The health promoter sets the scene and identifies the roles but doesn't force anyone to act any role in which they are uncomfortable. Clear instructions should be given to players about what to do.

During the role play the client acts out their own situation or that of another person. It therefore promotes involvement in a situation and helps them work through a problem or test a solution. Role play is a particularly useful method of changing attitudes. Following the role play the health promoter helps participants and observers analyse the situation by asking them to describe their feelings about the interactions. There may follow a general discussion on the participant's performance but this must be positive and constructive.

Story-telling is useful with children to explain situations or events such as admission to hospital, a course of treatment or 'going to the operating theatre'. The child can be further involved by the use of colouring books linked to the story.

LARGE GROUPS

The lecture is a commonly used method for larger groups. It can be particularly effective in conveying information to large numbers of people and it is therefore relatively cost effective. However, there is usually little audience involvement and participation and it is not effective for demonstrating skills because large audiences will have difficulty seeing. It may be possible to incorporate some of the small-group methods into a lecture by dividing large audiences into smaller groups. Other methods suitable for larger groups are films and theatre.

MASS-MEDIA CAMPAIGNS

These methods attempt to reach much wider audiences through such things as nationwide television and radio campaigns, advertising hoardings or closed-circuit TV. These will be discussed more fully in Chapter 19.

COMMUNICATION IN THE EDUCATION PROCESS

Helping people develop new behaviours regarding their health and lifestyle requires considerable expertise from the health educator. The intention is to empower individuals to make an informed choice. In order to do this they need knowledge about their health state, the things that affect it and skills to adopt modified behaviours if they wish to do so.

The education process requires effective communication skills and a systematic, planned approach. Webb (1985) believes that powerful communicators become powerful teachers so long as their subject matter is sound. The steps involved are the same whether they are applied to individuals, small groups or to larger populations (see Figure 11.3). The aims are to:

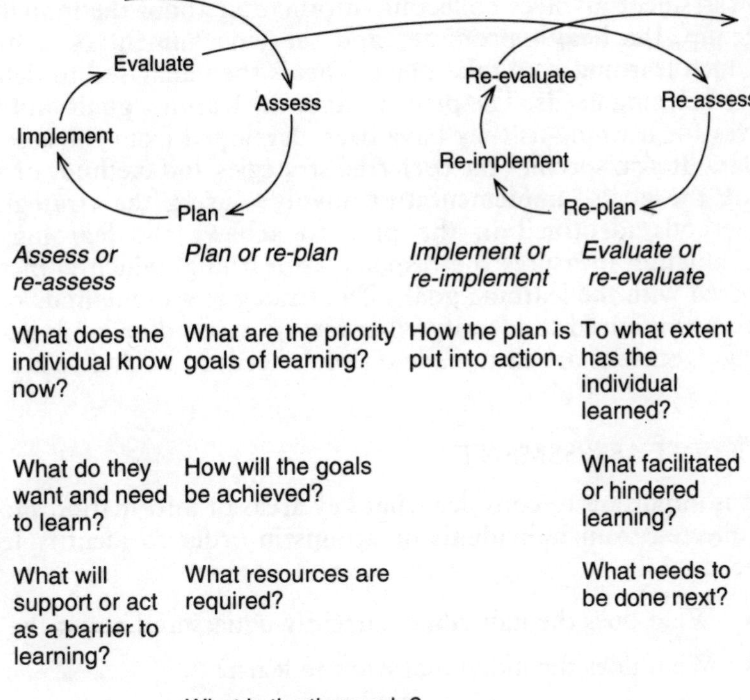

Figure 11.3 Using the teaching–learning process
The teaching–learning process rolls through repeated cycles of assess, plan, implement, evaluate.

1. identify the individual's or group's learning shortfall or needs
2. identify the learning goals or outcomes required
3. plan what is to be learned and the activities that will help the goals to be achieved
4. use learning and communication strategies to provide the activities identified in the plan
5. evaluate the effectiveness of the process and decide what to do next

Education thus becomes a problem-solving process involving four stages. Each stage is undertaken in partnership with the client:

1. assess
2. plan
3. implement
4. evaluate

Assessment involves collecting information about the individual or group, the health promoter and the environment or context in which learning is to take place. This is then analysed to determine the learning needs. The **plan** specifies the learning goals and objectives for learning as they have been developed from the assessment data. It also specifies the preferred strategies and methods of achieving the goals. **Implementation** involves using the strategies and methods identified in the plan to achieve the learning goals. **Evaluation** measures the response to learning, which is then compared with the learning goals. The strategies and methods used are also scrutinised to identify what factors assisted or inhibited learning. Decisions are then made on what needs to be done next.

CLIENT ASSESSMENT

It is important to consider what key areas of information should be collected from individuals or groups in order to identify learning needs. Ask:

- What does the individual currently understand about the topic?
- What does the individual want to learn?
- What does the individual need to know?
- What is the individual's preferred method of learning?
- Is the individual willing and able to learn?

CURRENT UNDERSTANDING

Finding out what individuals already understand about their health status or the topic is important for the following reasons:

- It provides a baseline from which to work. People learn more easily if new information and skills are linked to existing knowledge.
- It provides a level or gauge for future evaluation to show the extent to which learning has occurred.
- It highlights existing misunderstandings or misconceptions about the subject which must be resolved – otherwise confusion may occur later.
- It prevents time and energy being wasted on covering what is already known.

WHAT DOES THE INDIVIDUAL WANT TO LEARN?

People usually learn best when they see the relevance of learning, when they experience the need to know something, or when they have to put a new skill into practice (humanistic learning theory – see Chapter 6, page 97). Information or skills which are seen as irrelevant or unimportant may, at best, be ignored or may cause anger and frustration so that no learning takes place. Discovering what an individual wants to know is therefore essential.

Sometimes there are several reasons why people find it difficult to identify what they want to learn. They may not know the scope of what there is to learn or they may have difficulty putting it into words. They may be reluctant to ask for fear of appearing ignorant. The educator can help by providing cues and highlighting some of the things people commonly want to know about the subject. It must be remembered, however, that some people genuinely do not want to know about aspects of their health.

WHAT DOES THE INDIVIDUAL NEED TO KNOW?

The professional's expertise and knowledge of the health topic and situation should be used to balance what individuals want to learn and what they need to know.

Professional experience suggests aspects of a subject which an individual:

- **Must know** – for safety, survival and comfort
- **Should know** – useful but not essential
- **Could know** – knowledge and skills related to the subject but which do not fall into the above two categories

Getting the balance between what the individual needs and wants to know is not easy. Their learning needs may be over-estimated by a health promoter who is very knowledgeable and confident about a subject. On the other hand, learning needs may be under-estimated if the health promoter is not very knowledgeable on the subject or finds it sensitive or embarrassing.

PREFERRED METHOD OF LEARNING

People like to learn in different ways (see Chapter 6, Tables 6.1–6.3) and are more likely to learn if the methods that they prefer are chosen.

IS THE INDIVIDUAL WILLING AND ABLE TO LEARN?

Motivation, together with ability to learn, is commonly called 'readiness to learn' (Pohl 1965; Redman 1984). Understanding what makes individuals ready to learn is essential in assisting educators to plan and modify their teaching activities. Health behaviours do not exist in a vacuum (Davison 1994). Motivation to learn about possible modifications to behaviour depends upon daily experience of life. There may be many other competing issues in the individual's life which make learning for health a low priority.

For an individual to learn, firstly they must want to learn. Motivation varies with individuals, situations and topics. Usually people are motivated by seeing some benefit or reward for learning (see the discussion of learning theories in Chapter 6) or avoidance of punishment or problems. It is part of the educator's role to establish what factors motivate each individual and then plan learning experiences around this (see Chapter 7).

ABILITY TO LEARN

Closely linked with motivation is the ability to learn. Ability to learn relates to:

- **physical ability**

  strength, co-ordination, dexterity

  vision, hearing or speech
- **Intellectual ability**

  level of numeracy and literacy, reasoning

  problem-solving and communication skills

  existing knowledge and skills

  current health status

The learning experience has to be tailored to the individual's physical and intellectual ability and their preferred method of learning (see Chapter 6). It must also take into account existing knowledge and skills. For example, a client will have difficulty in understanding about a calorie-restricted diet if they don't know that food types have different calorific values.

CURRENT HEALTH STATUS

Current health status can motivate or hinder learning. A person with back disorders is likely to want to learn about posture and exercises that will help their situation. On the other hand, a person who is in pain or weak following surgery may be unable to concentrate sufficiently to learn.

Assessment of health status tends to focus on physical health. Armstrong (1993) highlights the importance of also assessing mental health needs, and identifies factors which can contribute, such as difficulties with relationships, bereavement, loss of employment, financial and housing problems, social isolation and personal and family history of mental illness.

COLLECTING INFORMATION FROM CLIENTS

A comprehensive assessment involves the collection of a large amount of information. However, there is often little time available so it should not be wasted in seeking information which has already been collected for other reasons. Critical information should be sought first. Pre-formulated checklists or questionnaires may be used to speed up the process though health promoters should use them flexibly so that important items not on the proforma are not overlooked (see Figure 11.4)

Information can be gathered in several different ways and it is often effective to use a combination of:

- asking questions
- observation
- reviewing records
- discussion with colleagues

When collecting information from the client by asking questions and observation the health promoter must first explain the purpose of the discussion and how the information will be used. They will need to be well prepared with questions that will help to elicit the information and then use all the active listening skills described above (page 175). The health promoter should make short notes of the main points and check their accuracy with the client.

CLIENT ASSESSMENT FORM

Confidential

1. **Demographic data**

   Name .... Age .... Sex ....

   Current or previous occupation ....

2. **Physical ability**

   Hearing .... Hearing aid ....

   Vision .... Glasses/Lenses ....

   Speech ....

   Co-ordination/Dexterity ....

3. What does the client **want** to learn about? ....

   ....

4. What does the client already know and feel about the subject?

   ....

5. Does he/she have concerns about how it might affect his/her lifestyle?

   ....

   ....

6. Are there any problems that might inhibit learning? ....

   ....

   ....

7. What is the client's preferred learning style? ....

   ....

8. What additional aspects does the client need to know?

   ....

THE PRIORITY LEARNING NEEDS ARE:

1. ....

2. ....

3. ....

Figure 11.4 Client learning-needs assessment form
A simple form like this helps health educators assess client learning needs.

Observation will add to the information about the individual's feelings, beliefs and thoughts. It is particularly important to observe facial expressions, gestures, posture and other body language as these may reveal whether the individual is anxious, frightened, confused, disinterested and lacks understanding or alternatively is keen and eager to learn more.

REVIEWING RECORDS

In some situations education will be part of treatment and care for health disorders or of an ongoing health programme – for example, a mother attending antenatal classes or a patient attending a clinic for treatment of hypertension. Patient records available in such circumstances contain information on current and previous illnesses and should provide details about health status and previous experiences. Other information may be obtained from referral letters and current documentation from other health care professionals. These can be supplemented by discussions if necessary.

Discussion/Activity 11.3 Assessment for learning

Choose an individual or group with whom you want to work. Using the principles and guidelines above, undertake an assessment. Identify what they want to learn and compare it with what you think they need to know.

ASSESSING YOUR SKILLS AS A HEALTH PROMOTER

Just as important as assessment of the client is assessment of the health promoter. In order to be able to facilitate learning they must have the ability and motivation to teach. The should have:

- knowledge and understanding of the subject
- competence in related skills
- effective communication skills
- basic teaching skills
- appropriate values and beliefs about health promotion
- appropriate feelings towards the individual
- appropriate attitudes towards the subject matter

When the health promoter lacks knowledge or understanding of a topic they may avoid teaching it or give inadequate or incorrect information. When teaching particular skills, the health promoter must be proficient in performing and demonstrating the techniques.

For example, a health visitor showing a child and its parents how to use a buzzer alarm for enuresis problems must know how the equipment works and then be able to demonstrate this. Health promoters can however still be useful when they are unsure of their knowledge or skills if they are willing to learn alongside the client. Indeed many clients may find this approach more helpful than the traditional approach.

Health promoters should be able to assess the individual's learning needs, plan and prioritise learning opportunities, use a variety of teaching techniques and strategies, and evaluate the effectiveness of teaching and learning. They must also be willing and motivated to help the individual learn.

The attitudes, beliefs and values of the health promoter are vital. They will not be effective in promoting attitudes or values that they do not themselves hold. They must also acknowledge that views and behaviours of others may conflict with their own and recognise that some people are easier to get on with than others. It is essential that the health promoter accepts that they and their client may hold different attitudes and values but still develops appropriate feelings towards the client.

Some subjects may be difficult to talk about. Health promoters must be able to recognise when this is the case for them. Help and advice should be sought from colleagues who may be able to suggest ways of coping or may take on the teaching role in that situation.

HEALTH PROMOTER'S SELF-ASSESSMENT

Health promoters need to judge whether they feel ready to teach a topic by undertaking a self-assessment of the areas identified in the list above. A pre-formulated checklist can act as an *aide-mémoire* and speed up the process (see Figure 11.5).

Discussion/Activity 11.4 Can you help people learn?

Working with the same client or group as in Discussion/Activity 11.3, and using the guidelines in Figure 11.5, critically assess your ability to help this person or group learn.

THE LEARNING ENVIRONMENT

Health promotion can occur in virtually any situation, from formal classrooms with groups of people to one-to-one events in an individual's home. There are several factors that will influence learning:

- privacy
- equipment
- room size
- psychological environment

	Excellent	Good	Poor
	(tick appropriate box)		
1. Knowledge			
Is my knowledge and understanding of the subject	☐	☐	☐
Rationale			
2. Skills			
Are my communication skills	☐	☐	☐
Rationale			
Are my teaching skills	☐	☐	☐
Rationale			
Are my technical skills	☐	☐	☐
Rationale			

3. Attitudes
How important is it that this individual achieve his learning goals?

What are my feeling about this individual?

What are my feelings about the subject?

4. Summarise
WHAT, IF ANYTHING, DO I NEED TO DO TO BE READY TO TEACH THIS PERSON?

Figure 11.5 Self-assessment checklist for health promotors
A short checklist like this will help you prepare yourself to help clients learn.

In some situations privacy will be essential, particularly if the topic is sensitive or embarrassing. Frequent interruptions or fear of being overheard may reduce concentration and raise anxiety. Sometimes however it may be extremely difficult to find a separate, quiet room, and an educator will have to be creative and resourceful in finding suitable areas free from noise, distractions and disruptions.

The right equipment and teaching materials (see Chapter 12) should be readily available. This may include materials such as leaflets, books, apparatus and audiovisual aids. If these are not to hand the educator will appear disorganised and unprepared so that learning is likely to be less effective.

An appropriate size room should be used if possible. It is difficult to develop a relaxed, comfortable atmosphere with one person in a large and sparsely furnished room. Similarly, rooms which are used for demonstrations to groups should be big enough so that all can see and hear in comfort. Heating, lighting and ventilation should be adequate whatever the situation, and blackout facilities should be available if necessary.

Ideal conditions are rarely available and the assessment of the individual's needs should help to determine the priority in terms of the learning environment. For example, in some situations privacy will be the overriding concern but in others it may be the opportunity to use specific equipment.

THE PSYCHOLOGICAL ENVIRONMENT

To be able to learn, individuals need to feel respected and valued and not threatened or judged. Educators have a responsibility to ensure that each individual's dignity, privacy and interests are safeguarded so that they feel relaxed, comfortable and confident that they will not be made to look silly. Clients should be encouraged to take as much responsibility for learning as they are able and develop a partnership with the educator.

THE PLAN

The next step in the education process is to develop a plan using the information from the assessment. The content and purpose of the plan are listed in Table 11.2.

THE LEARNING GOALS AND OBJECTIVES

The goals and objectives within the overall aims direct the learning experience. They should describe exactly what the client should do, how well they should do it and under what circumstances (see Chapter 6).

The learning goals and objectives should be developed with the client. They must be achievable. If they are set so high as to be unattainable the client becomes frustrated, threatened and demotivated. On the other hand, goals should not be so low as to be patronising.

Many people experience difficulty writing goals and objectives. The following checklist, using the mnemonic RUMBA (after Kitson 1990), may help. For each objective and goal, ask yourself if it is:

- **Relevant** Will it help the client learn what they want and need to learn?
- **Understandable** Is it precise and practical?
- **Measureable** How will you know if learning has occurred?
- **Behaviourally stated** Does it state what the client will do?
- **Achievable** Can it be done in the time available?

Table 11.2 Education plan

Learning needs	Identified from information collected in the assessment. Balance between what the client **needs** and **wants** to learn. Priorities identified: **must** know **should** know **could** know
Learning goals and objectives	Goals and objectives of learning agreed by client and educator **Goals** describe the learning outcomes or goals desired. **Objectives** describe in more detail the behaviours that will achieve the goal.
Activities	The activities which the client and educator are to carry out in order to achieve the goals are selected. The **educator** demonstrates, instructs, shows, informs, etc. The **client** reads, practises, watches, listens, discusses, etc.
Resources	The necessary resources are identified, e.g. leaflets, videos, equipment, models, etc. Which health care professional is responsible for helping the client learn?
Time-scale	When should learning occur by?
Demonstration of achievement	Method of assessing achievement identified, e.g. by the client explaining, demonstrating skills, etc.

THE ACTIVITIES

Having decided on the objectives and goals for learning, the activities to achieve them should be selected. These are likely to include the client in discussion, practice, self-instruction, role play, watching films and videos, reading leaflets and problem-solving (see page 177).

The activities chosen will depend on:

- the learning objectives
- the time available
- the age, gender and ethnicity of the client
- abilities and preferences of client
- physical resources available (room, equipment, etc.)
- the skills and preferences of the health promoter

RESOURCES

The activities that can be chosen may be limited by the teaching materials, equipment and rooms available to you. The choice will also be limited by the staff time and skills upon which you can call. The plan must identify what resources will be needed so that you can confirm that they are available.

TIME-SCALE

It is often helpful if the plan includes a time-scale, especially if several areas of knowledge or skills need to be learned before a particular event. For example, patients may need to learn self-care skills before the date set for their discharge from hospital. Time-scales help the health promoter co-ordinate education activities with other elements of care and space out learning over the period of time available. They also provide an indication of how quickly progress is being made and they act as motivators.

DEMONSTRATION OF ACHIEVEMENT

The final part of the plan identifies how the client's achievement of learning will be assessed. The methods chosen should relate to the learning objectives. For example, the client might demonstrate self-injection technique, or describe how they have progressed with their exercise regime, or choose the 'permitted' foods from a menu.

Progress towards achieving learning should be recognised and rewarded. Most people would say 'I like to know how I'm doing'. Highlighting progress and achievements, giving praise or material rewards will reinforce learning and motivate most individuals.

Feedback is essential to reinforcement. It should be constructive, given as soon as possible after learning and directed at behaviours about which the patient can do something.

CASE STUDY: LOSING WEIGHT

Joanne, aged 35, is 5 feet 5 inches tall and weighs 15.5 stone. She has been advised by her GP to lose weight to prevent her health from suffering in the long term. Following assessment by her GP, practice nurse and dietitian, Joanne has agreed to work towards achieving the following goal and objectives.

Goal: to lose weight at a rate of 6–8 lbs per month until her weight reaches 9 stone.

Objectives: Joanne will be able to:

- weigh herself accurately once a week
- explain which food groups make up a balanced diet
- identify which foods to
  1. try to eat
  2. try to avoid
  3. eat in moderation
- choose a daily menu suitable for her 1800 calorie/day diet
- perform agreed daily and thrice-weekly exercise plan

Achievement of these objectives can be checked at least in the short term. However, only over a period of time will it be possible to judge fully whether Joanne achieves them and actually 'weighs herself accurately once a week' or continues 'to perform the daily and thrice-weekly exercise plan'.

Discussion/Activity 11.5 Devising a learning plan

Using the same client or group identified in the previous exercises and using Table 11.2 as a guide, devise a plan to meet the identified learning needs. Ask colleagues or teachers for constructive criticism.

IMPLEMENTATION

Even the best plans are of no use unless they are implemented. Those caring for the patient will need to integrate the planned education process and ensure it is delivered.

EVALUATION

Evaluation of the education process involves collecting data and making judgments about the extent to which:

- the client has met their learning needs
- the health promoter has assisted learning
- the environment has supported teaching and learning

Although evaluation is presented here as the fourth phase in the education cycle it is also an activity that is undertaken throughout the cycle as formative or ongoing evaluation (see Chapter 10). This allows modifications to be made during any stage of the process in the light of the findings.

HAS THE CLIENT MET THEIR LEARNING NEEDS?

The learning goals and objectives provide a good basis for evaluation. If these have been developed and checked using the RUMBA mnemonic (page 188), the expected client behaviours are more easily identified. Evaluation may assess short-term learning or it may be longer term and assess whether clients have incorporated new behaviours into their lifestyle (see Figure 10.2).

Both client and health promoter should assess the client's learning against the goals and objectives. A short-term evaluation can be carried out soon after the learning experience – before a patient is discharged home for example, or at the end of antenatal or health promotion clinics. Decisions about whether the client has incorporated new behaviours into everyday life will take longer to judge. For example, it may need the time for three outpatient appointments at monthly intervals or for several months of visits from the GP or observation throughout a pregnancy.

HOW FAR DID THE HEALTH EDUCATOR ASSIST LEARNING?

This area of evaluation should focus on the processes of the learning experiences. Was the initial assessment adequate and accurate? Were the objectives set relevant, understandable, measurable, behaviourally stated and achievable? Were the methods appropriately chosen and were they effectively implemented?

In addition to examining the phases of the education process, it may be helpful to discover the perceptions of clients about the health promoter's performance, either in writing or directly through discussion. It may be wise to ask specific questions or seek comments relating to specific areas, otherwise only broad, general statements may be given.

Health promoters need also to reflect on their own performance and make notes on the techniques they used. They should record those that were successful and those that were less so, together with possible reasons. This will help to indicate helpful methods for the future. In some circumstances it may be possible to obtain the opinions of colleagues.

Evaluation of the learning process should also consider how well the learning environment supported learning. Were there adequate learning materials and equipment available or would further materials have been helpful? Did the leaflets, booklets, video and so on help the client learn and were they easily understood? Was the room comfortable and did it inhibit or support education? Was the timescale realistic? Was achievement appropriately identified?

SUMMARY POINTS

Effective communication is fundamental to the health education process.

Communication is a complicated cyclical process which involves the exchange of information between two or more people.

Effective communication is best achieved by keeping the message simple and straightforward.

Non-verbal communication plays an important part in sending information and supporting verbal messages.

Education is more likely to be successful if:

- ☐ a planned, systematic process is used which includes: assessment, planning, implementation and evaluation phases
- ☐ it is individualised according to the individual's needs, ability and motivation to learn

- ☐ the client wants to learn
- ☐ the client is actively involved in all stages
- ☐ goals and objectives are realistic
- ☐ priority needs are met first
- ☐ new learning is related to previous experiences/knowledge
- ☐ learning advances from the simple to the complex
- ☐ learning is related to life experiences – learning must be seen to be relevant
- ☐ client and educator work in partnership
- ☐ opportunity for practice is provided
- ☐ immediate feedback is given, coupled with appropriate positive reinforcement

REFERENCES

Armstrong E. (1993). Mental health check. *Nursing Times*, **89** (No. 33), 40–42.

Davison C. (1994). Conflicts of interest. *Nursing Times* **90** (No. 13), 40–42.

Kasch C.R. (1984). Interpersonal competence and communication in the delivery of nursing care. *Advances in Nursing Science* **6** (No. 2), 72, 75, 76.

Kitson A. (1990). *Quality patient care; the dynamic standard setting system.* RCN Standards of Care Project. London: RCN.

May C. (1990). Research on nurse–patient relationships: problems of theory, problems of practice. *Journal of Advanced Nursing* **15**, 307–315.

Parkin D.M. (1976). Survey of the success of communications between hospital staff and patients. *Public Health* **90**, 203–209.

Phillips J. (1992). Breaking down the barriers. *Nursing Times* **88** (No. 35), 30–31.

Pohl M.L. (1965). Teaching activities of the nursing practitioner. *Nursing Research*, Winter, **14** (No. 1), 4–11.

Porrit L. (1990). Communication: the basis of interaction. Chapter 1 in *Interaction strategies: an introduction for health professionals* (2nd edition). Edinburgh: Churchill Livingstone.

Redman B.K. (1984). *The process of patient teaching in nurse education.* St Louis MO: The C.V. Mosby Company.

Tones K. (1986). The methodology of health education. *Journal of the Royal Society of Medicine* **79**, Supplement 13, 5–7.

Webb P. (1985). Getting it right – patient teaching. *Nursing*, second series **2** (No. 38), 1125–1127.

Wilkinson S. (1992). Confusions or challenges? *Nursing Times* **88** (No. 35), 24–28.

FURTHER READING

Hubley J. (1993). *Communicating health: An action guide to health education and health promotion.* London: Macmillan.

CHAPTER TWELVE

Health education materials

GOAL

To obtain and use written, audiovisual and other teaching materials effectively to enhance health promotion activities.

OBJECTIVES

- to identify the range and types of materials available
- to assess the advantages and disadvantages of using different types of materials in a specific situation
- to review existing health education materials and evaluate their effectiveness for a particular group of people
- to plan, organise and produce new health education materials which will enhance learning
- to develop a system for storage and distribution of health education materials

INTRODUCTION

Health education is a very important part of health promotion (see page 31) . Although the materials described in this chapter may occasionally be used in other aspects of health promotion, we have referred to them as health education materials since this is the aspect of health promotion in which they are most frequently used.

Over the last decade there has been a proliferation of the types and range of health education materials available. These can be divided into three main categories:

1. written materials
2. audiovisual materials
3. other teaching materials

WRITTEN MATERIALS

Written materials such as leaflets, booklets and posters are widely available. They are to be found not only in hospitals, surgeries, health centres and clinics, but also in chemists, libraries, supermarkets and shopping centres. Some seek generally to raise awareness of health issues such as road safety, accident prevention and healthy living. Others seek to provide information on specific topics such as drug abuse, alcohol problems, effects of surgery, diabetes and high blood pressure. Health care professionals may use them as part of a planned learning programme. Alternatively they may be freely distributed for anyone to take and use as they want (Williams *et al.* 1987).

AUDIOVISUAL MATERIALS

Audiovisual materials such as videos, films, audio tapes, slides and computer programs are increasingly being used. They can be used as part of a planned learning programme and during organised health promotion events. They can also be used for opportunistic health promotion – shown in health centres and hospital waiting areas, for example. These types of materials are not as easily available to the public for home use unless they are broadcast on radio or television. As more people get home video machines and computers they may be more widely used in the future.

OTHER TEACHING MATERIALS

Other teaching resources are the equipment and materials which health care professionals use to enhance their teaching. They include such things as overhead projectors, flipcharts, models and toys.

SOURCES OF HEALTH EDUCATION MATERIAL

The Health Education Authority produces a wide range of written materials which is available free or at low cost. Materials on particular topics are also produced by government departments, voluntary organisations and professional organisations (see Table 12.1). These are often attractively produced and well suited to the needs of their target populations. The main disadvantage is that information is not necessarily geared to the local situation or conditions.

Pharmaceutical companies and commercial organisations with a particular interest in linking their product with health promotion also produce materials. Most of these materials are very

Table 12.1 Some useful sources of health education materials

Health Education Authority	
Government Departments	Department of Health Department of Energy Ministry of Agriculture, Fisheries and Food
Voluntary organisations (patients)	Arthritis and Rheumatism Council British Association of Cancer United Patients (BACUP) British Diabetic Association British Heart Foundation British Lung Foundation Chest, Heart and Stroke Association Leukaemia Research Fund Parkinson's Disease Society
Voluntary organisations (campaigning)	Action on Smoking and Health (ASH) Age Concern Alcohol Concern Coronary Prevention Group The Advisory Council on Alcohol and Drug Education (TACADE)
Trade organisations and firms	Flora Fruit and Vegetable Growers' Association Kelloggs National Dairy Council Sainsbury Tesco Pharmaceutical firms
Commercial producers	(whose commercial purpose is producing and selling health education materials)

professionally produced and provided free to health promoters. Many have excellent educational content but users must always be alert to the possibility that some bias may exist in favour of the company's product (Hodges 1993). Some of the material offered by commercial firms as health promoting is thoroughly misleading. For example, some baby-milk firms have in the past produced 'health promotion' materials which gave the impression that bottle feeding was generally preferable to breast feeding. General interest magazines frequently publish feature articles on health issues and these can be useful (Friend 1992).

Many health promotion materials have been produced by health service units and most are available for purchase. New health promotion materials are reported in the Health Education Authority newsletter *Healthline*. There will probably be health promotion materials which have been produced in your locality. The district health education/promotion department should be able to advise on what materials are available and how they can be obtained.

The advantages and disadvantages of in-house production are discussed later in this chapter (page 204).

THE USES OF HEALTH EDUCATION MATERIALS

Health education materials are used:

- to enhance learning
- to increase awareness

USING HEALTH EDUCATION MATERIALS TO ENHANCE LEARNING

If a leaflet, video or poster is being used as part of a planned learning experience, it must contribute to that learning in some way (Murphy and Smith 1992). The materials used should be well presented, easy to understand, accurate and contain the information the individual needs and wants to know. They should not be included merely as a gimmick as this may well just distract individuals attempting to learn. The following criteria will help you decide whether the materials you are considering will enhance learning. Will they:

- create and maintain interest?
- explain how something works?
- help understanding?
- show what something looks like?
- demonstrate a procedure or technique?
- encourage client participation?
- confirm and support what is being said verbally?
- deliver a message and help retention of learning?

If materials fail to accomplish at least one of the above then they are likely to be superfluous.

Once it has been established that materials will help, one must choose the right ones for the job. Table 12.2 describes the most frequently used types of materials and media.

USING HEALTH EDUCATION MATERIALS TO INCREASE AWARENESS

Posters and other health education materials are also used in a less focused way to create awareness of health issues and sow seeds that can be nurtured by further health promotion work. The expectation

Table 12.2 Health education materials

Materials	Uses	Examples
1. Written materials Leaflets, books handouts, pamphlets, etc.	For self-initiated and independent reading To supplement other health promotion activities As an *aide-mémoire* to read and to reinforce learning at a later time	Leaflets on diet, hygiene, smoking, etc. found in chemists, surgeries, health centres and clinics Booklet on diabetes given in addition to individualised education programme Checklist, e.g. discharge instructions, list of medications
Pictures, colouring books	To explain events and real-life situations To introduce a topic for further discussion To encourage client involvement and interest in subject	Colouring books related to seizures Admission to hospital Cancer treatment *Vegetables* cartoon to inform children of nutritional requirements
Posters and charts	To raise awareness To create interest in a subject To provide information for advertising	Posters on a range of health issues, dental health, HIV and AIDS Posters in GP surgeries and libraries advertising well-woman or family-planning clinics, with times, addresses or telephone numbers
2. Audiovisual materials Videotapes and films	To influence knowledge, attitudes and skills To re-create real-life situations To teach how to handle problems To introduce a topic for further discussion To present facts, experiences and places For self-initiated and independent viewing and teacher-led activities	Used to show admission procedures to clients on hospital waiting lists Exercise programmes

Advantages	Caution
Can be used repeatedly and shared with others Can provide additional information Are relatively easily produced	Some clients: are not able to read are not able to see well enough to read do not want to read do not understand the language Some materials are not suitable or acceptable
Popular with children	Children may concentrate on the activity rather than the message
Have the potential to be seen by large numbers of people Require little input once produced Easily stored if necessary	People may ignore the poster if it is: poorly displayed left in place for longer periods of time May be damaged or defaced
Popular media with most clients Useful for people with limited reading ability Used for small groups, individuals in health care settings or homes Can be used repeatedly Relatively simple to use	Should not be used instead of health care professional Review before use to check relevance and suitability Copyright laws Clients' attention span may be short Films require blackout Equipment requires maintenance and secure storage

(continued)

Table 12.2—*continued*

Materials	**Uses**	**Examples**
Slides	To promote understanding of facts and ideas To help clients imagine real situations To promote discussions To attract and maintain interest To demonstrate skills For self-instruction	Pictures showing examples of hazards in the home Pictures of food rich in different vitamins Pictures of happy parents and babies to go with child-care talk
Audiotapes and, cassettes	To reinforce and repeat facts To encourage client participation in activities To accompany slides or printed text For self-instruction To share real-life experiences between clients	Relaxation and stress-reduction exercises For children, story-telling related to health topics
Computer programs	To learn and review facts For problem-solving To assess client needs To keep track of client information	Programs which ask questions for participants to complete Assessment of calorific intake when clients input details of foods consumed over a given period Tutorials on drug abuse and pregnancy prevention
3. Other materials Overhead projector and transparencies	To convey facts To present ideas To show diagrams To encourage participation To simplify concepts	Used to show patients how heart attacks occur

Advantages	Caution
Easy to re-arrange if different sequence is required Easy to produce, maintain and store in-house Clients enjoy seeing pictures Clients can control the equipment Can be linked with audiotapes Can be used repeatedly	Blackout needed for viewing Equipment requires maintenance
Small and easy to transport Relatively cheap to obtain, run and store Can be used almost anywhere Useful for clients who cannot see or read	Difficult to produce material without studio facilities Some clients are unable to hear Clients may have short attention span in absence of visual stimulation
Popular with younger clients Can be used repeatedly	Problems of compatibility between hardware and software Some clients fear computers Expensive Secure storage may be difficult
Good for large and small groups Transparencies easy to make and prepare ahead of time Easy to transport and store Equipment widely available in health service	Diagrams and prints should be large enough to be seen Information should be kept to a minimum Bulb can fail at a crucial moment

(continued)

Table 12.2—*continued*

Materials	Uses	Examples
Flipcharts	To attract attention and interest To convey facts To show diagrams To collect group members' contributions and ideas (brainstorming) To simplify concepts	Summary points of subject to be covered in session List of situations suggested by group in which they are likely to drink too much
Toys, models equipment	To encourage clients to be actively involved – observing, handling, manipulating objects To teach skills Real-life experience Demonstrations and supervised practice	Teddy bear used to explain to a young child a visit to the operating theatre Food models used to explain nutritional and dietary requirements

is that these materials will be casually glanced at rather than studied in detail. They must first attract attention and then encourage attitudes and mental associations conducive to health.

QUALITY OF HEALTH EDUCATION MATERIALS

The quality of presentation and accuracy and the appropriateness of content varies tremendously in all types of health education materials. People are accustomed to very high standards of presentation in written or graphic materials, in films and on television. Materials which are not technically excellent can give all the wrong impressions.

Sometimes it is obvious that little consideration has been given to the client's ability to understand the material, as the following extract from an information sheet for patients with prostate gland enlargement shows :

> The aim of the prostate operation is to ensure an unobstructed outflow of the urine. The operation most frequently performed is a TURP. This stands for Transurethral Resection of the Prostate. This operation is done entirely by instruments passed up the urethra under either a general or spinal anaesthetic and no cuts

Advantages	Caution
Inexpensive	Not suitable in large groups
Easy to prepare	Diagrams and prints should be large enough to be seen
Readily available in many health service settings	
Encourage confidence	Are often expensive
Can be used repeatedly	May get lost or broken

or stitches are needed. Using a special telescope the bladder is inspected from the inside and most of the prostate is then removed in small chips.

Some commercially produced materials may look good but be inaccurate or biased in their content. Conversely, 'home-made' materials may contain straightforward, useful information but be poorly presented. However, some examples of both commercially produced and home-made materials are excellent in all respects.

To be effective, audiovisual materials must be of good quality and therefore well produced. This requires professional expertise and professional equipment, and both are expensive. In some large organisations these may be available in-house but in many situations outside assistance may be required. Information should be up-to-date and accurate, and should reflect current practices and objectives. It may be necessary to include information on alternative treatments and care that are on offer.

APPROPRIATE TO CLIENT

Clients differ in their verbal comprehension and recall skills. Some people are not very skilled at reading and will learn best from written materials with a simple reading level or from videos. People who are more verbally skilled may prefer health promotion materials suitable for independent learning.

Language and illustrations used in materials must be culturally appropriate so that the user recognises it as relevant to them. Particular care has to be taken to avoid inadvertently reinforcing ethnic or gender stereotypes. Nurses and health visitors are not necessarily female or white. Try (as we have tried in this book) to use words that are gender-neutral (i.e. could apply equally to males and females.)

It is also necessary to be sensitive to the feelings of the potential user. One hospital produced a leaflet for women undergoing a uterine prolapse repair and called it a 'Repairs manual'. It wouldn't be surprising if some patients became distressed at the analogy to a car repair manual, considering their likely emotional state.

REVIEWING EXISTING MATERIALS

Before planning to develop any new health promotion materials you must check if there are any existing materials appropriate for the use you have in mind. You will want materials that cover the relevant topics with an appropriate level of detail. The material should also be suitable for the client-group characteristics, including age range, language, culture and ethnic background. Existing material can then be evaluated for availability, content, educational level and language, style and presentation, using the guidelines in Table 12.3. Once this has been done, the material should be checked out by a sample of the client group who are going to use it.

Discussion/Activity 12.1 Evaluation of health promotion materials

Choose an example of written or audiovisual material available in your area of work. Using the guidelines in Table 12.3, evaluate its appropriateness for the client group with which it is currently being used.

LOCAL PRODUCTION OF HEALTH EDUCATION MATERIALS

You must ask yourself whether it is a good use of resources to produce yet more health education material. The final product will all too often look as though it has been produced by amateurs (which it has). Are you really sure that you will produce something which is better than any existing material? Would it not be cheaper to buy something produced by someone else? There can be no

Table 12.3 Guidelines for reviewing existing health education materials

Availability
- Does each client require a copy of the material?
- How many clients per week/month?
- Will the client have access to and be able to operate the equipment?
- Is the supply of materials readily available?
- What is the cost and are there funds available?

Content
- Is the content accurate and up-to-date?
- Does it cover what the client group needs and wants to know?
- Does it contain practical information that will help the client?
- Is it objective and unbiased?

Educational level and language
- Is the material simple to understand?
- Is it available in different languages?
- Does the written material use simple words, short sentences and correct grammar?
- Is the audiovisual material clear and easy to see and hear?
- Does it use a personal tone and conversational style to create interest?
- Is the reading level appropriate for the population concerned? (see table 12.4)?

Style and presentation
- Is there a logical flow of information?
- Does the sequence start with simple ideas and move towards more difficult ideas?
- Is there consistency in style and use of words?
- Are technical words kept to a minimum and explained?
- Is it attractively presented with content areas separated by headings and subheadings?
- Are key areas highlighted by boxes, bullet points or other symbols?
- Are there diagrams or drawings which enhance the visual appearance and assist in clarification?
- Is the technical quality of the material adequate?

doubt that health units up and down the country waste a great deal of resource by each producing their own materials. If only health promoters in different districts would co-ordinate their efforts, co-operate and share costs they could obtain much better and much cheaper materials.

Producing high quality health promotion materials is expensive and time-consuming. None the less there are some good reasons for producing your own materials. It may be that none of the existing material meets your needs. The exercise of producing new materials will be good for team building and developing commitment to health promotion. All of these are real advantages of local production.

You may wish to promote the corporate identity of your unit by having its name and logo on the health promotion material. It is often possible to customise existing leaflets and posters with the logo and name of your hospital unit or district, either with adhesive labels or by having them overprinted.

In some instances it will be necessary to develop new health promotion materials to meet a specific need. Producing good quality materials with limited resources is not easy. The process involves eight stages:

1. Planning
2. Costing
3. Allocating tasks
4. Designing (producing brief, text, illustrations, layout)
5. Pre-production testing
6. Editing
7. Reproduction
8. Evaluation

PLANNING NEW HEALTH EDUCATION MATERIALS

A number of factors should be considered before you attempt to develop the material:

- purpose of the material (topic and client group)
- type of material required
- quantity required
- funds available

The material should contribute in some way to helping the client learn. You must start with a clear understanding of the health topics to be covered, the characteristics of the client group, the information and behaviours the clients want to learn and the situation in which it will be used.

You can then choose the type of material (leaflet, video, overhead) in the light of these considerations:

- Is it appropriate for the purpose?
- Is it appropriate for the age group and type of client?
- Will it be used with individuals, small or large groups?
- Does it require equipment to operate it, e.g. video recorder, slide projector?
- Can it be used repeatedly in different situations?

- Does it require a special environment or conditions, e.g. blackout?
- Can it be used easily by the health promoter or client or does it require technical support?

For leaflets and posters the number of copies required must be calculated. Usually the greater quantity produced the lower the unit cost. The main cost in a printing job is setting up, and the cost of producing one thousand copies will be little more than the cost of producing one. However, large quantities may not be required and it is likely that some materials will need reviewing and updating after a year as new ideas or techniques are developed.

At an early stage you must find out roughly what funds are available for production of materials as this will influence the type and quantity chosen.

COSTING

Developing and producing materials is expensive in time and money. Accurate estimates of the cost of developing health promotion materials should be part of the planning process so that bids for funding can be considered as part of the overall business planning and resource allocation programme.

Consider the costs of:

- personnel time
  - to write, edit and test the material
  - to evaluate the effectiveness of materials
- specialist advice for layout, design, illustrations, photography and filming
- materials – paper, etc.
- typesetting and printing
- filming and developing
- storage, distribution
- equipment
- administration
- overheads – heating, lighting, etc.

It may be possible to recoup some of the costs of development and production by selling the leaflets produced to other units.

ALLOCATING TASKS (PREPARATION AND PRODUCTION)

Having decided what materials you want, you then have to decide how they will be prepared. The tasks are:

- **Design**
    - producing the brief
    - writing the text
    - adding illustrations
    - finalising layout
- **Production**
    - producing camera-ready materials (i.e. final stage before reprinting)
    - reproducing the materials

All these tasks can be done in-house or you can hand them over to an outside commercial firm at any stage. Obviously the more a firm is asked to do the more it will charge. Technical services in hospitals such as medical illustration departments will have many of the necessary skills and local health promotion units will be able to offer a great deal of advice.

PRODUCING THE BRIEF

The brief explains in detail what the leaflet or other health education material is intended to do, who are its intended users and what information it should contain. It is a good idea to interview several clients to obtain their views before drawing up the brief. How much information on what topics are needed to satisfy the educational need? For example, one leaflet on prevention of coronary heart disease may simply identify the risk factors and briefly cover the 'Dos' and 'Don'ts' related to them. Another leaflet on the same general topic could describe the effects of stress, excess weight, smoking, etc., and go into great detail about how to avoid these.

WRITING THE TEXT (STYLE AND READABILITY)

The potential user should be kept in mind when the text is being written and appropriate vocabulary and language used. Health worker's jargon, abbreviations and technical terms should be avoided if possible but if they have to be used they must be explained.

The following extract from a leaflet given to patients who have had a hysterectomy illustrates the danger of using jargon:

> With hysterectomy there is always a chance of complications such as infection, post-operative bleeding or wound separation.

> In addition there may be damage to the bladder or ureters, bowel adhesions and risk of pulmonary emboli and thrombophlebitis caused by the slowed circulation during and immediately following surgery.

This description may be acceptable to a minority of patients but it is more suited to a textbook for health care professionals.

Short sentences using simple words which are in common use will be most easily understood. Paragraphs should be kept short and cover only one idea. Grammar and punctuation should also be correct. People often find it helpful if a personal, conversational style is used rather than a more formal, impersonal tone.

Written material should be checked for its readability (how easy it is to read). The reading skills of clients are variable. Twenty six per cent of the adult population in England have insufficient literacy skills to cope with materials more complicated than papers such as the *Sun* or the *Mirror* (Nichol and Harrison 1984). All too often health promotion materials are suitable only for those with well-developed literacy skills.

Albert and Chadwick (1992) found that GPs were more concerned with the quality of printing and presentation of their practice leaflets than with the importance of focusing on clients' needs and using good, simple, written communication. If the reading level of written materials is beyond the skill of the client's comprehension, recall and motivation to continue using them will be reduced.

There are a number of methods or formulae which can be used to predict the readability of written health promotion materials (Gunning 1952; Fry 1968; Flesch 1974). These are usually based on the length of words and sentences. One of the most frequently used in health services is the FOG formula by Gunning (1952) (see Table 12.4). This has been adopted by the Plain English Campaign.

ILLUSTRATIONS

Illustrations, charts and diagrams can be used in all types of health promotion materials to assist understanding and enhance learning. Many clients remember information better if it is presented in pictures or diagrams. Rohret and Ferguson (1990) report on a number of studies which show that illustrated materials result in better recall. They argue that many illustrations are included on the basis of cost, ease of availability and to increase attractiveness rather than for an educational purpose.

An illustration should be used for specific purposes. It should be:

- **Essential** Is it essential for the reader's understanding of the topic? Does it help to clarify the facts?

Table 12.4 Steps in calculating the FOG formula for readability

1. Count the number of words (W) in a passage of approximately 100 words (excluding titles and ending at the end of a sentence).
2. Count the number of complete sentences in the passage (S).
3. Divide the number of words by the number of sentences to give the average sentence length (W/S).
4. Count the number of words with 3 or more syllables and express as a percentage of the total number of words (A).
   Do not count:
   (a) verbs ending in *-ed* or *-es* if these make the third syllable
   (b) Proper nouns
   (c) combinations of simple words, e.g. *screwdriver*
5. Use the formula to calculate the reading level:
   (W/S) + A = reading level
6. Sometimes the score is multiplied by 0.4 to give an approximate 'reading age'.

Example

You get free National Health Service (NHS) prescriptions automatically while you are pregnant and for a year after your baby's birth. Also you do not have to pay for any prescriptions for your baby or for any other child who is under 16.

If you are pregnant, get form FW8 from your doctor, midwife or health visitor. If your baby was born less than a year ago and you did not apply for free prescriptions while you were pregnant, fill in form A on leaflet P11 NHS prescriptions. Send form FW8 or form A (from leaflet P11) to your Family Health Services Authority, or Health Board if you live in Scotland. They will send you an exemption certificate.

Words (W)	118
Sentences (S)	6
Average number of words per sentence (118/6)	19.7
Words with 3 or more syllables	10
Percentage of 3-syllable words (A) (10 × 100/118)	8.5
FOG score (19.7 + 8.5)	28.2

- **Clear** Is the illustration of an appropriate size for the material? Is it distinct and easy to recognise? Is the labelling clear and unambiguous?
- **Concise** Is the illustration simple or does it contain too much information? Are there any distracting elements?
- **Correct** Is it the correct type of illustration to convey the content?

FINALISING LAYOUT

The layout or sequence of the material is important. Materials that are attractively presented in a logical sequence will not only raise the users' interest but also contribute to their understanding and subsequent learning. The style of presentation can be enhanced by using headings and subheadings, numbers or bold print. Key elements should be emphasised by using boxes, asterisks, symbols or large and bold print (see Figure 12.1). Avoid using too many different fonts as this will only make the page look messy and confusing.

Use **bold** print to emphasise points.
Underline key points within the text.
Use italic type to emphasise *comments* or *spoken* text.

Choose your main point of issue and emphasise it by using clear type and allowing extra space to surround it.

DRAW INTEREST
TO MAIN POINT

The use of different fonts *can make the message more readable or attractive.*

Use indent to make paragraphs stand out and make the page look more interesting.
Use UPPER or lower CASE to draw attention.

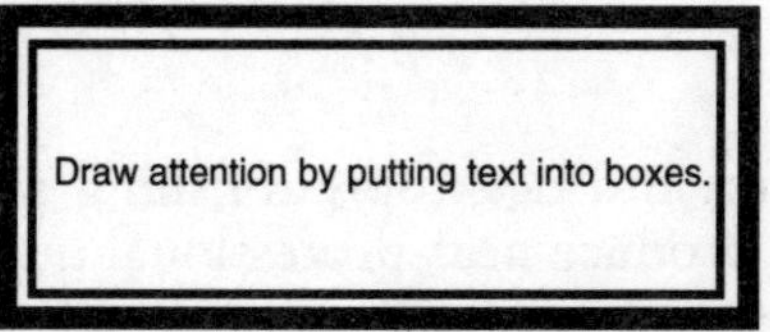

Use simple graphics to add interest.

To emphasise lines:
use an *
or a bullet ●
or the hash sign #
or any other symbol
✤ ✦ ✧ ★ ✪

Figure 12.1 Some tips to improve the appearance and impact of written material
Modern word-processing and desktop-publishing packages make it relatively easy to produce written materials that are eye-catching and clear.

In all types of materials key information should be summarised and repeated periodically to increase users' understanding of the subject and help them focus on the most important parts.

Do not overcrowd the page, wide margins and spaces will make it more attractive and easier to read. Colour can be helpful but adds to the cost of printing. Skilled page design can make all the difference to a leaflet.

Discussion/Activity 12.2 Writing a leaflet for patients

Consider the extract from the hysterectomy leaflet on pages 208 and 209. Calculate the FOG readability score. Re-write it in a form that you think would be more helpful to a patient. Would you want to use any illustrations? If so, what would they be? Make a rough sketch of what you would want the finished leaflet to look like (i.e. plan the layout).

PRE-PRODUCTION TESTING

Testing of the material should take place frequently and involve both peer review and testing by potential users. Use a number of independent reviewers who come fresh to the work. Ask them to examine the format, organisation, grammar, writing style, clarity, content and technical quality. However, the best test of the suitability of the material is to get the views of the potential users.

EDITING

Word-processing and desktop-publishing packages have made it much easier to produce near-professional quality written materials. They make it simple to use a range of different fonts and to mix text and graphics. Producing excellent health promotion materials in-house has become a more feasible proposition.

At each stage all materials must be carefully edited, checking the material and making necessary changes so that the messages given are exactly what was intended. This may involve a number of re-drafts. Editing also involves looking for errors such as omissions and inaccuracies in content, inconsistencies between headings, titles, abbreviations used, typing mistakes and trying to achieve consistency in styles. Once the final draft is prepared it must be carefully proof-read.

REPRODUCTION

Photocopying is a simple way of reproducing a small number of copies. Using coloured paper can make materials more attractive. For larger numbers of leaflets printing will be a more practical proposition. Professional printers can usually work from 'camera ready' material. This means they will exactly reproduce the original that you gave them (including any mistakes that you did not spot). Alternatively they can work from your rough design and typescript to produce the finished product. In this case before printing they will produce proofs which they will ask you to check.

The more work the printer is required to do the more expensive it will be. Printing using several colours is much more expensive than one colour. Remember most of the cost comes in setting up the job so that two thousand leaflets may cost very little more than one thousand.

EVALUATION

Evaluation of the material should attempt to determine its effectiveness in helping people understand and learn new information and behaviours. Information which will assist in the evaluation includes:

- number of times the material is used
- clients' level of satisfaction with the material
- what clients have learned
- level of staff satisfaction

You will also want to consider the cost and so decide if there might have been more cost-effective ways of achieving the same objectives.

FILMS AND VIDEOS

Films and videos are useful for demonstrating skills. They are also an excellent way of offering information to people who are not comfortable with written materials. Clear, well-paced and interesting voices should be used. Subtitles can be used to reinforce the introduction of new ideas and key elements can be emphasised by tone of voice, use of tables, charts and diagrams. It is easy to cover a great deal of information in a video but members of the audience will only be able to retain a small proportion of this.

The development of camcorders and equipment suitable for amateur use has apparently made it much easier to produce videos. However, the good technical quality which people expect requires a high degree of skill in scripting, filming, lighting, recording and editing, which very few amateurs possess.

MATERIALS FOR A MULTICULTURAL SOCIETY

Many cities now have sizeable communities of different ethnic groups and this must influence the design of materials. Materials should be suitable for as wide a range of people as possible. You should therefore check that different ethnic groups are included in any illustrations used.

Materials for use by people who are not fluent in the English language present further problems. When a leaflet is intended for general distribution there are powerful arguments for using several languages on the same leaflet. This means that it will be accessible to speakers of the different languages and one leaflet can be used for all. There are however important drawbacks. The requirement to print everything in several languages will limit the space available for any message. Furthermore, typesetting and printing in characters other than English will add greatly to the printing costs. The alternative is to print several versions of the same leaflet in different languages. This may be easier but means that you have to find a way of getting the appropriate language leaflet to each individual.

Preparing leaflets for use by people from different cultures involves far more than language translation. Translation itself is not easy. The translator has to translate the concepts conveyed by the words rather than the words themselves. This is often particularly difficult for ideas related to health and illness. As well as obtaining appropriate translation of written material, you must also ensure that the illustrations and ideas are appropriate to the intended audience. Leaflets about nutrition need to refer to the foodstuffs and dishes which are normally eaten by the intended readers.

It is still difficult to find health education materials for different ethnic groups but the range available is steadily increasing (Bhatt and Dickinson 1992; Lethbridge 1993).

APPROVAL OF MATERIALS

Before any material is used it should be checked to ensure it is good quality and meets the clients' needs. The guidelines in Table 12.3 and the checklist in Table 12.5 will assist in this process. Approving materials in this way will prevent duplication and so ensure some consistency of information. It will also be less confusing to health promoters who may have difficulty in knowing what to use.

ORGANISING AND CATALOGUING

There are a very large number of health education materials and there should be a co-ordinated policy as to which of these are used. A medical unit of a medium-sized general hospital was recently found to have over 200 different leaflets on a variety of subjects. There was no consistency in the use of the leaflets. Some were felt to be useful for patients and were used frequently. Others were little used and

Table 12.5 Steps in the approval process

Step	Ask	Comments
• Identify need for material	Who will use this item? How will it improve learning?	
• Check if existing materials meet need	Has catalogue been checked?	Yes/No
• Review for accuracy of content	Has the content been checked by experienced professionals?	Yes/No
• Review for educational level	Is the material suitable for intended audience?	Yes/No
• Review for reading/ listening/viewing ease	Is it clear, concise, grammatically correct? Has readability test been performed? Has it been tested on a sample audience?	Yes/No
• Review for style and presentation	Is the material well organised, interesting and attractively presented?	Yes/No
• Make recommendations	Approve as it is Minor revisions Major revisions	
• Process and catalogue	Has it been entered in catalogue?	Yes/No

were only there because they had been given by pharmaceutical representatives or provided by the hospital. An approval system is required to ensure effective use of materials and to avoid use of unsatisfactory ones. This will need to be supported by a system of cataloguing, ordering, storing and distribution of materials.

These activities are best carried out by the group of professionals concerned with the particular aspect of health promotion, who act as a clearing house. This group might consist of members of the primary health care team in a health centre, staff in a medical unit or a patient education committee. Members of the district health education department will be able to help such a group.

A catalogue of approved materials is a valuable resource to health promoters. The following information is helpful and can be stored in a loose-leaf file or on index cards to allow for additions and removals:

- title of material
- initiator/author/source of material

- type of material – booklet, video, tape, etc.
- intended client group
- brief description of content
- equipment required
- approval date
- location

ORDERING, STORING AND DISTRIBUTION

It is essential that there is a supply of materials readily available for use. In many health care settings in this country ordering materials is done on a haphazard basis. A co-ordinated approach is more likely if a designated individual is given responsibility for maintaining stocks in locations where they are required. In hospitals in the USA this role is often carried out by volunteers who deliver health promotion materials and equipment to clinical areas in response to requests. A simple referral form could be used (see Figure 12.2).

Department *Ward 2 Cardiology*

Material requested

Title *Back to Normal – Heart Information Series No. 1*

Source *British Heart Foundation*

Type *Booklet*

Quantity *30*

Equipment required *None*

Date required *25.4.95*

Date of referral *18.4.95*

Referred by *S. Churchfield*

Designation *Staff Nurse*

Figure 12.2 Referral form for health education materials

SUMMARY POINTS

There are many health promotion materials available:

- ☐ written
- ☐ audiovisual
- ☐ teaching

Materials should be carefully reviewed for suitability for a particular client group before use.

Materials should only be used if they will enhance learning in some way.

Clients differ in their verbal, reading, comprehension and recall skills and in their cultural background. Therefore they will benefit from different types of material.

Developing new health promotion materials is both a time-consuming and costly process and should involve careful:

- ☐ planning
- ☐ designing and costing
- ☐ production
- ☐ testing
- ☐ evaluation

Health promotion materials should be:

- ☐ accurate in content
- ☐ interesting
- ☐ attractively presented
- ☐ at the right level
- ☐ appropriate to the clients' needs
- ☐ cost-effective

A system for cataloguing, ordering, storing and distributing health promotion materials in health centres, surgeries, hospitals and other settings will facilitate an organised approach.

REFERENCES

Albert T. and Chadwick S. (1992). How readable are practice leaflets? *British Medical Journal* 305, 1266–1268.

Bhatt A. and Dickinson R. (1992). An analysis of health education materials for minority communities by culture and linguistic group. *Health Education Journal* **51**, 72–77.

Flesch R. (1974). *The art of readable writing*. New York: Harper & Row Publishers, pp. 184–186, 247–251.

Friend B. (1992). Healthy reading. *Nursing Times* **88** (No. 36), 16–17.

Fry E. (1968). A readability formula that saves time. *Journal of Reading* **11**, 514–517, April.

Gunning R. (1952). *The technique of clear writing*. New York: McGraw-Hill Book Co., pp. 29–39.

Hodges C. (1993). A healthy balance. *Nursing Times* **89** (No. 14), 44–45.

Lethbridge J. (1993). Health promotion and education for black and ethnic minority groups. Chapter 15 in Hopkins A. and Bahl V. (eds), *Access to health care for people from black and ethnic minorities*. London: Royal College of Physicians.

Murphy S. and Smith C. (1992). An examination of the use of health education leaflets by Health Promotion Officers. *Health Education Journal* **51**, 166–170.

Nichol A. and Harrison C. (1984). The readability of health care literature. *Developmental Medicine and Child Neurology* **26**, 596–600.

Rohret L. and Ferguson K.J. (1990). Effective use of patient education illustrations. *Patient Education and Counselling* (15) 73–75.

Williams J., Ashcroft B., Carter A. and Comyn C. (1987). Using printed materials effectively in health promotion. *Health Education Journal* **46**, 165–167.

SECTION 3

Specific settings

CHAPTER 13

Health promotion in schools

Joe Harvey
Health Education Adviser, Birmingham LEA Health Education Unit

GOAL

To appreciate the opportunities for and limitations of health promotion in schools.

OBJECTIVES

- to list characteristics of good practice in schools health promotion
- to understand what makes a school health-promoting
- to describe the aims of health education in schools
- to understand how health education fits into the school curriculum
- to appreciate the importance of the school nurse in schools health promotion
- to understand how the school nurse can support health education in school

ISSUES IN SCHOOLS HEALTH PROMOTION

The subject of health promotion in schools raises a mixture of enthusiasm and frustration, hopes and fears, certainty and confusion. The questions debated will fall into one or more of these categories:

- Who does it?
- What do they do and when?
- To whom do they do it?
- Who supports whoever does it?
- Who says it is OK to do it?
- Who pays?

People have always expected schools to respond to concerns about children's health and behaviour and usually had quite unrealistic expectations of what could be achieved by that response. Governments have also had similar expectations but have failed to provide schools with the time, resources and expertise needed for them to respond. They have also failed to set any national framework for the support of local delivery.

There has always been a limit to what schools can achieve in health promotion. However, in the last ten years schools have moved a long way in recognising the value of health education and their obligation to provide it.

GOOD PRACTICE IN SCHOOLS HEALTH PROMOTION

Listing features of good practice in health promotion is a good exercise for school staff training sessions. One can be sure that most of the following would be mentioned:

- an educational philosophy that values health
- appropriate health policies and programmes
- headteachers and governing bodies with positive attitudes towards health education
- active participation of young people in their own learning experiences about health with a concomitant growth of autonomy
- a teacher with designated responsibility for health promotion throughout the school
- appropriate training for teachers and other staff in a broad range of health education issues
- co-operation with the community and outside agencies
- a collection of suitable curriculum support material
- a 'whole school' approach to health promotion

The school should develop policies and programmes that meet both the statutory requirements of the National Curriculum and the particular health needs of the diverse groups among their pupils. The whole ethos of the school must convey health messages consistent with those promoted through curriculum teaching. A designated teacher acting as the focal point for the development and coordination of health education and other health promotion activities helps to achieve these things.

As a result of this the school enables young people to:

- gain a wide understanding of health matters
- feel good about themselves and respect others

- acquire the skills necessary to live a full and healthy life
- make informed and responsible decisions about their own health and that of their community

---

Discussion/Activity 13.1 Your experience of schools health promotion

Think back to your own school days. Did you and your school friends want any health promotion? Did the schools you attended make any effort to be health-promoting? What did they get right? What did they get wrong? How could the school have done better?

If you have school-age children of your own, compare their experience of health promotion at school with yours. Is it better or worse?

THE HEALTH-PROMOTING SCHOOL

The 'whole school' approach to health promotion requires that classroom health education be set in a wider framework, thereby creating a health-promoting school (Nutbeam *et al.* 1987; Smith *et al.* 1992).

The health-promoting school:

- supports and promotes attitudes, practices and understanding conducive to good health (HMI 1984)
- promotes quality of life and the physical, social and mental well-being of the individual (NCC 1990a)

Health promotion activities include not only health education but all other activities which seek to promote positive health through changes in physical, social or political environment (Birmingham LEA 1991).

The health-promoting school should seek to develop:

- positive relationships between
  - pupils and staff
  - staff and parents
  - school and community
- positive patterns of behaviour through role-modelling
  - courtesy, concern, respect
  - appropriate systems of reward and punishment
- organisational and management structures which encourage self-confidence and build the self-esteem of pupils and staff
- a pleasant and stimulating physical environment

Health education in schools does not begin and end in the classroom. The subtle messages that pupils receive about health from the daily life of a school are as important as those given during lessons. The messages thus conveyed should be consistent. Classroom teaching on smoking is supported if smoking is prohibited for all on school premises (Harvey and Flannagan 1993). School catering needs to be consistent with what is taught on healthy eating (National Forum for CHD Prevention 1994). National guidance on the whole curriculum refers to the importance of the spirit and ethos of a school (NCC 1990b). The aims, attitudes, values and procedures of a school are fundamental to the success of any health education programme.

The relationships between staff and pupils and those among staff themselves are important elements of health education. Standards, attitudes and patterns of behaviour can convey powerful messages and their significance is often underestimated. Lessons which promote courtesy, concern, respect and acceptance of responsibility for self and others will be more effective if these qualities are valued consistently in every aspect of school life. Health messages will have more impact if they are supported by appropriate systems of reward and punishment. Health skills learned in the classroom need to be reinforced by opportunities to practise them.

Young people who are happy with their self-image are able to take more control of their lives, including decisions relating to healthy lifestyles. The organisation and management structures of a school can do much to encourage the development of self-confidence and self-esteem. For example, open communication can make an individual feel wanted and valued. A strong pastoral system can support personal development as well as being a mechanism for responding to crises or misdemeanours.

The quality of relationships between a school and the local community is also important. Health promotion is a responsibility which schools share with others. School health education activities should include opportunities for involving governors, parents, families and the community so that what is learned at school can be supported by appropriate experiences at home and in the community. The community also hears new ideas about health from the children so that the school becomes a channel for community health promotion. The school also needs good links with local health services. Local health promotion units can provide planning and teaching resources and contribute to training sessions and workshops.

The physical environment of a school can do much to promote effective health education. While some environments have insurmountable structural problems, it is usually possible to create classrooms, corridors and staffrooms which are pleasant, stimulating places in which to be. Such environments encourage high work levels, healthy functioning of the body and promote self-esteem. They help to reduce stress, alleviate tension and encourage the development of positive working and social relationships. The school environment can also be a practical demonstration of ecological principles (Bachman 1986).

HEALTH PROMOTION POLICY

Schools will find it helpful to formulate a policy for each health promotion topic on which they wish to make progress. A schools health promotion policy and guidelines on its implementation should be drafted by a concerned group and discussed as widely as possible within the school. These policies and guidelines will need to be reviewed at regular intervals. Policies are of little use unless they are widely known and acted upon so they need to be explained to pupils, staff, governors, parents and everyone else concerned with the school.

A policy should contain the following elements and answer the following questions:

- Why have a policy?
- Who wrote the policy?
- Aims of the health education programme, including desired outcomes.
- Where and how will health education be taught, and by whom?
- How will parents and governors be involved?
- Implications for staff training.
- Other areas considered important.
- Recommendations for change.
- How, when and by whom will the policy and programme be reviewed?

The introduction to the policy should mention relevant legislation and reports (e.g. Curriculum guidance No. 5 (NCC 1990a), Children Act, Sex education at school (DES 1994)). It should spell out what is meant by health education and why it is considered important.

Guidelines are likely to be fuller than a policy statement. They will include suggestions for a sequenced programme of health education. In addition to all the items to be found in a policy, guidelines will contain:

- year-by-year content of the programme
- examples of teaching methods related to content

- resources for teaching, including local resources
- some local and national agencies
- examples of good practice

AIMS OF HEALTH EDUCATION IN SCHOOLS

Health education in schools should seek to:

- impart factual, balanced information about health
- explore attitudes, values, beliefs and feelings about health
- promote the development of pupils' personal skills related to health, e.g. decision making, assertiveness
- foster the development of pupils' self-esteem and encourage a positive self-image
- enable pupils to understand and respond effectively to peer pressure related to health
- increase pupils' understanding about choices related to health and widen the range of choices open to them
- reinforce or change behaviours, so that ultimately pupils live healthier lives
- promote the choice of healthy lifestyles

EDUCATION FOR HEALTH

Section 1 of the Education Reform Act 1988 places a statutory responsibility upon schools to provide a broad and balanced curriculum which:

(a) promotes the spiritual, moral, cultural, mental and physical development of pupils at the school and of society
(b) prepares pupils for the opportunities, responsibilities and experiences of adult life

Health education is seen as part of the broad process of socialisation. Emphasis is placed on empowering young people to make informed choices and decisions on matters relating to their health (Kalnins *et al.* 1992). As such, health education must be concerned with allowing pupils to explore attitudes and feelings, to acquire and practise skills such as decision making, and to receive relevant information on which to base their decisions. If young people are to accept some responsibility for their own health then it is vital that they develop a positive self-image.

> Education for health begins in the home, where patterns of behaviour and attitude influence health for good or ill

> throughout life and will be established before a child is five. The tasks for schools are to support and promote attitudes, practices and understanding conducive to good health. In so far as they are able to counteract influences which are not conducive to good health, they should do so with sensitive regard to the relationship which exists between children and their families.

Health education cannot be left to chance. A coherent health education programme is required if pupils are to be encouraged to establish healthy patterns of behaviour and to contribute to the development of a healthy population.

TOPICS FOR HEALTH EDUCATION

The National Curriculum lists a series of topics which should be covered in years 1 to 11 (ages 5–16) (NCC 1990a):

- substance use and misuse
- sex education
- family life education
- safety
- food and nutrition
- personal hygiene
- environmental aspects
- health-related exercise
- psychological aspects

Substance use and misuse

The acquisition of knowledge, understanding and skills which enable pupils to consider the effects of substances such as tobacco, alcohol and other drugs on themselves and others and to make informed and healthy decisions about the use of such substances.

Sex education

Sex education provides an understanding that positive, caring environments are essential for the development of a good self-image and that individuals are in charge of and responsible for their own bodies. It provides knowledge about the processes of reproduction and the nature of sexuality and relationships. It encourages the acquisition of skills and attitudes which allow pupils to manage their relationships in a responsible and healthy manner. The statutory basis is described in Table 13.1.

Table 13.1 Statutory framework for sex education in schools

For county, controlled and maintained special schools, Section 18(2) of the Education (No. 2) Act 1986 requires that:

> The articles of government for every such school shall provide for it to be the duty of the governing body:
> (a) to consider separately (while having regard to the local education authority's statement under Section 17 of this Act on their policy in relation to the secular curriculum in maintained schools) the question whether sex education should form part of the secular curriculum for the school; and (b) to make and keep up to date a separate written statement of their policy with regard to the content and organisation of the relevant part of the curriculum; or where they conclude that sex education should not form part of the secular curriculum, of that conclusion.

Section 46 requires that:

> The local education authority by whom any county, voluntary or special school is maintained and the governing body and headteacher of the school, shall take such steps as are reasonably practicable to secure that where sex education is given to any registered pupils at the school it is given in such a manner as to encourage those pupils to have due regard to moral considerations and the value of family life.

DES (1994) gives further guidance on sex education at school.

Family life education

The principal objective of family life education is that pupils understand and value the central role of the family as an institution and the important part it plays in the development of attachment, love and concern. This covers the need for good child care, effective parenting and the changing nature of relationships within the family.

Safety

The acquisition of knowledge and understanding of safety in different environments, together with the development of associated skills and strategies, helps pupils to maintain their personal safety and that of others.

Food and nutrition

Education about nutrition covers the effects of diet on health, the nutritional quality of different foods and food safety. It encourages pupils to make healthy choices. National Curriculum attainment targets for food and nutrition are shown in Table 13.2.

Table 13.2 Attainment targets for key stages in teaching Food and Nutrition

Key stage 1
- Know that there is a wide variety of food to choose from and that some foods are better that others.

Key stage 2
- Know that diet is a combination of foods each with a different nutrient content.
- Know that different nutrients have different effects on the body, and the amounts in the diet, and balance between them, can influence health, e.g. sugar and dental health.
- Know how to handle food safely and recognise the importance of additives in food safety.

Key stage 3
- Know that individual health requires a varied diet.
- Understand malnutrition and the relationships between diet, health, fitness and circulatory disorders.
- Understand basic food microbiology, food production and food processing techniques.

Key stage 4
- Be able to analyse and evaluate diet and recognise suitable adjustments which take into account a range of factors such as the availability of food and social, cultural and financial influences.
- Know that various types of diet promote health for different groups, acknowledging cultural and ethnic variations.
- Understand consumer aspects of food hygiene; shopping for food; legislation; including the current food labelling system.
- Understand the relationships between food, body image and self-esteem.
- Have accurate information to distinguish between fact, propaganda and folklore in dietary matters.

Personal hygiene

Acquisition of the knowledge and practices needed to promote personal cleanliness helps to reduce transmission of communicable diseases and encourages pride in body maintenance.

Environmental aspects of health education

An understanding of environmental aspects of health education, including social, physical and economic factors which contribute to health and illness, helps to raise awareness of environmental health issues, avoid unnecessary risks and promote good health.

Health-related exercise

Recognition of the role of exercise in promoting and maintaining good health encourages pupils to make positive choices about their own activities.

Psychological aspects of health education

The acquisition of knowledge and understanding of the factors that affect mental health help to promote emotional well-being. Development of self-awareness, stress-coping skills and healthy attitudes further support mental health.

FITTING HEALTH EDUCATION INTO THE TIMETABLE

Health education is most likely to be successful when it is built on the best of current practice and does not require schools to adopt an unfamiliar pattern of teaching. Six different timetabling arrangements based on existing practice are:

1. permeating the whole curriculum
2. as a separately timetabled subject
3. as part of a Personal and Social Education (PSE) course or programme
4. as part of a pastoral or tutorial programme
5. through opportunities arising from other activities
6. timetabled in long blocks

The list is not exhaustive nor are the options mutually exclusive. Some schools may choose to combine elements of different approaches, and to use varying combinations at different key stages. Each arrangement has advantages and disadvantages. These are compared in Table 13.3. Some approaches, for example 1, 5 and 6, are particularly relevant to primary schools. Others are more relevant to secondary schools, which are likely to favour combining 1 with one or more of the other approaches.

For younger pupils (key stages 1 and 2) many schools currently teach health education as part of their topic work. This usually takes the form of a separate theme and is done at a particular age or time of year. Topic-based health education like this may lack coherence, continuity and progression. It may depend too much on the interests of the individual class teacher. Few primary schools have extensive curriculum guidelines for health education and many have none at all apart from the sex education statement, which is a requirement under the Education (No. 2) Act 1986.

For older pupils (key stages 3 and 4) many schools teach health through other subjects such as science. These subjects have their own priorities and health education is often no more than an incidental consideration. Thus while pupils might learn about the reproductive system in science they might not be required to consider wider aspects of their sexuality or personal relationships.

Many schools have resolved this dilemma by providing timetabled courses such as Personal and Social Education (PSE) which build on learning acquired elsewhere and which tackle a range of topics that do not fit easily into other subjects. However, elements of health education taught through PSE, science and other subjects are often poorly co-ordinated.

Health education is an essential part of the whole curriculum. The most effective form of provision is a carefully planned programme across the whole school career which embraces all the formal and informal arrangements that schools use to promote positive health behaviour. Teaching health education through a number of subjects and, where appropriate, through separately timetabled provision offers pupils the best opportunity to receive a broad programme of health education. This pattern of teaching allows schools to provide opportunities for pupils to acquire knowledge, understanding and skills through the programmes of study and attainment targets of National Curriculum subjects. If the agreed syllabus allows, elements of health education may also be covered in religious education, offering pupils additional time in which to practise skills and to clarify attitudes, values and beliefs.

Discussion/Activity 13.2 Learning about healthy eating

Look at the attainment targets for food and nutrition in Table 13.2. Are there things you think should be added to these? How would you fit teaching of these subjects into the curriculum? How could the 'health-promoting' school reinforce the messages learnt in the classroom?

TEACHING APPROACHES

The teaching approach should start by exploring the child's own attitudes, clarifying their starting point and recognising their previous experiences and knowledge. A health education session might follow this pattern:

- **Explore feelings and attitudes**, e.g. children's feeling about smoking; food likes and dislikes; attitudes to risk and danger.
- **Give information** – new facts and knowledge – e.g. about the effects of smoking on the body; nutrition facts; safety procedures.
- **Practise skills**, including social skills, e.g. response to offer of cigarette; planning meals; crossing the road.

Table 13.3 Advantages and disadvantages of different timetabling arrangements for health education

ADVANTAGES	DISADVANTAGES
1. Permeating the whole curriculum	
• secures a place for health education within the statutory curriculum • ensures all teachers take some responsibility for aspects of the work	• may be difficult to ensure appropriate teaching and learning methods • may be regarded as a peripheral element within subjects • may be difficult to give sufficient time to consider sensitive and controversial issues • may be difficult to co-ordinate theme that lacks sharp definition
2. As a separately timetabled subject	
• secures a firm place in the curriculum for health education • likely to be taught by specialists • facilitates progression and continuity • augments knowledge, understanding and skills gained elsewhere	• may focus on the cognitive and medical aspects of health education to the detriment of work relating to attitudes and behaviour • difficult to find space in an already crowded curriculum • isolates health education from other elements of the whole curriculum
3. As part of a PSE course or programme	
• has the potential to be taught by a specialist team • enables links to be established between health education and other cross-curricular themes • flexibility can be provided by use of modular structures but these will need to be provided at relevant times • facilitates progression and continuity	• competition between cross-curricular themes may restrict time given to any one theme • may become isolated from other elements of the whole curriculum
4. As part of a pastoral or tutorial programme	
• most teachers will have some responsibility for health education • teachers are in touch with the needs and emotional development of the pupils in their care.	• multitude of administrative tasks may leave little time for health education • teachers may not have received appropriate training and may lack the necessary knowledge, skills, confidence and commitment to teach about health matters, particularly the sensitive issues

Table 13.3—*continued*

ADVANTAGES	DISADVANTAGES
5. Through opportunities arising from other activities	
• provides a variety of contexts for health education which relate to pupils' lives outside school, e.g. topics which are the focus of current media interest, events which have formed part of the personal experience of pupils, school visits and visitors to school	• inappropriate for teaching some aspects of health education • needs to be part of a planned programme of health education
6. Timetabled in long blocks (e.g. 'sixth day' timetabling, activity week)	
• provides opportunities for a range of activities, e.g. health week, external visits • supports individual resource-based learning and it is community-linked • short, intense periods of learning may aid pupil motivation	• inappropriate for teaching some aspects of health education • needs to be part of a planned programme of health education.

- **Digestion of new learning** – the opportunity to use and assimilate new learning – e.g. discussion, decision-making/choice situations, role play.

RESOURCES FOR TEACHING

There is a wide range of resources available to schools. Some general features of using resources were discussed in Chapter 12. The following may be useful in schools:

- videos
- training packs
- leaflets/posters
- games (cards, boards, computer)
- photographs
- equipment (e.g. models)

The perfect resource does not exist! Materials have to be carefully reviewed to ensure that the information they contain is up-to-date and appropriate to the age ability and needs of the pupils (see Table 12.3). This is particularly true for materials provided free by some commercial firms. Resources can be obtained from the Health Education Authority, commercial publishers, local health promotion/education units and the School Library Service (see Table 12.1, for other suggestions).

USE OF OUTSIDE SPEAKERS

Many schools invite speakers from outside the school to cover selected health education topics. This has advantages but must always be done as part of a planned teacher-led programme and not as 'one-off' events. Such talks must always be consistent with the school's philosophy and policies of health promotion. The content of the talk and the approach to be used should be carefully discussed with the speaker and approval obtained from the headteacher and governors as appropriate. This is especially important if the talk is to cover sensitive issues such as HIV and sex education and in some cases it may also be necessary to notify parents as well. It must be emphasised that talks by outside speakers are no substitute for a developmental health education programme.

THE SCHOOL NURSE

The first school nurse was appointed in 1892 and since then school nurses have shown how much they can contribute to the health of the school (Vine 1991). The headteacher and governors will look to the school health service (nurse and doctor) to guard the health of pupils in a number of ways:

- to provide support for children in school who have special medical needs such as diabetes or asthma
- to liaise with a child's health visitor before school entry
- to liaise with parents about their child's health
- to screen for vision and hearing defects
- to perform medical examinations of selected children in accordance with school health service policies
- to provide advice and training for teachers and other school staff to ensure a better understanding of specific medical conditions
- to advise school staff when they are concerned that a child may have a health problem
- to provide medical care for children who are 'statemented' (i.e. have been identified as having special educational needs)
- to advise on the provision of suitable arrangements for first aid
- to check immunisation status to ensure that children are fully protected
- to counsel children on health and personal problems
- to make contributions to health education

School nurses must balance the different components of their job. Enthusiasm for health education must not lead to neglect of the other health-promoting tasks which the schools rely on them to perform. In the past there has been a regrettable tendency to expect school nurses to be all things to all people. Because their role was not defined they were often asked to give support in ways for which they were not trained.

THE SCHOOL NURSE AS HEALTH EDUCATOR

The headteacher and governors of the school are responsible for delivery of health education just as they are responsible for all other aspects of the operation of that school. Other local authority or health authority staff may give support through training, resources and advice on policy and programme planning. Like all health professionals in schools, the school nurse should see her role as supporting not supplanting the teacher. The school nurse should help with planning an integrated health education programme and contributing in a way that complements other health promotion in the school (Bagnall 1993).

To do this adequately requires:

- appropriate training
- relevant experience
- a clear knowledge of the legislation
- a good understanding of the 'politics' of school structure and process

School nurse training should equip them to understand the differences between reducing disease and promoting positive health in schoolchildren. Their training needs to prepare them for a role which straddles school and health service. This will best be achieved if training is jointly planned and jointly delivered by school and health staff.

Headteachers and governors also need to be trained to appreciate the importance of health and to make the best use of such skilled support. There have been too many examples in the past of headteachers using a school nurse to give one-off 'talks' (for example to girls on menstruation). This allows the school to escape its obligation to deal adequately with the subject with a carefully structured health education programme for all the children.

SCHOOL NURSES AND 'SENSITIVE ISSUES'

Sensitive issues such as contraception and sexual activity present school nurses with a considerable dilemma. Adolescents at schools may well turn to the school nurse for counselling on these matters.

Many children may feel unable to seek support elsewhere and this type of service is clearly needed (Macfarlane and McPherson 1992). However, it should only be offered after the most careful consideration. Procedures for instituting such support should be agreed with the local education authority. Under no circumstances should such counselling take place without the prior approval of the headteacher and governors or the full knowledge and understanding of both pupils and parents or guardians. This caution protects the interests of the school and the school nurse.

In some situations where the school feels unable to allow such counselling to be offered on its premises, the health service may have to make alternative arrangements to give children access to the service.

Discussion/Activity 13.3 A sensitive problem

You are the school nurse for the Sacred Heart Secondary School. At your weekly drop-in session, Maxine, who is 14, comes to see you ostensibly to talk about a skin-care problem (acne). In the course of the conversation she mentions that she is having sex with her boyfriend Jim. When you ask her she also tells you that she is not using any method of contraception. She has not and will not talk about this to her parents or her family doctor.

What are your responsibilities to Maxine? What are your responsibilities to the school (which teaches that artificial methods of contraception are morally wrong)? What will you do?

GOVERNMENT SUPPORT FOR SCHOOLS HEALTH PROMOTION

The *Health of the Nation* document acknowledged the importance of schools and the education service in attaining the national targets (DoH 1992). Unfortunately this has not yet been matched by interdepartmental support at a national level. The Department of Health and the Department of Education have not produced a well coordinated policy in matters of young people's health, nor is there adequate funding at a local level.

The National Curriculum (NCC 1990a) outlines a fairly detailed content for health education in schools, thereby including it within the statutory element of a school's programme. However, it does not go so far as to make health education an entitlement. In addition, government school league tables based on academic achievements encourage schools to place less emphasis on personal and social education.

Various government funding programmes have been helpful in supporting schools health promotion work at a local level. The most important of these was the Education Support Grant (ESG), begun in 1986. Originally this was set up to support drug education but it was recently replaced by the Grants for Education Support and Training (GEST), with a wider brief to cover all health education. This grant helped create a national resource of locally based advisory teachers who could assist with the development of health education policy and programmes in schools. These advisory teachers were also able to supply training and resources to support schools.

The GEST scheme, which was seen as 'pump priming' by the Department of Education, ended in 1993. Unfortunately this happened at a time when control of school budgets was being moved from the Local Education Authority (LEA) to the local school governors (Local Management of Schools (LMS)). As a result, LEAs have found it difficult to continue paying for the advisory teachers. In deprived urban areas these difficulties have been compounded by the withdrawal in 1993 of Inner City Partnership Grants, which previously funded some health education in many schools.

Health education has also benefited in the past from the activities of Her Majesty's Inspectorate (HMI), a respected independent agency which could monitor quality, increase awareness and speak out for higher standards. Recently the powers of HMI were reduced and many of its duties given to a new agency called the Office for Educational Standards (OFSTED).

SILVER LININGS

Despite these reservations there is little doubt that the *Health of the Nation* and the introduction of the National Curriculum have had a beneficial effect on health promotion in schools. There are increasing signs that the importance of collaboration, sound planning, clear guidance and appropriate resourcing for schools health promotion is becoming understood at national and local levels. The reorganisation of the health service allows District Health Authorities to co-operate with Local Education Authorities in complementary purchasing of health promotion for young people. Inspections organised by the new OFSTED can stimulate health education in schools. They can focus on quality of pastoral care and examine the link between a school's written health education policies and what actually happens. There are encouraging moves towards making use of the previously untapped but huge resource of parent support.

Minimum levels of entitlement sit at the heart of civilisation and democracy. As the gap in income between rich and poor grows, so does the gap in health. There can be few more important gifts that education can bestow on a young person than:

- the knowledge of themselves as they grow
- an awareness of their own attitudes and how these affect their behaviour
- a range of skills to enable sound decisions to be taken about the way they live their lives

These should be an entitlement for all our children and we are all challenged to ensure that they receive it.

SUMMARY POINTS

All schools should have an educational philosophy which encourages pupils to value health. The school should help its pupils to:

- ☐ understand health matters
- ☐ feel good about themselves and others
- ☐ acquire skills necessary for health
- ☐ make informed choices about behaviour

The whole school should be health-promoting so that messages learned in the classrooms are reinforced by all aspects of the school's life. The school environment should promote health.

There should be written policies and programmes defining how the school deals with important health issues.

Health education should have a defined place within the curriculum. Topics covered include substance use and misuse, sex, family life, safety, food and nutrition, personal hygiene, environmental aspects, health-related exercise and psychological health.

The school nurse is an important health resource for the school. They do health surveillance for the school and care for the health of pupils. The school nurse can play a valuable part in helping teachers fulfil their responsibility to provide health education. Health education and counselling by school nurses must always be compatible with the school's philosophy and policies.

Government has included health education as part of the school curriculum but there is little identified funding to support health education.

REFERENCES

Bachman R. (1986). Ecology in the school environment. *Health Promotion* **1**, 325–334.

Bagnall P. (1993). Health promotion, school nursing and the school age child. Chapter 6 in Dines A. and Cribb A. (eds.), *Health promotion concepts and practice*. Oxford: Blackwell Scientific.

Birmingham LEA (1991). *Heading for health*. Birmingham: Birmingham Health Education Unit.

DES (Department of Education and Science) (1994). *Sex education at school*. Circular 5/94.

DoH (Department of Health) (1992). *Health of the Nation: a strategy for health for England*. London: HMSO.

Harvey J. and Flannagan M. (1993). *Smoking in schools*. Birmingham: Birmingham Health Education Unit.

HMI (Her Majesty's Inspectorate) (1984). *Curriculum matters 6: Health education from 5 to 16*. London: HMSO.

Kalnins I., McQueen D., Backett C., Curtiss L. and Currie E.D. (1992). Children, empowerment and health promotion: some new directions in research and practice. *Health Promotion International* 7, 53–59.

Macfarlane A. and McPherson A. (1992). Sex and teenagers. *Health Visitor* **65**, 18–19.

National Forum for CHD Prevention (1994). *Food for children*. London: National Forum for CHD Prevention.

NCC (National Curriculum Council) (1990a). *Curriculum guidance No. 5. Health education*. York: National Curriculum Council.

NCC (National Curriculum Council) (1990b). *Curriculum guidance No. 3. The whole curriculum*. York: National Curriculum Council.

Nutbeam D., Clarkson J., Phillips K., Everett V., Hill A. and Catford J. (1987). The health promoting school: organisation and policy development in Welsh secondary schools. *Health Education Journal* **46**, 109–115.

Smith C., Nutbeam D., Roberts C. and MacDonald G. (1992). The health promoting school: progress and future challenges in Welsh secondary schools. *Health Promotion International* 7, 171–180.

Vine P. (1991). Ninety nine and counting. *Health Visitor* **64**, 150–151.

ACKNOWLEDGEMENT

Rosie Higgins and Martin Donovan are thanked for their help with this chapter.

CHAPTER 14

Health promotion in hospitals

GOAL

To develop the skills and knowledge required to organise, co-ordinate and deliver health promotion in hospitals.

OBJECTIVES

- to identify the factors which influence health promotion practice in hospitals
- to recognise the contribution of different health care workers in health promotion
- to explore the opportunities for health promotion in hospitals
- to discuss the potential barriers to successful health promotion in hospitals
- to utilise a number of devices which will enhance the co-ordination and delivery of health in hospitals

PRESSURES FOR HEALTH PROMOTION IN HOSPITALS

Hospitals should be not only places which cure and care but also places which promote health (Spiros and Sol 1991). Three influences have combined to produce a new awareness of the need for health promotion in hospitals:

1. political
2. consumer
3. professional

The political pressure for health promotion is illustrated in the recent NHS and Community Care Act (HMSO 1990), which stated the government's concern 'to deliver improved health for the population and secure better health services for individuals' over the next decade. Hospitals were listed as one of the 'settings for action' for achievement of the targets in the *Health of the Nation* document (DoH 1992) (see Chapter 1, page 16). Hospitals, as the most visible part of the health service, were expected to play their part in preventing ill health, promoting good health and ensuring individuals have the necessary information to exercise choice.

Pressure for health promotion also comes from consumers. The welcome increased awareness by patients and relatives of their rights to information requires hospitals to respond with better health education. The rights of every citizen to receive clear explanations about proposed treatment and any risks or about alternatives available are laid out in the Patient's Charter (DoH 1991). Hospital stays are getting shorter due to changes in service delivery, advances in surgical techniques and more effective treatments. These shorter stays mean that patients themselves and family members are required to take more responsibility for their own care and need adequate preparation to do this effectively and safely (Markanday and Platzer 1994).

The third pressure for health promotion comes from health care professionals. Greater emphasis is being given to health promotion in the role of each profession. The codes of conduct or professional practice produced by statutory and governing bodies either identify explicitly the role of the professional in health promotion and education, or else infer the role and responsibility. For example, registered nurses are expected to be able to identify the health-related learning needs of patients and clients, families and friends, and to participate in health promotion (HMSO 1989).

OPPORTUNITIES FOR HEALTH PROMOTION IN HOSPITALS

Health promotion in hospitals concerns:

- in- and outpatients
- visitors
- hospital staff

Each year about 8% of men and 11% of women are admitted to hospital as inpatients and many more will attend outpatients or casualty (OPCS 1990). These patients will in turn be visited by an even larger number of visitors. The NHS is one of the largest employers in Europe and many of its employees work in hospitals. This means that a very high proportion of the population can be reached by health promotion through hospitals.

Hospital health promotion as well as reaching a very large proportion of the community is likely to be effective. The situation favours learning (see Chapter 6) since health is likely to be salient in the minds of people attending hospital as patients or visitors and the hospital staff are likely to be seen as credible sources. Furthermore, since patients inevitably spend some time waiting while they are in hospital, they also have the time to consider health education messages. All these circumstances make the chance for health promotion in hospital too good to be missed.

HEALTH-PROMOTING HOSPITALS

The health-promoting hospital is a hospital which takes every opportunity for health promotion with patients, visitors and staff (Milz and Vang 1989). Health promotion comes not only from the staff taking opportunities for formal (planned) or informal health promotion but also from a whole environment that supports and reinforces health education messages. Checklists showing how a hospital can be health promoting have been published (Health Promotion Authority for Wales 1989).

The health-promoting hospital develops a systematic and co-ordinated approach to health promotion. Ways in which this could be done are:

- safe work practices
- environmentally friendly work practices
- policies to promote healthy lifestyles (smoking, food, exercise, etc.)
- health information readily available from leaflets, posters, etc.
- opportunities for staff to promote their own health
- patient support groups

Hospital work includes such risks as infection, back and other injuries and exposure to hazardous substances. Healthy work procedures recognise these risks and minimise them. Hospital procedures should not damage the environment by improper disposal of waste or wasteful use of resources (Wider 1991).

In health-promoting hospitals information on health matters is made available to patients, visitors and staff. Posters on the walls remind them of health issues. Should they want more information, leaflets and other materials are readily obtainable. Special events such as healthy eating days, accident prevention exhibitions and exercise happenings can also be used to stimulate interest among the staff.

All the information is supported by a whole range of hospital policies to promote healthy lifestyles. Non-smoking would be promoted by the provision of a smoke-free environment and support for those who need help in giving up (Batten 1988). Policies on alcohol would encourage healthy attitudes to drink, making information on sensible drinking available to all and not making alcohol available to staff who are on or about to go on duty. The policies would also encourage early recognition of staff who might be developing a drinking problem so that help could be offered. Healthy eating policies ensure that hospital catering gives people the choice of healthy eating while not unduly limiting the choice for those who wished to eat less healthy diets. Exercise can be encouraged by providing changing and other facilities.

HEALTH PROMOTION AND HOSPITAL STAFF

There is a danger in hospitals of concentrating so much on improving the health of and caring for patients that the staff are forgotten. However, employers have a responsibility to ensure they provide a healthy workplace and opportunities for their staff to maintain and improve their health. Making hospitals and NHS workplaces healthy workplaces has belatedly been recognised as a priority for NHS management (NHS Management Executive 1992). Health promotion for staff is essential firstly because healthy staff are more productive staff; and secondly because if staff do not think it worth promoting their own health they are unlikely to be effective as health promoters for patients.

Some of the many possibilities for health promotion with hospital staff are listed in Table 14.1.

DIAGNOSIS- AND NON-DIAGNOSIS-RELATED HEALTH PROMOTION

Health promotion for patients in hospital frequently focuses on the diagnosis or specific problems for which they have been admitted. This is essential to help the patient understand their illness and treatment and participate more effectively in their care (Fair 1994). For example, a newly diagnosed diabetic will want to learn about the effects of diabetes on the body, their diet, insulin, blood-sugar levels, skin and foot care. Often there is only enough time to help patients learn what they need to know about their current condition and no time to cover other topics. There are also times when a patient's lifestyle is obviously relevant to their condition, such as the patient with peripheral vascular disease who smokes, or the patient with liver disease who drinks heavily. In these examples no

Table 14.1 Health promotion initiatives for staff in hospitals

Promoting fitness
- corporate or reduced membership rates for gyms and swimming pools
- on-site facilities – gyms, jogging trails and swimming pools
- fitness assessments and exercise programming
- keep-fit and aerobics classes – lunchtimes and evenings
- hospital sports tournaments

Promoting healthy eating
- provision of healthy food choices in staff restaurant

Screening and health checks
- breast screening clinics
- cervical screening
- healthy heart checks

Reducing health risks
- slimming support groups
- stop-smoking initiatives – provision of counsellors and self-help support groups

Health education
- raising awareness of a variety of health issues by poster presentation, notice-boards, newsletters
- putting on health promotion events

one could deny that health education is a vital part of the patient's care (Roemer 1984).

However, there are many other hospital situations where health promotion does not focus directly on patients' diagnoses. For example, when a patient is admitted for repair of a hernia it may be appropriate to raise other health issues such as smoking or diet. The hospital visit represents an opportunity to reinforce healthy behaviours in patients and to encourage them to question less healthy behaviours.

In some situations it is wise to restrict health education to issues closely related to the patient's condition. Introducing other elements of health promotion unrelated to their health problem may be confusing and unhelpful. The health care worker has to decide (with each patient) how far-reaching the health promotion agenda should be. The process of educating for health was discussed in Chapter 7.

Discussion/Activity 14.1 Non-diagnosis-related health promotion

What health promotion activities are there in your hospital or health centre that focus on non-diagnosis-related issues? At whom are they aimed and what effect do they seem to have? What other health promotion opportunities could be introduced and at whom should they be aimed?

TEAM APPROACH TO HEALTH PROMOTION

Many hospital staff have a contribution to make to promoting health and, as with any element of patient care, interdisciplinary, collaborative working is essential. Each professional group has a contribution to make:

- physiotherapist
- occupational therapist
- chiropodist
- speech and language therapist
- ward clerk
- nurse
- doctor
- midwife
- many others

Traditionally, professional groups have tended to work in isolation. Poor communication about who is doing what has led to problems for both staff and patients. If patients are given varying information about the same topic by different staff, they may well become confused. There may be boring repetition, omission of essential areas and contradictory messages.

Lack of collaboration between staff groups leads to a lack of understanding of each other's role. Late referrals may mean there is not enough time for teaching. Staff feel undervalued and underutilised when they are not given the opportunity to use their special skills in health promotion. Alternatively staff become stressed when they are expected to teach skills which they are not competent to perform.

A team approach can be enhanced by:

- having adequate knowledge and understanding of the roles and expertise of those in other disciplines
- effective communication between professional groups
- having a common goal and a positive attitude

The team approach can be developed by having multidisciplinary training events to prepare staff for health promotion. Working together to produce leaflets and design education programmes, multidisciplinary team meetings and team teaching are other ways of building the team. Team working has many benefits for patients and clients (see Table 14.2).

Table 14.2 Benefits of a team approach in the hospital setting

- ensures continuity of health education
- identifies clear areas of responsibility
- breaks down barriers between professional groups, resulting in mutual respect and recognition of expertise
- develops commitment and involvement of staff
- improves the quality of health education
- improves patient and client satisfaction because a co-ordinated approach reduces confusion and frustration
- leads to staff satisfaction
- results in staff development as individuals learn from each other

Discussion/Activity 14.2 Your contribution to the health promotion team

What can your profession contribute to health promotion? Are there things which only your profession can do? What does your professional code of conduct say about health promotion?

How does your professional contribution fit into a multidisciplinary team? What things could be done by a member of your profession but could also be done by a team member from some other discipline? How effectively are you and your colleagues able to work as a multidisciplinary team in delivering health promotion? What would you like to improve?

BARRIERS TO HEALTH PROMOTION IN HOSPITALS

There are many barriers to successful health promotion in hospitals. In the past, attempts at educating patients have often been haphazard. Health care professionals have not been properly prepared to teach patients and incorporate education activities into care provision. In consequence, they have lacked the knowledge and ability to overcome communication barriers. Unco-ordinated events have not always been successful at meeting patients' needs (Jenny 1978; de Haes 1982; Holland 1986). Professionals working in isolation may assume that others have responsibility for health promotion with the result that it is not provided at all.

Education activities may be frustrated by lack of human, financial and other resources. An enthusiastic individual may develop education but it is not sustained when they leave. Clinical practitioners may give it low priority in their work. Managers may fail to encourage their team to do their part or fail to support health education when it happens. Health promotion may not be sufficiently specified in contracts and business plans (Close 1992).

ORGANISING, CO-ORDINATING AND DELIVERING HEALTH PROMOTION IN HOSPITALS

Organisation and co-ordination are the key to overcoming many of the barriers to the delivery of health promotion in hospitals. Ways of doing this are:

- improved preparation of staff for health promotion
- strategic planning in health promotion and patient education
- patient education committees
- patient education co-ordinators
- protocols, guidelines and standards
- educational programmes for specific patient groups

IMPROVED PREPARATION OF STAFF FOR HEALTH PROMOTION ACTIVITIES

The extent to which professional staff groups are prepared for health promotion at both pre- and post-qualifying levels is variable. Although most health care professions see health promotion as part of their professional role, many feel they have been inadequately prepared (Latter *et al.* 1993; HEA 1994).

In order to perform well as health promoters, health care professionals need to be able to:

- assess the health promotion needs of individuals and groups
- plan and co-ordinate health promotion activities
- recognise opportunities for health promotion
- identify priorities
- deliver effective health promotion to individuals and groups
- use different teaching aids – flow sheets, models, demonstrations, leaflets, posters, etc.
- evaluate health promotion activities
- act as role models

Discussion/Activity 14.3 The adequacy of your training

Think about your professional training. How adequate was your pre-qualifying/registration training in preparing you for health promotion activities? How have you developed your skills further since qualifying?

From your colleagues identify someone who provides a good role model for health promotion. What attributes do they have that make them a good role model?

STRATEGIC PLANNING IN HEALTH PROMOTION AND PATIENT EDUCATION

Chapter 10 described overall planning of health promotion. Strategic planning is a management tool which is used to ensure the long-term continuation and growth of health promotion and patient education activities in any organisation such as a hospital, community unit, GP surgery or health centre. It follows a cyclical process which links four main elements (see Figure 14.1).

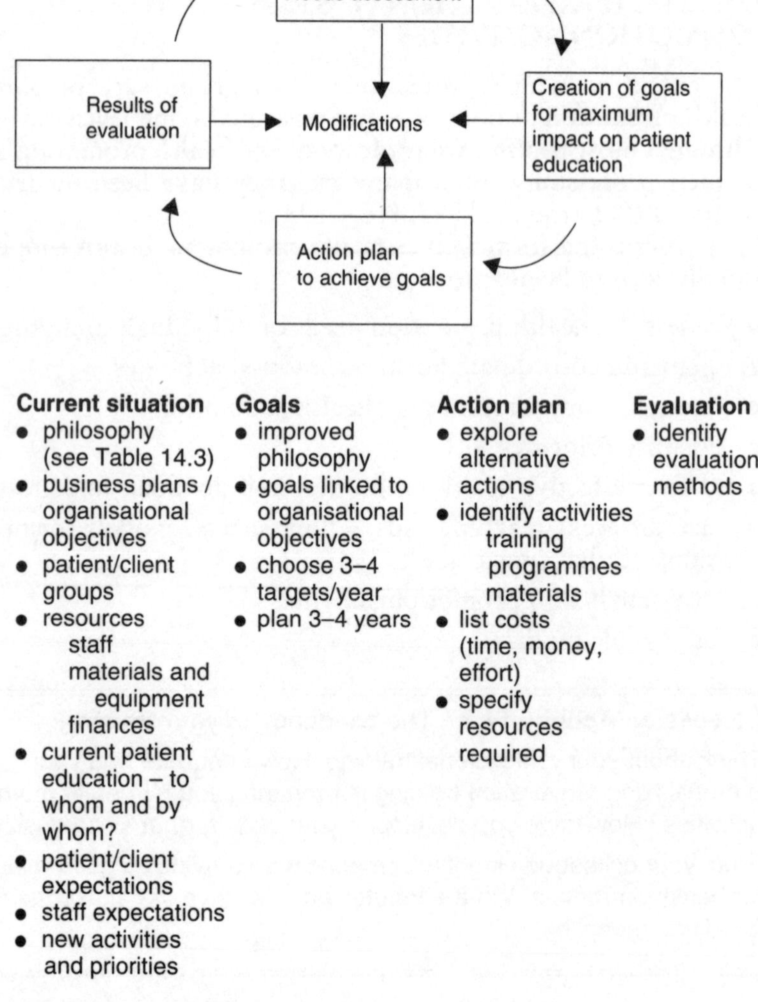

Figure 14.1 Strategic planning in patient education

These four elements answer the following questions:

- **Where are we now?** Assess the current situation in the hospital regarding patient education.
- **Where do we want to be?** Set goals designed to have maximum impact on patient education.
- **How are we going to get there?** Develop an action plan which identifies exactly how the goals will be achieved.
- **How will we know when we get there?** Evaluate and monitor results in order to readjust the strategic plan.

The advantage of using this approach is that new information can be exploited as it is acquired. In addition, a formative (ongoing) review of progress allows the plans to be modified while the programme is under way.

ASSESSMENT OF THE CURRENT SITUATION: WHERE ARE WE NOW?

In order to plan effectively it is necessary to assess the current provision of patient education. This assessment highlights both existing strengths, and areas of unmet need where further developments or resources should be focused. A comprehensive assessment of the situation in all parts of a hospital will be a very lengthy task. It may be more appropriate to work within different directorates, departments or teams as the situation will differ in each setting. However, the overall assessment must be drawn together to identify common problems, and resources that can be shared. The information to be collected is summarised in Table 14.3.

Information should be sought from a wide range of people, both inside and outside the hospital, who will be able to provide different perspectives on requirements for patient education and health promotion in hospital. The people consulted should include:

Within the hospital

- staff undertaking direct clinical care, managers, support staff, technicians, administrators, educationalists and others
- inpatients and outpatients and their relatives

Outside the hospital

- staff working in the community, voluntary, private and social service sectors
- past and potential patients, clients and their relatives
- bodies such as the Community Health Council who represent patients' interests

Table 14.3 Patient education – strategic plan
Questions to be answered in the assessment of the current situation

Philosophy
- What do staff/patients understand by the term 'patient education'?
- Whose responsibility should it be?
- What should it achieve?
- How should it be put into operation?
- How important is it as a part of care?
- Is there a formal philosophy which highlights patient education?
- How do views compare with this formal philosophy?

Business plans/organisational objectives
- What if anything does the unit business plan say about patient education?
- Do any of the activities mentioned in the business plan imply patient education activity without explicitly mentioning it?
- How is patient education included in organisational objectives?

Patient/client groups
- What are the most common diagnoses and health problems patients present with?
- What are the average lengths of stay?
- What are the age ranges?
- What is the ethnic and cultural mix?
- What languages are used?

Resources available: staff
- Do any members of staff have particular responsibility for patient education (e.g. Stoma therapist, HIV educator)?
- Are patient education activities included in job descriptions, responsibilities and performance appraisal?
- What preparation have staff had in patient education activities during initial qualifying courses, induction programmes and post-qualifying courses?
- What skills do staff have in patient education activities (including planning, organising, delivery and evaluation)?

Resources available: equipment and materials
- What equipment and materials are currently used for patient education?
- How is it obtained?
- Where is it stored?
- How is it maintained?
- What does it cost?

Resources available: finances
- What finances are available for:
  staff development?
  patient education programme development?
  equipment purchase and maintenance?
  development of media and materials?
  overheads?

Current patient education
- What patient education activities are currently being implemented?
- Is there a core plan available with:
  learning objectives?
  pre-determined objectives?

Table 14.3—*continued*

identified content?
materials (videos, leaflets, etc.)?
- Can the programme be individualised?
- How are activities:
  documented?
  evaluated?
- How are staff prepared in order to participate in specific education activities?
- What factors contribute to successful patient education?
- What problems have acted as barriers and how frequently were they seen in practice?

Patient/client expectations
- What do patients/clients/relatives want to know about?
- How do they expect to be involved?
- How do they like to learn?
- Who do they want to help them learn?

Staff expectations
- What do staff expect to achieve through patient education?
- What support do staff expect to receive for patient education?

New activities and priorities
- What new activities need to be addressed and in what priority?

These enquiries should be supported by an examination of relevant documents:

- in the hospital – patients' records, business plans, health reports, audits and contract agreements
- more general – national, regional, local and government policy statements such as the Patient's Charter (DoH 1991) and *Health of the Nation* (DoH 1991)

A variety of methods should be used to collect the information, including:

- one-to-one and group interviews
- focus groups
- questionnaires
- formal and informal discussions (individuals and groups)
- document analysis and evaluation

When the assessment is complete, a summary of the current patient education situation should be made, with the main issues and recommendations highlighted.

Table 14.4 A philosophy of patient education: an example from a medical unit

We believe:

Educating patients, their relatives and carers is an essential part of care and treatment. It involves providing information about their condition, related factors, treatment and care and how it will affect their lives. Patients have a right to know, and information can help them come to terms with their current situation.

Patients need to be actively involved in their care, and education enables them to understand what is happening, to make choices, to help themselves and to take on more responsibility for their health care.

Patient education should be the responsibility of all members of the multidisciplinary team. Those who have a close relationship with patients and are in frequent contact with them have an ideal opportunity. Good communication between professional groups will assist collaborative working and the development of a uniform and consistent approach. This will enhance patient education and enable patients to have more choice and influence in relation to the care they receive.

SETTING GOALS: WHERE DO WE WANT TO BE?

The information collected during the assessment is used as a baseline to help the institution decide its future goals for patient education and health promotion. The philosophy of the hospital or department should be the starting point. This philosophy is often summarised in a mission statement. Sharing beliefs and values with colleagues is the first step to ensuring that patient education and health promotion become an important priority in care. The philosophy directs the entire patient education process and influences the choice of goals. It is important that staff should own the philosophy and be involved with developing any new philosophy. Groups should work together to identify the key concepts involved in patient education. They should clarify their beliefs about these key concepts and the relations between them (see Table 14.4).

Goals for health promotion should address the needs of patients and staff, make full use of the resources available and be fully compatible with the philosophy. The hospital's business plan and service agreements must be analysed to identify where health promotion and education activities will fit. These business plans may not state explicitly what health promotion activities should occur but even so the health promotion goals should be linked into them.

The number of key goals in a strategic plan should be limited to 3 or 4 in each year and it is usual to plan for 3–4 years. Goals for the first year's plan will be firmly set but goals for later years must be subject to the changing needs of the institution.

Discussion/Activity 14.4 Health promotion in the business plan

Examine your unit/department business plan or service agreement. Identify what opportunities it provides for patient education and health promotion.

ACTION PLANNING: HOW ARE WE GOING TO GET THERE?

The next step is to identify activities through which the goals can be achieved. Alternative courses of action should be considered. An estimate of the time, effort and cost required should be made, together with the benefits that are likely to be produced. The most cost-effective action that best meets the goals can then be decided on. An action plan which states target dates and responsibilities is then drawn up and carried out.

EVALUATION: HOW WILL WE KNOW WHEN WE GET THERE?

Evaluation is an essential part of the strategic planning cycle. It is useful to review each stage as it occurs so that adjustments and modifications can be made. Early corrective intervention may save valuable resources.

Evaluation of the overall plan should be based on a review of the goals and targets identified in the second stage ('Setting goals'). In addition, the evaluation plan will also include:

- the tools or methods to be used
- who will conduct the evaluation
- when it will be done
- how it will be communicated

Evaluation reports should provide a summary of progress, highlight achievements and identify difficulties, and should be the basis for the next cycle of the strategic planning process. Evaluation also allows more to be gained in return for the considerable costs involved in developing programmes. Programmes which are shown to be successful can be reused several times and this gives greater benefit for the costs incurred in their development.

Table 14.5 Functions of a patient education committee

1. To determine the needs for health promotion and patient education in the hospital.
2. To prioritise the needs and make recommendations.
3. To organise the development of patient education and health promotion programmes by producing guidelines for:
   programme development
   developing and reviewing teaching and learning materials
   costing programmes
4. To develop a catalogue of health promotion and patient education resources available in the hospital.
5. To introduce mechanisms for distribution of health promotion and patient education materials.
6. To approve education programmes as they are developed.
7. To advise on staff training in health promotion and patient education.
8. To communicate information regarding patient education between PEC and Trust Management Board, directorate and outside agencies.
9. To evaluate the overall health promotion and patient education strategy.

PATIENT EDUCATION COMMITTEES

Many hospitals in the USA have Patient Education Committees (PEC) which co-ordinate and support patient education activities. A similar concept may be helpful in the UK. Ideally the group should consist of a variety of people from across the hospital, including members of different groups and levels of service (Close 1992). For example:

- representatives of clinical practitioners from different professional groups
- general managers responsible for human and financial resources
- patient and carer representatives who can provide the consumer perspective
- senior and junior employees
- others with expertise in marketing, learning resources, audio-visual aids and printing and publishing

The functions of a PEC are listed in Table 14.5. It acts as a steering group responsible for co-ordinating each stage of the strategic planning cycle. Careful choice of membership for the group should ensure that it is representative and communicates effectively with individuals and groups within the organisation. The membership should also include others with the ability, resources, influence and enthusiasm to implement patient education activities.

PATIENT EDUCATION CO-ORDINATORS

Some hospitals in the USA also employ patient education co-ordinators in place of or in addition to the Patient Education Committees. Rankin and Duffy (1990) describe a co-ordinator as, 'a person responsible for facilitating and co-ordinating the design, implementation, monitoring and evaluation of a system of patient education and teaching programmes'.

The scope of the patient education co-ordinator in hospital is potentially very wide. Their role may include:

- setting up the co-ordinating committee
- leading the strategy development
- involvement in the development, co-ordination and distribution of teaching materials and resources
- the orientation and preparation of staff for health promotion and education activities
- face-to-face teaching of staff
- quality assurance (Close 1991)

Education co-ordinators in hospital settings should have a background in one of the health care professions as a considerable amount of education relates to patients' diagnoses and the problems which they present. Experience in education will also help to provide the co-ordinator with appropriate skills and knowledge to organise and deliver patient education and enable the staff to do the same.

PROTOCOLS, GUIDELINES AND STANDARDS

Protocols, guidelines and standards are other tools for improving the quality of health promotion and patient education activities in hospital. They will help provide practitioners with:

- a common goal – it is essential that health care professionals agree on what they are attempting to achieve and how they are going to do it
- an understanding of the areas of responsibility of each professional group
- the basis for auditing activities

Protocols and guidelines for health promotion and patient education specify:

Table 14.6 Example standard (1): Preparing patient education materials

Standard statement
Written leaflets and handouts for a specific patient group are prepared to enhance learning experiences for patients.

Structure	Process	Outcome
1. There are staff with the technical knowledge and skills to produce leaflets. 2. These are health care practitioners with knowledge of and expertise in caring for the patient group. 3. There is an adequate budget for the production of leaflets. 4. There are guidelines for: (i) developing leaflets (ii) costing of leaflets	Relevant health care practitioners 1. assess the need for new leaflet 2. identify the characteristics of target patient group 3. calculate the number of leaflets required and cost of production 4. prepare the leaflet according to guidelines 5. review content in conjunction with colleagues and patient family representatives 6. check readability/ reading ease of leaflet	1. Health care professionals state that leaflets reinforce essential information. 2. Patients and relatives state that the leaflet: (i) is easy to read and understand (ii) provides them with essential information

- the resources required, such as the types of staff, knowledge and skills, the equipment, learning resources, leaflets and documentation
- exactly what the health care professional must do to help the individual learn what is necessary
- the results or what is expected in terms of behaviour change
- who is responsible for doing what

Standards specify a level of performance that staff are aiming to achieve when educating patients and promoting health. Protocols, guidelines and standards can be developed for many areas of health promotion in hospital. Standards can be written for broad areas such as the preparation of leaflets (see Table 14.6) or the planning of education programmes. Alternatively, standards may describe the education activities for specific groups of patients with a particular problem (see Table 14.7).

Table 14.7 Example standard (2): Teaching keyboard skills to children

Standard statement
Children with fine-motor/perceptional problems will be taught keyboard skills in order to improve finger agility, performance, stamina, spatial perception and to give an alternative method of recording work when legibility and speed are required.

Resources	Process	Outcome
	Therapist...	Child...
1. Electric typewriter and electrical socket, paper supply	1. assesses the need for keyboard skills training	1. manages the technicalities of the typewriter independently
2. Keyboard skills protocol	2. uses 'Keyboard Skills Protocol'	2. uses each separate finger of both hands as shown
	3. checks learning at beginning of each new session	3. achieves finger agility without conscious recall to visual prompting
	4. provides time for supervised practice	4. monitors and self-corrects own work
	5. teaches child to monitor own work for mistakes	5. achieves a typing speed equivalent to own handwriting speed
	6. evaluates progress and gives positive feedback	

ADAPTING CORE PROGRAMMES

While education programmes need to be adapted to the needs of specific groups or individuals, it is helpful to base them on core programmes. Having core programmes as a base encourages a unified approach to teaching patients and consistency among different health care professionals. Being based on a satisfactory core programme ensures that all programmes specify learning objectives, content, teaching and learning strategies, who is responsible for teaching each part of the programme, the methods of documenting activities and how learning will be evaluated.

PROGRAMMES FOR SPECIFIC GROUPS

The steps to be followed in developing a specific programme are shown in Figure 14.2. The first step is to identify the target group and situation for which the programme is needed. This might be children on a pre-admission visit to a surgical ward, carers of relatives following a stroke, patients on a cardiac rehabilitation pro-

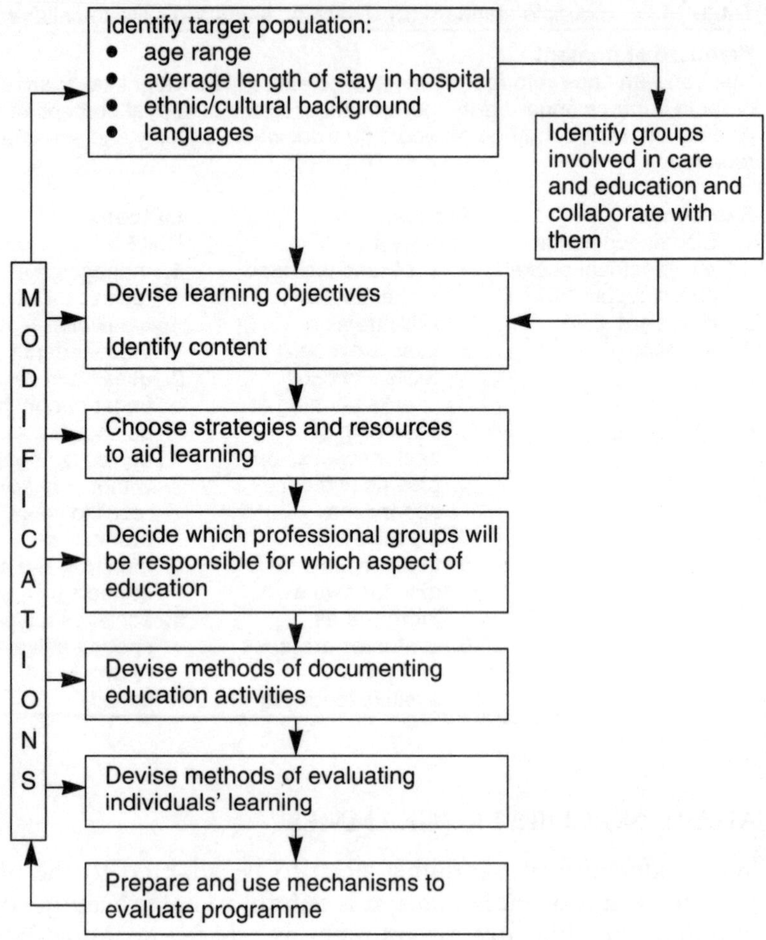

Figure 14.2 Steps involved in developing an education programme

gramme or some other group. The age range, how long they stay in hospital or frequency of contact, ethnic and cultural backgrounds and languages spoken should be identified. This information will enable you to choose the most appropriate information content and teaching methods and the resources that will be needed.

The professional groups involved with the care and education of the patient should be identified at an early stage so that they can participate in programme development. Representatives of these groups now work together with patients to identify what the

OLDTOWN HOSPITAL
Form 26/8/1991

Female Patient's Intermittent Self-Catheterisation

Name: *Sheila Smith*

Goal: The patient will be able to undertake self-catheterisation safely when required.

Objectives	Information Given/Observed	Supervised	Information Understood/Independent	Signature
1. The patient is able to explain the reasons for undertaking intermittent self-catheterisation	1.3.94	N/A	Able to explain why she requires self-catheterisation	J. Jones Staff Nurse
2. The reasons why asepsis is necessary.	1.3.94	N/A	Able to explain consequences of sepsis.	J. Jones Staff Nurse
3. What equipment is required.	1.3.94	Observed 1.3. 94	Able to name and identify equipment required	J. Jones Staff Nurse
4. How frequently the procedure is required.	1.3.94	N/A	Able to state when procedure required.	J. Jones Staff Nurse
5. The patient is able to demonstrate: (a) correct hygiene procedure	1.3.94	2.3.94	3.3.94	P. Bryan
(b) safe preparation of the environment and equipment	1.3.94	2.3.94	3.3.94	P. Bryan
(c) visualisation of the urethra using a mirror	1.3.94	2.3.94 3.3.94	4.3.94	P. Bryan
(d) the introduction of the catheter into bladder neck, drainage of urine and removal of catheter	1.3.94	2.3.94 3.3.94	4.3.94	P. Bryan
(e) the safe disposal of used equipment and urine	1.3.94	2.3.94 3.3.94	4.3.94	P. Bryan

Figure 14.3 A checklist for patient education
This checklist is used for a female patient who needs to learn to perform intermittent self-catheterisation. It ensures that she has learned the knowledge and skills that will enable her to perform this procedure with confidence.

Table 14.8 Education programme for children with newly diagnosed asthma

Target population: children (aged 6 months to 16 years) and their parent or carer

Learning objective The child and their parent or carer is able to:	**Content**	**Strategies and resources**	**Professional responsible**	**Evaluation of learning by child and parent/carer**
Explain what asthma is and its effect on them as an individual and on their family	Narrowing of airways in asthma How it affects breathing and speaking How it causes anxiety How its symptoms of wheeze, cough, breathless on exertion, and nasal stuffiness are caused	Verbal explanation with diagram to show airways constriction	Doctor	Are they able to explain what asthma is? Can they describe its effects on breathing anxiety and level of anxiety? Do they understand enough about disease to have basis for further learning?
Identify factors which precipitate asthma	Precipitating factors: atmosphere temperature change exercise night time infection allergy psychological stress	Verbal explanation Explore child's own circumstances and history	Doctor	Have they been given leaflet and given an opportunity to discuss it? Are they able to identify precipitating factors in relation to their own circumstances?
Explain how to avoid precipitating factors	What to do in situations where asthma likely to be precipitated	Discuss what they could do in particular circumstances	Doctor	Are they able to suggest actions that will minimise exposure to precipitating factors?

Demonstrate which drugs they should take to prevent attacks and when to take them	Preventive drugs: sodium chromoglycate inhaled steroids long-acting theophylline antihistamines	Verbal explanation for each drug: its purpose how it works its side effects how to use it safely	Doctor Pharmacist	Are they able to explain which drugs to take, when and in what dose and how the drugs will help them? Have they been observed taking the prescribed dose of drug safely on two or more occasions?
Explain which drugs to take for relief during asthmatic attacks	Treatment drugs: beta stimulants oral steroids inhaled steroids antibiotics oxygen nebulised drugs subcutaneous adrenaline	Written list of individual's own medication Demonstration and supervised practice of taking drugs Verbal explanation about drugs Questions and answers	Nurse Pharmacist	Can they explain how they will obtain further prescriptions? Are they confident about continuing medication at home?
Use inhaler correctly	How to use inhaler	Demonstrate use Supervised practice	Physiotherapist Nurse	Have they been observed using inhaler correctly?
Use peak flow meter correctly	How to use peak flow meter	Demonstrate use Supervised practice	Physiotherapist Nurse	Have they been observed using peak flow meter
Maintain and store equipment	How to do it Reasons why important	Demonstrate maintenance and storage of equipment Supervised practice Explain reasons	Physiotherapist Nurse	Can they demonstrate how to maintain and store equipment? Are they able to explain why this should be done?
Use recording and self-management chart	How to use chart	Supervised self-recording in self-management chart	Physiotherapist Nurse	Have they completed self-recording section of self-management chart?

(*continued*)

Table 14.8—*continued*

Target population: children (aged 6 months to 16 years) and their parent or carer

Learning objective	**Content**	**Strategies and resources**	**Professional responsible**	**Evaluation of learning by child and parent/carer**
The child and their parent or carer is able to:				
Recognise deteriorating signs and symptoms of asthma and know when to seek doctor's advice	Significance of wheeze, cough, breathless on exertion and low peak flow rate Assessment of symptoms using self-management chart and ready reckoner	Review signs and symptoms of asthma Question and answer with child and parent/carer Use self-management chart for assessment working jointly with child or parent/carer	Doctor	Can they describe the signs and symptoms which indicate they should contact the doctor?
Complete symptom diary appropriately	What to record in diary and why it is important	Verbal explanation and supervised practices	Nurse	Have they completed diary as instructed?
Explain what follow-up arrangements have been made	OP clinic GP liaison Local asthma society/club School Prescribe medication and repeat prescriptions Nurse asthma clinic	Provide written list Verbal explanation Question and answer	Nurse	Have they been given a written list of follow-up arrangements? Are they able, using the list, to explain what follow-up arrangements have been made and what they are expected to do?

patients want and need to know and how they will learn. Learning objectives, content of the education programme, teaching strategies and resources to aid learning can then be planned. Flow sheets, checklists and other documentation can be written for the education plan (see Figure 14.3). Finally the programme should include the methods for evaluating:

1. what the individual has learnt or can accomplish as a result of the programme (see Chapter 6)
2. how well the programme works

Each education programme for a specific group of patients will need to be evaluated to establish its effectiveness in helping that group to learn. The results of a programme can also be used to improve future education provision. Staff morale will be boosted when a programme is shown to be working well and when their competency in delivering it can be demonstrated.

Table 14.8 shows an education programme for a child during their first admission for newly diagnosed asthma. The programme was developed for children aged 6 months to 16 years or their carers. The children are likely to stay 2–5 days in hospital. The local population for whom this was intended was largely white and English speaking. A modified programme might be needed for children from other ethnic groups.

SUMMARY POINTS

Many factors affect the practice of health promotion in hospitals:

- ☐ political influences
- ☐ consumer influences
- ☐ professional influences

A large proportion of the population comes in contact with hospitals – as patients, visitors or employees. The opportunity for health promotion is therefore immense and should be exploited.

All health care professionals have an individual contribution to make but health promotion is more effective when a co-ordinated team approach is used.

A number of strategies can be used to enhance the organisation and delivery of health promotion in hospitals:

- ☐ improved preparation of staff
- ☐ strategic planning approach
- ☐ patient education / health promotion committees
- ☐ patient education / health promotion co-ordinators

- ☐ standards, protocols and guidelines
- ☐ core education programmes
- ☐ programmes adapted for specific groups of patients

REFERENCES

Batten L. (1988). The NHS as an agent of change: creating a smoke free environment in hospital. *Health Trends* **20**, 70–75.

Close A. (1991). Necessity or luxury? *Nursing Times* **87** (No. 28), 36–38.

Close A. (1992). Strategic planning in patient education. *Nursing Standards* **6** (No. 43), 32–35.

de Haes W.F.M. (1982). Patient education a component of health education. *Patient Counselling and Health Education* **4**, 95–102.

DoH (Department of Health) (1991). *The Patient's Charter*. London: HMSO.

DoH (Department of Health) (1992). *The Health of the Nation*. London: HMSO.

Fair P.A. (1994) Hygiene for health. *Nursing Times* **90** (No. 5), 71–72.

HEA (Health Education Authority) (1994). Smoking and pregnancy survey. *Midwives' Chronicle and Nursing Notes* **107** (No. 1273), 53.

Health Promotion Authority for Wales (1989). *Healthy hospital competition: criteria and guidelines*. Health Promotion Authority for Wales.

Holland S. (1986). Teaching patients and clients. *Nursing Times* **82** (No. 49), 34–37.

HMSO (1989). *Statutory Instrument for nurses, midwives and health visitors. No. 1455. Nurses, midwives and health visitors (Parts of the Register) Amendment (No. 2) Order*.

HMSO (1990). *NHS and Community Care Act 1990*. London: HMSO.

Jenny J. (1978). A strategy for patient teaching. *Journal of Advanced Nursing* **3**, 341–348.

Latter S., Maben J., Macleod-Clark J. and Wilson-Barnett J. (1993). Perceptions and practice of health education and health promotion in acute ward settings. *Nursing Times* **89** (No. 21), 51–54.

Markanday L. and Platzer H. (1994) Brief encounters. *Nursing Times* **90** (No. 7), 38–42.

Milz H. and Vang J.O. (1989). Consultation on the role of health promotion in hospitals. *Health Promotion* **3**, 425–427.

NHS Management Executive (1992). *Priorities and planning guidance 1993–1994*. EL(92) 47, 20 July. London: Department of Health.

OPCS (Office of Population Censuses and Surveys) (1990). *General Household Survey 1988*. London: HMSO.

Rankin S.H. and Duffy K. (1990). *Patient education, issues, principles, practices*. Philadelphia PA: Lippincott.

Roemer M.I. (1984). The value of medical care for health promotion. *American Journal of Public Health* **74**, 243–248.

Spiros C.I. and Sol N. (1991). Health promotion in hospitals. In Bandura B. and Kickbusch I. (eds.), *Health promotion research: towards a new social epidemiology*. WHO European Regional Publications No. 37.

Wider P. (1991). Environmental care in the NHS. *Nursing Standard* **6** (No. 3), 33–36.

CHAPTER 15

Health promotion in general practice

GOAL

To develop the skills and knowledge required to organise, co-ordinate and deliver health promotion in general practice.

OBJECTIVES

- to identify the opportunities for health promotion in general practice
- to describe the process of health checks in general practice
- to recognise scope for nurse-run health-check and disease-management clinics in general practice
- to recognise the importance of teamwork within the primary care team
- to discuss the potential for health gain and health loss in screening

OPPORTUNITIES FOR HEALTH PROMOTION IN GENERAL PRACTICE

General practice is the point at which most people come into first contact with the health service. General practices see 65 per cent of the population registered with them each year and 90 per cent over the course of five years. Many of the groups for whom health promotion might be most beneficial, such as children, young mothers and older people, are particularly frequent attenders of general practice. People usually attend their general practice at a time when they are worried about and therefore conscious of their health. For all these reasons general practice offers a great opportunity for health promotion (Fowler 1986).

General practice health promotion should not be restricted to lifestyle issues. The members of the primary care team are well placed to assess the effect of environment on their patients' health and they can be effective advocates on matters such as housing and road safety. Recent experiments with offering benefits advice in a general practice setting have proved highly successful (Paris and Player 1993).

THE SCOPE FOR HEALTH PROMOTION

The health promotion activities which can naturally be undertaken in general practice cover the whole life span, from preconception to death. Some of them are listed in Table 15.1. Many of these are already being done by most practices.

OPPORTUNISTIC HEALTH PROMOTION

Stott and Davis (1979) identify four potential activities in every primary care consultation:

1. management of presenting problems
2. management of continuing problems
3. modification of help-seeking behaviour
4. opportunistic health promotion

While the patient may well have come expecting treatment and advice for a particular complaint, the consultation offers opportunities for health education both on making most effective use of services (help-seeking behaviour) and on other matters related to the patient's health.

In doing opportunistic health promotion one must however be very careful not to overstep the patient's right to define the agenda for a consultation (see Chapter 2, page 31). For example, a patient might attend the practice for treatment of a cut hand and find them-

Table 15.1 Health promotion activities in general practice

- pre-conceptual advice
- health care in pregnancy
- advice on infant feeding, safety, etc.
- immunisations
- child accident prevention advice
- advice on safe sex and contraception
- cervical screening
- self-care advice for patients with diabetes, asthma, etc.
- advice on safe drinking
- advice on stress management and mental well-being
- stop-smoking advice
- assessment of coronary risk factors
- accident prevention in older people

selves being asked about their smoking and drinking habits and then invited to consider changing them. Is it right for the health care worker to shift the agenda of the consultation to issues not raised by the patient? Studies have shown that, far from objecting, most patients welcome this sort of enquiry (Hughes 1988; Sullivan 1988).

EFFECTIVENESS OF HEALTH PROMOTION IN GENERAL PRACTICE

Health promotion in general practice appears to be remarkably effective. The process of asking about lifestyle is often sufficient to encourage the patient to contemplate change (Skinner *et al.* 1985). Randomised controlled trials have shown that focused consultations and other brief interventions in general practice are effective in helping smokers give up smoking (Jamrozik *et al.* 1984) or heavy drinkers cut down on their drinking (Wallace, Cutler and Haines 1988). Cost–benefit analysis (Williams 1987) suggests that advice from GPs to stop smoking is one of the most cost-beneficial activities undertaken by the health service (see Table 15.2).

Most of the trials of effectiveness of health promotion in general practice have looked at doctors. There are reasons for thinking that other members of the primary care team would be as effective, if not more so (Robson *et al.* 1989) though some trials have been disappointing (Sanders *et al.* 1989).

HEALTH CHECKS

The success of opportunistic health promotion led many to suggest that health promotion in general practice should be provided more systematically rather than be subject to the vagaries of practice workload. Health promotion could be the subject of a dedicated consultation rather than tacked onto the end of a consultation arranged for some other purpose. Such health promotion consulta-

Table 15.2 Cost per QALY for health gain from different health service activities

QALY stands for Quality Adjusted Life Year. A health gain of one QALY is the equivalent of giving a patient one extra year of life in full health.

Activity	Cost per QALY
Advice by GPs to stop smoking	180
Pacemaker implant for heart block	700
Heart valve surgery for aortic stenosis	900
Coronary artery graft for severe angina	1040
Heart transplant	8000

Source Williams A. (1987), p.103.

tions are usually focused on one particular topic, such as well-woman, well-man, health of older people, and so on.

HEART HEALTH CHECKS

One topic for which health checks have been widely used is heart health. This type of health check is often known as the 'Oxford' model since this was the district where it was developed. It is also often referred to as an MOT check by analogy with the annual check on motor vehicles. The main features of this health check are:

- patients are invited to attend
- risk of cardiac disease is assessed
- the consultation is based on a standard protocol
- the patient is offered lifestyle counselling
- results are recorded
- patients are followed up

INVITING PATIENTS

Patients can be opportunistically or systematically invited to attend a heart health check. Opportunistic invitations are given when the patient contacts the practice for some other reason. Tagging the notes of patients who should be offered health promotion makes it easy to take action when the patients come to the practice. Posters in the waiting areas can be used to encourage patients to ask for appointments for the heart health check. These and similar techniques can ensure that opportunistic invitations reach nearly everyone on the practice list. The high proportion of the practice list who attend within a given period means that opportunistic health promotion is generally quite satisfactory.

Systematic invitations involve writing to all patients on the practice list. Very little is gained from the much greater organisational effort needed to operate systematic calls. Now that doctors are required to offer a health check to patients on their list who have not attended in the previous three years, systematic calls are difficult to justify.

THE CONTENT OF THE HEART HEALTH CHECK

Information collected in a heart health check usually includes the following:

- personal history of angina, heart attacks, stroke or other evidence of cardiovascular disease

- any history of diabetes
- medications
- family history of cardiovascular disease, especially premature death from heart disease or stroke in close relatives
- smoking history
- drinking habits
- measurement of height and weight
- measurement of blood pressure
- testing of urine

Other items of information which are collected in some practices include measurement of blood cholesterol, dietary habits, exercise habits, tetanus immunisation status and (in women) contraceptive use and when they last had a cervical smear.

Measurement of blood pressure (British Medical Journal 1987) and other measurements are done by carefully standardised methods. Body mass index or degree of obesity is estimated from height and weight using a chart.

ASSESSMENT OF RISK

All this information is used to assess coronary risk. This can be done informally (by reviewing all the information) or more formally by using one of the coronary risk scores devised by Shaper (Shaper *et al.* 1987) or by the Dundee group (Tunstall-Pedoe 1991). The Shaper risk score can be calculated from a simple formula, and an easy-to-use disk device is available to calculate the Dundee risk score. Risk depends on several different factors (see page 70) rather than on any single factor and the risk scores have the advantage of taking a range of factors into account.

When the risk has been assessed, it is discussed with the patient, with particular emphasis on those factors that are modifiable. It is important to avoid frightening the patient and to remember that risk scores are only a very rough indication. Even people in the highest risk band are unlikely to suffer a heart attack in the few years following the risk assessment.

MODIFYING RISK

The purpose of assessing risk factors is to reduce risk. This may entail:

- referral for further medical investigation
- lifestyle counselling

Some risk factors such as moderate or severe hypertension or newly recognised glycosuria (sugar in the urine) will require referral for further medical investigation. A protocol for risk factor checks will give guidance on when this is appropriate. Figure 15.1 shows one such protocol for checking blood pressure.

However, most risk factors such as smoking, heavy drinking and overweight can be lowered by simple measures. The health education skills described in Chapter 7 are required to help the patient consider making changes. A practical manual on lifestyle counselling has recently been distributed to all practices in the UK (Anon. 1993). The primary health care worker will discuss the different risk factors with the patient, clarifying the options for and the barriers to change. The patient is then able to decide whether they wish to modify their lifestyle to reduce risk. The patient and

Blood pressure to be measured at least 5 minutes after patient has come into room when patient is relaxed and at ease. The patient should be comfortably seated. Blood pressure to be measured on left arm using 4″-width cuff. Cuff to be inflated to 20 mm above point where pulse disappears. Systolic taken as first appearance of sounds, diastolic as disappearance of sounds (Korotkoff 5).

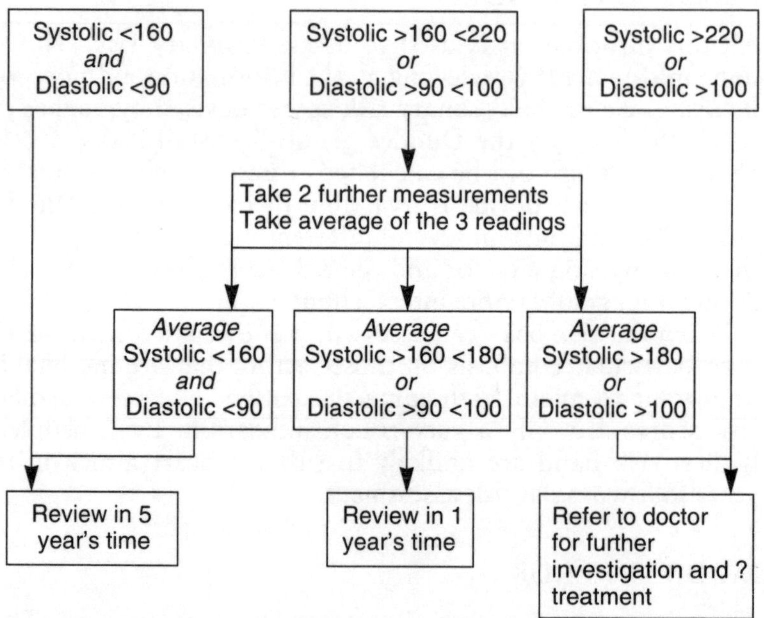

Figure 15.1 Protocol for blood pressure measurement
Source Adapted from Fullard E., Fowler G. and Gray M. (1987), Promoting prevention in primary care: a controlled trial of low technology low cost approach, *British Medical Journal* **294**, 1080–1082.

health professional together can plan any behavioural changes. Where some change is planned, the patient will be given follow-up appointments to give them support and monitor progress. In some cases referral to another agency such as a weight-reduction group, an exercise and fitness centre, a stop-smoking group or an alcohol advisory centre may be appropriate.

THE RECORD

The findings of the risk assessment, any targets for change negotiated, and follow-up plans are recorded on a special record. This is convenient for collecting the information and acts as an *aide-mémoire* during the check (see Figure 15.2). This special record can then be filed with the main patient records. It can be used to organise follow up and as a basis for audit of the health checks. Where records are computerised, the standard record card simplifies data entry. Computerisation makes calculation of risk scores and subsequent analysis of records much easier.

Discussion/Activity 15.1 Attending a general practice health check

You have just received a letter from your general practice inviting you to attend for a well-woman/well-man health check. Will you accept the invitation? What are the factors that made you accept or reject it? If you go, what will you expect and what aspects of the health check would make you say 'I am glad I went' after you had been?

DISEASE MANAGEMENT CLINICS

Special clinics may be set up along similar lines for the management of common chronic conditions such as hypertension (Jewell and Hope 1988), diabetes (Murphy, Kinmonth and Marteau 1992), and asthma (Charlton *et al.* 1990). In common with the heart health checks, these clinics have a major health education element and are based on carefully written protocols. Clinics may also be devoted to immunisation for travel (Fox and Jones 1993) or to supporting particular aspects of behavioural change such as stopping smoking, weight control and sensible drinking.

HEALTH PROMOTION FOR INFANTS

Mothers with young children attend general practice frequently so there are great opportunities for health promotion with this group. Developmental assessment, immunisation and advice on child

Entered on computer 1/4/94

Name JONES GP KENT

Address John Robert Check date 30/3/94

Sex (M)/F

Date of birth 12/3/44 Age 50

Occupation Self Fitter Spouse H/wife

Self-defined ethnic group

1.	White UK	(2.)	White Irish	3.	White other
4.	Black Carib	5.	Black African	6.	Black other
7.	Indian	8.	Pakistani	9.	Bangladeshi
10.	Other				

History	Self	Family	Other history
Prem CHD	Yes/(No)	Yes/(No)	
CHD	Yes/(No)	Yes/(No)	Father hypertensive & diabetic
Hypertension	Yes/(No)	(Yes)/No	
Hyperlipid	Yes/(No)	Yes/(No)	Current medication
Diabetes	Yes/(No)	(Yes)/No	
Stroke	Yes/(No)	Yes/(No)	
TIA	Yes/(No)	Yes/(No)	

Oral contraceptives Yes/(No) Urinalysis ....

Last smear date ..../..../.... Last tetanus inj ..../..../....

Smoker (Yes)/No

Smokers No. cigs per day ..... Cigars Y/N Pipe Y/N

Years smoked ....

Non-smokers (Ex-smoker)/Never Years stopped 20 yrs

Blood pressure Syst Diast

1. Date 30/3/94	BP 145/85	Syst	(1)	2	3	4
2. Date / /	BP /		<160	160–179	180–199	200+
3. Date / /	BP /	Dias	(1)	2	3	4
Mean	BP ..../....		<90	90–99	100–109	110+

Figure 15.2 Record card for heart health checks
This record card acts as an *aide-mémoire* and provides easy-to-use record for heart health checks. It folds into a size that will fit into the patient's notes wallet. It is designed to hold a lot of information in a small space, but still be reasonably easy to read. Data are collected in a way that makes it easy to enter on a computer. Information on blood pressure, serum cholesterol, BMI (body mass index) and alcohol is stored both in actual measurements and in grouped form.

Cholesterol Date ....../....../........ Value .... mM

(0.) Not measured 1. <5.2 2. 5.2–6.4 3. 6.5–7.8 4. > 7.8

Triglycerides ....

Height *176* cm Weight *121* kg BMI *29.7* kg/cm^2

BMI 1. <20 2. 20–24 (3.) 25–29 4. 30–34 5. 35+

Alcohol *15* units/wk

Drinking cat	1	(2)	3	4	5
Men	<1	1–21	22–34	35–50	>50
Women	<1	1–14	15–20	21–35	>35

Exercise *Very little exercise*

Needs to do more

Diet

Fruit/Vegetables *2* per day

Starchy foods *4* per day

Fried foods *3* per week

Fish *1* per week

Wholemeal bread Yes/(No)

Milk type (Full)/Skim/Semi

Other diet comments

Eats lunch in works canteen

Risk Score ....

Problem follow-up negotiated

None	Y/ N	Personal history	Y/(N)	Family history	Y/(N)
Smoking	Y/(N)	Blood pressure	Y/(N)	Cholesterol	Y/(N)
Weight	(Y)/N	Alcohol	Y/(N)	Exercise	(Y)/N
Diet	Y/(N)	Other	Y/(N)	....	

Investigations ordered ....

....

Comments ....

....

Figure 15.2 (*continued*) Reverse side of record card.

rearing are all health promotion activities. The mothers expect advice on nutrition, child hygiene, home accident prevention and numerous other aspects of child care.

General practice offers an ideal setting for all these activities. The mothers are interested and highly motivated to do their best for their child. They are in a familiar setting with people they know and trust. They will be with other mothers who are their friends, who give mutual support and with whom they can share their problems and solutions. Health promotion in general practice should be offered in a way that makes the most of these advantages. The waiting area and consulting rooms should be warm, comfortable and decorated in a child-friendly way. There should be toys for the children and perhaps hot drinks for the mothers. All these things will make health promotion at the mother and baby clinic an experience to be looked forward to and enjoyed rather than a duty to be performed.

Immunisations are a vital contribution to disease prevention (DoH 1990). Children need no longer be exposed to the risk of death or serious disablement from diseases such as paralytic polio, diphtheria, pertussis, measles and mumps. Nor should mothers need to fear the tragedy of a child severely disabled by congenital rubella. Nowadays when these diseases occur in the UK they should be regarded as an avoidable failure of disease prevention rather than an unavoidable misfortune. While most mothers will bring their children for immunisation with little prompting, health care workers must play their part to ensure that as many children as possible are protected. They can do this by:

- ensuring every mother is invited to have their child immunised
- giving accurate and factual information on immunisation to mothers
- following up mothers whose children are not immunised
- reassuring mothers who are anxious about immunisation

NURSE INVOLVEMENT IN HEALTH PROMOTION

The different members of the primary care team all have their part to play in health promotion. Very often the practice nurse takes the lead, running heart health checks and other checks. They are increasingly involved in disease-management clinics (Cant, Killoran and Calnan 1993) as well as taking smears and blood samples for screening programmes (Jeffree 1990). The practice managers and record staff are also essential members of the team organising systems to invite people for immunisation, health checks and screening.

Surveys suggest that nurses enjoy health promotion work and extending their role beyond treatment room work. They find that increased responsibility and autonomy within the team improves job satisfaction. Role conflict with doctors and inadequate job descriptions were often mentioned as factors which limited nurse involvement. These difficulties could be overcome by developing teamwork within the practice. Lack of a suitable room for health promotion work, lack of time and lack of supporting resources were also mentioned as barriers to good health promotion work. Many practice nurses also expressed a wish for further training in aspects of health promotion skills (Cant, Killoran and Calnan 1993; Robinson and Robinson 1993).

Discussion/Activity 15.2 Doing health checks in general practice

Imagine you are working in a general practice. At the practice meeting it is agreed that the practice should be offering well-woman/well-man health checks. It is further suggested that you might take responsibility for organising and providing these. Would you enjoy this task? If so, why? If not, why not? What further training would you want to equip you for this work? What support would you expect from the other members of the practice team?

ARE CLINICS A GOOD THING?

Health promotion in general practice has been increasingly separated off in clinics. This has happened to a large extent because of the way general practice is paid for rather than for more solid health reasons. Putting health promotion in clinics has the advantages of giving it a defined place in practice work and means it cannot be forgotten. It also allows the practice staff to timetable their work efficiently. On the other hand, it may be less convenient for the patient who has to make a special appointment. The health promotion activity has to fit into a time slot and is split away from the patient's other medical needs. In some practices, health promotion clinics may have replaced opportunistic health promotion. On balance, health promotion clinics are probably a very useful addition to health promotion activity in general practice but they are not a solution to all health problems. There is a need to think carefully as to what work is best done in clinics and what is better integrated into the everyday work of the practice.

PRIMARY CARE FACILITATORS

Recent years have seen the development of a new post: the primary care facilitator (Astrop 1987). This worker, who is often a nurse by training, has the task of encouraging primary care teams to become involved in health promotion. They help with advice on training and organisation for health promotion. The role was pioneered in Oxford by Fullard (1992) and has subsequently been extensively developed and copied.

A NOTE OF CAUTION ABOUT HEALTH CHECKS

Health checks in general practice are a relatively new idea and as with other new ideas it took longer to recognise the drawbacks than to see the advantages. With further experience it is becoming clear that even in the best-run practices uptake may be lower than expected and the extra work generated considerable (ICRF OXCHECK Group 1991). On average three-quarters of patients attending may need some further intervention and follow up. Furthermore, the reduction in risk is less than first hoped for (ICRF OXCHECK Group 1994; Family Heart Study Group 1994). The patients who take up offers of health checks tend to be those at lower risk. There is a very real danger that health checks could divert attention away from the most deprived patient towards the relatively favoured (Gillam 1992), thereby adding to inequity.

SCREENING

The rationale for screening is that if disease is detected at an early stage treatment will be more effective in curing or preventing the disease and less unpleasant for the patient (see the definition of secondary prevention in Chapter 2). Diseases and conditions routinely screened for are listed in Table 15.3.

Undertaken wisely, screening can produce a great deal of health gain and avert much suffering. Undertaken unwisely, it can cause a lot of harm. All screening procedures will produce some false posi-

Table 15.3 Conditions screened for in the UK

Breast cancer (age: 50–65)
Cervical cancer (age: teens–65)
Foetal congenital defects (neural tube defect, Down's syndrome, phenylketonuria (PKU))
Congenital dislocation of hip
Hearing and visual disorders in children
Developmental delay
Risk factors for coronary heart disease

Table 15.4 Criteria for screening

A screening programme for any particular condition is only justified if the following criteria can be satisfied:

1. The condition causes serious distress.
2. The condition can be cured or ameliorated if detected early.
3. Early treatment produces better results than later treatment.
4. The natural history (course) of the disease is known and a pre-symptomatic phase can be recognised.
5. There is a test with an adequately low rate of false positives and false negatives.
6. The test is acceptable to the population.
7. It is possible either to screen all the population or to identify a high-risk group and screen all of them.
8. The cost of the programme is reasonable.

It will be easier to satisfy these criteria for commoner conditions than for very rare ones.

tives (people who according to the test might have the disease but in reality do not) and some false negatives (people who according to the test do not have the disease but in reality do). People who are falsely positive have to suffer unnecessary anxiety and the inconvenience of further and possibly more unpleasant investigation (Marteau 1989). People who are falsely negative receive unwarranted reassurance which may lead them to delay treatment when the disease becomes apparent. Even people who are true positive only benefit if the subsequent treatment is effective. If treatment is unsuccessful, the only effect of screening has been to make them aware of their disease at an earlier stage and so prolong the time that they were distressed by it. It is therefore essential that screening is only undertaken in situations where it produces health gain. The criteria for deciding whether screening is helpful are listed in Table 15.4 (Hakama 1991).

QUALITY CONTROL OF SCREENING

The damage which can be done by ill-advised or badly implemented screening has already been noted. Quality control of all stages is essential. This entails ensuring that:

- there is a comprehensive list of the target group
- a very high proportion of the target group is screened
- the test is properly administered or sample properly taken
- the patient is notified of and understands the result
- any further investigations required are done promptly
- any patient with a positive or uncertain result receives support

General practice provides an excellent framework for organising screening because this quality control can be done (Mant 1992). The cervical screening system is built around general practice (Austoker and McPherson 1992). Even when the test has to be done away from the practice premises, as with breast screening (mammography) the primary care team can control the quality of the process. The use of the general practice list to invite people for screening means that nearly everyone can be covered. People are more likely to take up invitations to be screened if they are endorsed by their primary care team and if they can turn to the team for advice and explanation should they want it. If further investigation or treatment is required after screening, this can be co-ordinated with their other health care through the practice.

BLOOD CHOLESTEROL SCREENING

Blood cholesterol screening provides a good example of some of the problems around screening. Machines have been developed which make it possible to measure blood cholesterol in the local health centre and give a reasonably accurate result in a few minutes. Many general practices started to include blood cholesterol measurement in their health checks. However, further experience has lead most UK authorities to conclude that this is not a good idea.

First, there are difficulties of quality control. While the machines can certainly give good results when used exactly according to instructions, they are unreliable when used less carefully. Unless great care is taken to test everyone in the target group one may test the 'worried well' rather than those who could benefit most. Furthermore, blood cholesterol by itself is a poor predictor of risk of heart disease. There is a danger that the primary care team ends up worrying about the blood cholesterol rather than the patient. There is little evidence that lifelong treatment of moderately raised blood cholesterol with expensive lipid-lowering drugs prevents much heart disease, let alone improves patients' quality of life. For all these reasons, most authorities now recommend that blood cholesterol testing should be used selectively on patients where there is reason to think it is important for making decisions about their care rather than be applied to all regardless of their risk (O'Brien 1991).

Discussion/Activity 15.3 Which diseases to screen for

Look at the list of diseases for which screening is offered in the UK (Table 15.3). Screening is not generally offered for blood cholesterol, lung cancer and osteoporosis. Think of some other diseases for which screening is not offered.

Why do you think we screen for some diseases and not for others? Are there any diseases which you think ought to be added to the list of diseases screened for? How well do these diseases measure up to the criteria in Table 15.4?

THE CONTRACTUAL SETTING OF GENERAL PRACTICE

General practitioners in the UK are independent contractors. They contract with the Family Health Service Authority (FHSA) to provide medical services to all the patients registered with them. The general practice is responsible for hiring and paying most of the members of the team and is in turn paid by the FHSA. The payments from the FHSA depend on the number of patients registered with the practice, the services provided and the staff employed.

Arrangements for paying general practices for health promotion have changed frequently. At first there was no payment for health promotion. Later payment was made for certain health promotion activities such as cervical screening and immunisation. Subsequently payments were introduced for 'health promotion clinics' and these have recently been replaced by payments determined by the 'band' of health promotion services provided by the practice. The best practices have always provided health promotion but the new financial incentives are greatly increasing the numbers involved. In an ideal system the organisation of 'health promotion' that gave maximum health gain would also give maximum practice income. The present system falls short of this ideal. There is a danger that in a few practices members of the primary care team will be frustrated in their desire to give maximum health gain by the desire of other team members to maximise practice profits.

There can be no doubt that best health promotion practice would see close co-operation between practice staff and community (district) staff employed by the local community trusts. Current arrangements with fund-holding practices and activities of community staff defined by contracts may make such joint working difficult. It is to be hoped that future funding arrangements will remove this unfortunate barrier to effective health promotion.

SUMMARY POINTS

General practice offers numerous and effective opportunities for health promotion.

Good general practice health checks invite all patients to attend, assess risk of disease, use a protocol-based consultation, offer patients lifestyle counselling, record the results and follow up the patients.

Health checks and disease-management clinics can be run by the practice nurse.

Work with mothers and children is another vital part of health promotion in general practice.

Health promotion in general practice is a team activity, with each member of the primary care team having a role to play. Team members need training in health promotion to optimise their effectiveness.

Screening to detect disease early – at a stage when treatment is more effective – is a valuable activity. If done unwisely screening can cause a great deal of worry and harm. General practice offers opportunities for doing screening well, with careful quality control of all stages.

The contractual setting of general practice influences the way in which health promotion is delivered and sometimes makes co-operation more difficult.

REFERENCES

Anon. (1993). *Better living – better life*. Henley on Thames: Knowledge House Ltd.

Astrop P. (1987). Facilitator – the birth of a new profession. *Health Visitor* **61**, 311–312.

Austoker J. and McPherson A. (1992). *Cervical screening* (2nd edition). Oxford: Oxford University Press.

British Medical Journal (1987). *ABC of hypertension*. London: British Medical Association.

Cant S., Killoran A. and Calnan M. (1993). *Preventing heart disease: the role of the community nurse*. London: Health Education Authority.

Charlton I., Charlton G., Broomfield J. and Mullee M.A. (1990). Evaluation of peak flow and symptoms only self management plans for control of asthma in general practice. *British Medical Journal* **301**, 1355–1359.

DoH (Department of Health) (1990). *Immunisation against infectious disease*. London: HMSO.

Family Heart Study Group (1994). Randomised controlled trial evaluating cardiovascular screening and intervention in general practice: principal results of British family heart study. *British Medical Journal* **308**, 313–320.

Fowler G. (1986). The role of the primary health care team. *Journal of the Royal Society of Medicine* **79**, 633–636.

Fox A. and Jones M. (1993) Travel precautions. *Nursing Times* **89** (No. 38), 58–59.

Fullard E. (1992). The Oxford prevention of heart attack and stroke project. In Williams K. (ed.), *The community prevention of coronary heart disease*. London: HMSO.

Gillam S.J. (1992). Provision of health promotion clinics in relation to population need: another example of the inverse care law? *British Journal of General Practice* **42**, 54–56.

Hakama M. (1991) Screening. Chapter 6 in Holland W., Detels R. and Knox E.G. (eds.), *Oxford textbook of public health* (2nd edition), vol. 3. Oxford: Oxford University Press.

Hughes M. (1988). Patient attitudes to health education in general practice. *Health Education Journal* **47**, 130–132.

ICRF (Imperial Cancer Research Fund) OXCHECK Group (1991). Prevalence of risk factors for heart disease in OXCHECK trial: implications for screening in primary care. *British Medical Journal* **302**, 1057–1060.

ICRF (Imperial Cancer Research Fund) (1994). Effectiveness of health checks conducted by nurses in primary care: results of the OXCHECK study after one year. *British Medical Journal* **308**, 308–312.

Jamrozik K., Vessey M., Fowler G., Wald N., Parker G. and Van Vunakis (1984). Controlled trial of three different anti-smoking interventions in general practice. *British Medical Journal* **288**, 1499–1503.

Jeffree P. (1990). *The practice nurse: theory and practice*. London: Chapman and Hall.

Jewell D. and Hope J. (1988). Evaluation of a nurse-run hypertension clinic in general practice. *Practitioner* **232**, 484–487.

Mant D. (1992). Screening adults in general practice. Chapter 8 in Fowler G., Gray M. and Anderson P. (eds.), *Prevention in general practice* (2nd edition). Oxford: Oxford University Press.

Marteau T.M. (1989) Psychological costs of screening. *British Medical Journal* **299**, 527.

Murphy E., Kinmonth A.L. and Marteau T. (1992). General practice based diabetes surveillance: the views of patients. *British Journal of General Practice* **42**, 279–283.

O'Brien B.J. (1991). *Cholesterol and coronary heart disease: consensus or controversy?* Studies of Current Health Problems No. 98. London: Office of Health Economics.

Paris J. and Player D. (1993). Citizen's advice in general practice. *British Medical Journal* **306**, 1518–1520.

Robinson H. and Robinson A. (1993). A survey of practice nurses in Northern Ireland: identifying education and training needs. *Health Education Journal* **52**, 208–212.

Robson J., Boomla K., Fitzpatrick S., Jewell A.J., Taylor J., Self J. and others (1989). Using nurses for preventive activities with computer assisted follow up; a randomised controlled trial. *British Medical Journal* **298**, 433–436.

Sanders D., Fowler G., Mart D., Jones L. and Marzillier J. (1989). Randomised controlled trial of anti-smoking advice by nurses in primary care. *Journal of Royal College of General Practitioners* **298**, 1360–1362.

Shaper A.G., Pocock S.J., Phillips A.N. and Walker M. (1987). A scoring system to identify men at high risk of a heart attack. *Health Trends* **19**, 37–39.

Skinner H.A., Allen B.A., McIntosh M.C. and Palmer W.H. (1985). Lifestyle assessment: just asking makes a difference. *British Medical Journal* **290**, 214–216.

Stott N.C.H. and Davis R.H. (1979). The exceptional potential in each primary care consultation. *Journal of the Royal College of General Practitioners* **29**, 201–205.

Sullivan D. (1988). Opportunistic health promotion: do patients like it? *Journal of the Royal College of General Practitioners* **38**, 24–25.

Tunstall-Pedoe H. (1991). The Dundee coronary risk disk for management of change in risk factors. *British Medical Journal* **303**, 744–747.

Wallace P., Cutler S. and Haines A. (1988). Randomised controlled trial of general practitioner interventions in patients with excessive alcohol consumption. *British Medical Journal* **297**, 663–668.

Williams A. (1987). Screening for risk of coronary heart disease: is it a wise use of resources? In Oliver M., Ashley-Miller M. and Wood D. (eds.), *Screening for risk of coronary heart disease*. Chichester: John Wiley and Sons, pp. 97–106.

CHAPTER 16

Health promotion in the community

GOAL

To develop a greater understanding of the opportunities for health promotion in the community and the ways in which it can be delivered.

OBJECTIVES

- to recognise the contribution of different groups of people to health promotion in community settings
- to identify the settings in which health promotion takes place and highlight the opportunities and potential barriers these may create
- to explore the best approaches and methods of delivery that can be used in particular locations
- to discuss user involvement in planning and provision of health promotion and other services for the community

WHAT IS 'THE COMMUNITY'?

Community is another of those words which mean different things to different people. A community is a self-defined group which has common interests and recognises people as being members or non-members. The boundaries defining a community may be geographical or cultural and frequently do not coincide with any official boundaries. Members of a community tend to look to other members for advice and support. Health care workers may or may not be members of the communities they seek to serve.

The word community is also used to describe settings outside the bounds of the health service. Working in a hospital or health centre the health care professional is on home territory and the patient is not. In the community it is the client or patient who is at home and the health care professional who is generally the visitor. Community care refers to care in or close to the patient's own home as opposed to care in NHS hospitals.

MODELS OF WORKING IN THE COMMUNITY

Health care workers in many communities rapidly become aware that big issues such as unemployment, poverty, loneliness, bad housing, fear of crime, and family disputes have an overriding influence on people's health, swamping any effect of lifestyle issues such as smoking, eating and exercise. This challenges health promoters to make health promotion relevant to members of the community. They may react by adopting different models of working:

- knowledge – attitude – behaviour (KAB) model ('medical' model)
- empowerment model
- community action model

(See Chapter 2 for a description of these models.)

Many health professionals feel most comfortable with the KAB model, concentrating on health behaviours. They may prefer it because it allows them to retain the position of 'health expert'. Provided they take care to make the knowledge and skills taught relevant to the condition of the community, this can be useful. However, many would feel it fails to recognise the real health problems of many communities.

The empowerment model aims to build up the capacity of individuals to make choices and give them more control over their own lives. The health professional adopts the role of friend, advocate and counsellor. The logic of empowerment will lead the health care worker to become involved in much more than lifestyle issues.

The community action model aims to mobilise deprived communities to reduce the inequities that damage their health (Watt and Rodmell 1987). A health care worker adopting this model will be left with little time to spend on lifestyle issues. The shift of focus away from the individual may also raise uncomfortable questions about whose interests and health are being promoted.

CASE STUDY: A CHILD WHO IS NOT THRIVING

Sharon is a two-year-old girl who has had numerous health problems in her short life. She has had frequent respiratory infections and recurrent diarrhoea since she was a baby. Her growth is slow (weight below the third centile) and her speech development is delayed. She lives in a sixth-floor flat in a tower block with her parents Phillip (20 years old) and Jane (19 years). The family has very little money and is behind with the rent. Jane works as a shelf stacker at a local supermarket. When Jane is at work Sharon is looked after by Phillip, who is unemployed. Both parents smoke heavily. The family's meal patterns are erratic, and biscuits, crisps and take-away hamburgers form a large part of Sharon's diet.

The health visitor calls regularly to keep an eye on Sharon. She has discussed with Phillip and Jane how their smoking might make Sharon's chest problems worse. The health visitor has also talked over the nutritional needs of young children and is trying to arrange a place for Sharon at a toddler's group.

Discussion/Activity 16.1 Health priorities for Sharon and her family

What do you think are Sharon's health problems? Do the parents also have health problems? Do you think that the health visitor's advice on smoking and nutrition will be helpful? What else could be done to improve Sharon's and her parents' health?

HEALTH PROMOTERS IN THE COMMUNITY

Many agencies help promote health in the community, as shown in Table 16.1. (Compare this with Figure 1.3.) Nurses, midwives and health visitors have a significant contribution to make (White 1983; Magill-Cuerden 1993; Gane 1994). They enable people to make choices about healthier lifestyles, and to access screening and treatment services. They help by advice and advocacy to ensure safe and healthy environments in the home, workplace and wider community. Ways in which nurses, midwives and health visitors can contribute to health in the community have been described in a recent Health of the Nation handbook (DoH 1993). Several excellent community programmes have been concerned with promoting heart health (Evans 1993). Health promotion officers offer a wide range of services both directly helping individuals in the community as well as helping others to be health promoters (see Chapter 1, page 12). Nurses, midwives and health visitors doing health promotion with individuals or groups often work as separate professional groups. However, there are many occasions when the best health promotion work is done by different disciplines working together (Cassidy 1994; Siney 1994).

COMMUNITY HEALTH EVENTS

Community health events can be very effective in raising interest in health issues. An example of such an event was an 'Age Concern

Table 16.1 Agencies promoting health in the community

Health service	**Local authority**
Health Authorities	council
Trust Boards	social services department
hospitals	environmental services department
health centres	housing department
health education departments	parks and leisure department
ambulance service	engineers department
	planning department
Government bodies	libraries
Health Education Authority	schools
Department of Health	colleges of further education
Ministry of Agriculture, Fisheries and Food	
Department of Environment	**Independent sector**
Department of Education	chamber of commerce
Health and Safety Executive	commercial organisations
	industry
Voluntary bodies	shops
community groups	unions
charitable organisations	press, radio and TV
self-help groups	
churches	**Others**
	police service
	prison service
	probation service
	Community Health Council

Week' organised in one district which was intended to promote services for older people. The activities that took place included:

- the production of a directory of services for the elderly and how to find them, by the Primary Health Care Team
- fix your walking stick clinic, by physiotherapists
- accident prevention workshop, help and advice by occupational therapists
- joint session between young people and elderly with story-telling and reminiscence
- crime prevention seminar by police
- an amnesty for return of borrowed health service equipment (sticks, crutches, commodes, wheelchairs, etc.)
- town-centre exhibitions featuring the work of wheelchair services, home-loan schemes, day centres, dental health services, equipment and aids, leisure opportunities and social services

The organisation and running of this event required joint planning by the different agencies and then co-operative working. Collaboration in this way not only helps promote the event but also has spin-offs as each group comes to understand more of the services offered by their colleagues. Many of the people involved in the 'Age Concern Week' were health service staff, but voluntary organisations, social services staff from the local authority, police, fire services and of course the local residents were also prominently involved. Developing healthy alliances with other groups is an important by-product of these events.

Often local events may be linked to national campaigns such as 'No Smoking Day', 'Drinkwise Day', 'World Aids Day' and 'Look after your Heart' (see Chapter 19). The local health promotion department frequently takes a lead in co-ordinating such events.

Health visitors or community nurses might also set up and staff stalls concerned with health topics at local fêtes or carnivals. Informal talks to leisure organisations, women's groups and mother and baby groups can also be arranged. A slightly different sort of health event aimed at opinion-formers is described in Chapter 18.

HEALTH PROMOTION IN PEOPLE'S HOMES

Health workers visiting people in their own home often find opportunities to do health promotion. Groups of the population that are commonly visited by health professionals and other agencies include:

- families with small children visited by health visitors
- elderly people and people with physical disabilities visited by community nurses and social workers
- people with physical and learning disability or mental-health problems visited by community psychiatric nurses, therapists and social workers
- pregnant mothers visited by midwives
- people of all ages who require further help after discharge from hospital visited by district nurses, specialist nurses (e.g. stoma therapist) and other therapists

The home is a place where people can be themselves. Health promoters have a chance to work with and observe their clients in real situations. They are able to adapt their advice and skills teaching to reflect the client's needs and to choose examples relevant to the client's home environment. When you are working in people's homes it is particularly important to remember that the client's priorities may not always coincide with your professional priorities.

CASE STUDY: A DEPRESSED, UNEMPLOYED MAN LIVING ALONE

John, aged 23, lives alone in a small flat in an industrial town in the Midlands. He has been out of work most of the time since he left school and recently there have been a number of problems with the benefits that John receives. The flat is extremely dirty and untidy. The kitchen is littered with dirty pans and crockery and decaying food. John appears dirty and unkempt. He eats mostly fried foods and suffers from stomach problems. He is depressed and has talked about committing suicide.

Because John also had a mild learning disability he was seen by a community nurse who was qualified as a CNMH (Community Nurse Mental Handicap). Although the nurse was aware of the conditions under which John was living, he felt the most important thing to do was to develop a positive relationship with John to build up trust. Without this trust nothing else would have been achieved as John would have told the nurse to leave. Only when a positive relationship had been built, could counselling and other therapeutic interventions begin. Advice and help with benefits were then given. Information and education on diet and food and domestic hygiene were less important and would be left till later.

Discussion/Activity 16.2 Promoting John's health

What are the factors that threaten John's health? Which of these factors are amenable to change? How might your approach to John have differed from that described in the case study? Would you have tackled the problems in the same order?

PROMOTING THE HEALTH OF CARERS

The vast majority of health care in the home is provided by informal carers such as spouses, family members, friends and volunteers (Graham 1992). Their care may be supplemented by visits from a health professional whose primary focus is on the needs of the patient. However, carers themselves are often at risk of a breakdown in their health as a result of caring for the patient. Health professionals must recognise the needs of these informal carers and take opportunities to promote their health as well.

Situations with carers need to be handled sensitively so that the health professional is not seen as a busy-body. Care must be taken to avoid unwelcome intrusions. However, there are a number of ways in which health professionals can enhance the health and wellbeing of carers. For example:

- Teaching carers techniques for lifting and moving people and helping carers obtain lifting aids. This reduces the risk of injury to both carer and client and promotes the comfort of both.

- Providing information on and help in obtaining short-term respite care, sitting services and other support mechanisms.
- Providing opportunities for carers to discuss their own anxieties. Identifying stress-relieving techniques for carers.
- Using situations within the home to encourage safe practices and reduce the risk of accidents.

COMMUNITY HOMES

Over recent years many people with mental-health problems or learning disabilities have been successfully resettled from long-stay institutions into supported housing in the community. Changes to the way services are provided mean that many more will be similarly resettled in the future. In the setting of a community home people can enjoy a much better quality of life. Smaller units encourage more individualised care. There is evidence to suggest that people living in a group home are generally more comfortable and happy (Shepherd 1984). Quality of life is enhanced by staff who promote the philosophy of ordinary life and utilise the principles of normalisation. These principles aim to create living conditions and lifestyles that are as normal as possible for the person concerned. Individualised learning programmes can be developed for each resident. These help them improve their self-care skills and develop leisure interests and employment opportunities, which enhance both physical and mental health.

CASE STUDY: FOUR MEN IN A COMMUNITY HOME

Four men with learning disabilities live in a bungalow in a small town. They all moved there together from a long-stay hospital six months previously. Staff have initiated a number of activities aimed at promoting the health of the individuals and of the group. For example, the local general practitioners annually make a full physical examination and review of medication. Each of the four men has an annual flu vaccination and one man attends the local epileptic association. There is a no-smoking policy in the home as none of the residents smokes. The residents are currently trying to help some of the staff who do smoke to stop.

One particular project has been aimed at promoting healthy eating, not only for the men but also for the staff who eat with them. The men when they lived in hospital had little involvement in buying, preparing and cooking food. Home staff felt they all had the ability to participate in some way and believed they should have the opportunity. After six months, staff had a good idea of everyone's likes and dislikes. They found pictures of most of the foods the residents enjoyed and used these to help them choose a set of menus. The dietitian was asked to check the meal plans and recommended reducing the fat content by using low-fat spreads, oil and fat-reduced crisps. Pictures are also being used to prepare shopping lists and help the residents buy their own food (Richardson 1993; Spooner and Rudge 1993).

CLINICS AND HEALTH CENTRES

Clinics and health centres provide a range of opportunities for health promotion activities. Health promotion in general practice was described in the previous chapter (Chapter 15).

For midwives, health promotion is a vital part of care, involving education from the first antenatal contact through to the last postnatal visit. Ideally it should begin long before pregnancy occurs and it can be provided by midwives working in conjunction with school nurses, health promotion staff and teachers. Midwives are increasingly doing their health promotion in the community – working in clinics, surgeries and the client's own home. Table 16.2 shows the range of issues covered.

'DROP-IN' CENTRES, HEALTH SHOPS AND HELP-LINES

There is an increasing demand for health advice without the more formal setting of a clinic or family doctor surgery. Drop-in centres may be very effective in reaching younger people who may not wish to discuss their worries with their family doctor, school staff or their parents. Drop-in centres are also widely used to provide services for people with drug or alcohol problems. Mobile drop-in units have been used to make services and advice accessible to travellers (Reid 1993; Tyler 1993). The informal, unstructured setting may attract people who want to discuss their problems but do not feel comfortable in more conventional health settings.

Health shops are similar to drop-in centres. They are usually located in a shopping street with a prominent shop-front designed to encourage people to come in. They provide the community with easy access to support services on a range of issues without the need for referral. Support, counselling, advice and information may be available from health services, social services and voluntary agencies (Hick 1991; Malin and May 1992).

Telephone help-lines are another way in which one can try to make information easily accessible. Many users of telephone help-lines value the fact that they can remain anonymous. Help-lines on subjects such as HIV/AIDS and drug problems have proved very popular. The Samaritans and Childline are two other examples of help-lines which have proved valuable.

Table 16.2 Health promotion issues relating to midwifery

Pre-conceptual period
To prepare parents physically, mentally and socially for pregnancy and family life.

- general health screening and related advice
- immunisation
- family planning and contraception
- developing positive relationships
- menstrual history and cycles
- parenting skills
- information on midwifery services
- sexual health

Antenatal period
To equip mothers with sufficient knowledge and skill to enable them to maintain and improve their health during pregnancy; to enjoy pregnancy and prepare for the birth; to obtain the services to which they are entitled.

- nutrition during pregnancy
- physiological and psychological changes in pregnancy and how to cope
- labour and delivery – expectations and preparation
- dental care
- information on support services and benefits
- effects of alcohol, drugs and smoking on the individual and the newborn
- safety and prevention of accidents
- immunisation
- personal hygiene
- the newborn child and its needs
- the postpartum period – in relation to the parents and to the newborn
- baby feeding
- parent-couple issues – relationships and intimacy

Postnatal period
To equip mothers with sufficient knowledge and skill to have the confidence to look after themselves and their babies.

Mother
- hygiene
  - personal
  - preparing feeds
- abdominal and pelvic exercises
- nutrition
- breast care
- family planning

Baby
- hygiene
- feeding
- sterilisation of equipment
- cot death prevention
- transporting baby
- screening
- immunisation
- individual issues, e.g. twins, abnormalities

YOUTH SERVICES

The health of adolescents is a good indicator of the health of the community. This group is not only one of the most vulnerable but also one of the most difficult to influence. Making contact with young people and those who work with them is important. Young people are likely to reject anyone whom they feel fails to see things from their perspective. Health care professionals forget this at their peril (Scally 1993; Thompson 1993).

A forum that brings together youth workers, voluntary agencies, teachers, youth workers and those involved with the leisure services will help better networking. Health care workers may find it useful to join such a forum or create one if it does not already exist. The forum can discuss issues important to young people such as drug misuse, smoking, and sexual health and relationships.

Health promotion for any group of people must be accessible. Specific services such as advice on HIV/AIDS and drug counselling can be provided through youth centres and clubs. Young people are one group for whom an empowerment approach is essential. With this group attempts to preach or use authoritarian approaches will at best be useless and more likely worse than useless. Young people tend to be greatly influenced by peer pressure. Effective health promotion uses peer opinion leaders, and recruits the young themselves as health promoters.

The potential for health promotion in schools is considerable, as described in Chapter 13. School health services must work in collaboration with other community services.

CASE STUDY: A HEALTH PROBLEM IN AN INFANT-SCHOOL PUPIL

Michael, aged five, is due to start school. His mother has received a questionnaire, from the school nurse, which asks about Michael's health. One question relates to bowel and bladder control and is specifically about bedwetting. Michael's mother has been concerned during the past year that Michael is still wetting the bed even though he remembers to go to the toilet during the day and rarely has any accidents.

A week or so after she returned the questionnaire, Michael's mother received a helpful letter from the school nurse acknowledging Michael's problem and explaining she would be following this up in a year's time if he was still bedwetting. The letter explained that bedwetting is common in 12–15 per cent of five-year-olds, and that many children achieved bladder control by the time they were six or seven without specialist treatment. A leaflet explaining how normal bladder control was achieved was enclosed.

By the following year Michael was still bedwetting and the school nurse discussed with his mother his referral to the enuretic clinic held jointly by the school nurse and the community paediatrician. Michael and his mother were sent an appointment and asked to complete a chart to indicate when Michael was wet and when he was dry.

At the first appointment a history and examination were performed to decide on the treatment. As Michael liked to draw, he was asked to complete a chart colouring in pictures for the nights he was dry. He was seen regularly in the clinic and his progress monitored by the school nurse.

Although there was some improvement after several months, it was decided that Michael would probably benefit from an enuretic alarm. Its use was explained to Michael and his mother and the school nurse made a follow-up visit at home to make sure he was using it correctly. Within a month Michael was consistently having dry nights.

DRUG PREVENTION TEAMS

In some areas drug prevention teams have been established with the help of Home Office funding. Team members may come from a variety of backgrounds, including youth and social workers, psychiatric nurses, the probation service and others. Such teams have to work closely with education authorities, schools, local councils, police, parents and families, tenants' groups, local youth workers and voluntary groups. This is essential as the members of the team need to develop relationships with the community. They can then increase the community's power to resist drug taking by raising awareness, increasing self-help skills and providing clear information.

LIBRARIES

Libraries are an important focal point of the community and used by many people. They have a wealth of information on all sorts of things in books, magazines and specialist journals as well as in other media. Librarians are trained to help people access the information they want. Members of a community will often turn to the library first when they want information on any subject.

Health promoters cannot ignore such a useful ally. Libraries often put on displays about health and social issues affecting that particular community. People may also look to the local library for addresses of societies and groups that provide help for people worried about particular health problems. For example:

- Association for Stammerers
- British Heart Foundation
- Chest, Heart and Stroke Association
- Health Education Authority

CHEMISTS' SHOPS

Chemists are increasingly ready to provide health advice (Smith 1992; Todd 1993). This may involve advising customers on appropriate off-the-shelf medicines. It may concern the side-effects and contra-indications of prescribed medications and how to take these medications effectively. It could cover sugar-free baby foods and medicines (Manley, Sheiham and Eadsforth 1994). They also provide advice on when it would be more appropriate to seek the doctor's advice. Pharmacy staff can play a major part in prevention of diseases such as skin cancer by advising customers when they buy suntan lotions and sunscreens. Customers may receive advice on smoking-related problems when they buy nicotine patches and gum. Providing health promotion in this way expands and adds value to the role of counter staff in chemists.

HEALTH PROMOTION IN THE HIGH STREET

There are many activities which are not usually thought of as health promotion but which none the less support health promotion in the community. Many companies link their products to health as a marketing strategy and they therefore provide information about health. For example:

- supermarkets promoting low-fat products and giving out leaflets on low-fat foods
- TV advertisements for high-fibre cereals stressing the importance of fibre in our daily diet
- advertisements for sports equipment emphasising the pleasures and advantages of exercise

Stories and features in newspapers, magazines, TV and radio are a further source of information. For example:

- programmes on TV about HIV and safer sex
- a newspaper report of a road traffic accident which reinforces the need for people to wear seat belts
- feature article about some personality who has had alcohol problems and overcome them

These reminders of health issues are to be found in every community. Whether individuals see the information, understand it or decide to act on it is unpredictable. Certainly commercial interests will have designed their marketing and advertising with the intention that it will reach a specific target audience. Health workers need to be aware of this background health information and seek to build on it. For example, if a story in the local media has raised interest in fires, it may be a particularly good time to raise the issue of fire safety with clients. Equally it may be possible to increase the impact of a local health event if local retailers can be persuaded to tie in a relevant promotion at the same time. For example, if you have organised a healthy eating display at the health centre, the local supermarket might be willing to make a special offer on healthier food lines.

Discussion/Activity 16.3 Incidental activity supporting health promotion

Think back over the last week. Have you seen any advertisements or sales promotions in local shops that might influence your health and lifestyle? Have there been any stories or features in magazines or papers that you have read or programmes on TV or radio that might influence your health behaviour? What were the motives of the people who produced these things that you have seen or heard?

COMMUNITY SELF-HELP

Health promoters in the community must recognise that the community's greatest resources for health are its members. The role of the health promoter is to help people in the community to recognise how their health could be improved and then to assist them in pressing for the necessary changes. The solutions may lie wholly within the community, or its members may have to lobby outside the community to obtain funds or other resources. Events in one large village illustrate how health care workers can help. A large number of mothers with pre-school children lived in the village but there was no nursery or playgroup in the vicinity. The health visitor became aware that many of the mothers wanted to set up a playgroup. This would give them a chance to meet other mothers and children and allow them to do the shopping or just have a break while someone else cared for the children.

The health visitor acted as a catalyst by bringing the mothers together to co-ordinate their efforts and helping them to hire the church hall, raise funds to buy toys and equipment and draw up rosters.

TENANTS, AND SIMILAR COMMUNITY GROUPS

Tenants, and similar community groups can be channels through which the community expresses its wants and through which one can engage in discussion with the community. The health promoter needs to seek out such groups and develop positive relationships with them. Groups which run well will control their own meetings and agenda, and some health professionals may find this relationship uncomfortable (Hunt 1990). The health worker may seek the permission of the group to attend some meetings. They can then listen to the group's views of the community's problems and needs and possible solutions. This approach will help identify the issues that are important to the community as opposed to those that the health professional considers important. Developing effective communication in this way is vital to achieving health promotion.

When the health worker consults members of the community, they run the risk that the people consulted get unrealistic expectations and then become disillusioned when these cannot be fulfilled. In order to avoid this, community health workers have to be honest about what they can and cannot deliver. One also has to remember that some sections of the community may not be represented by community groups. For example, a residents' association may be dominated by one ethnic group and fail to represent the views of members of other ethnic groups.

The range of health issues that might be raised by community groups are enormous. Some examples, together with possible solutions, are listed in Table 16.3

Developing close links with community groups will also provide health promoters with opportunities to become involved. They might be invited to contribute to local events such as fêtes and carnivals or to discuss health issues with other groups.

Table 16.3 Community health concerns and solutions

Health concern	Community action solution
• unemployment increasing physical and mental ill health	• set up factories and businesses in the locality to provide jobs
• speeding traffic increasing risk of accidents	• speed humps and traffic-calming measures
• drug and solvent abuse	• police to arrest and prosecute dealers
• contaminated rivers and streams where children play	• force local industry to stop polluting watercourses
• lack of pre-school child care facilities	• provide nursery class
• long waiting times for hospital appointments	• improve health services
• broken and uneven footpaths have caused several falls	• council to repair footpaths
• dog excrement in the children's play areas	• enforce by-laws on dog fouling
• increasing smoking, particularly in teenagers	• more health education in schools

Discussion/Activity 16.4 Community health concerns

Consider the community or locality in which you live. What do you think are the major health concerns? Has anything been done about them? Who could do anything about them? What do you see as the priorities?

COMMUNITY PARTICIPATION IN SERVICE PLANNING

Residents should be involved in planning and implementing health care and other services for their community (NAHAT 1992; Bowling, Jacobson and Southgate 1993). A pioneering exercise in consultation was attempted in the state of Oregon in the USA in order to decide what services the state should provide for its population. The problems encountered and the controversies engendered by the Oregon experiment hold many lessons for the National Health Service in the UK (Bowling 1992).

At a more local level, people might be asked what facilities they wanted and to comment on the plans for a new health centre. Members of the community should have the opportunity to influence the types of services provided and the relative priorities given to – for example – physiotherapy, chiropody and dental services. Other ways in which participation can be encouraged include user groups (e.g. patients from a particular general practice or patients who have used a particular hospital service) so that local consumers can comment on the running of local health services. The difficulties of making participation work are further discussed in Chapter 18.

COMMUNITY DEVELOPMENT

Community action occurs when members of communities work together to demand changes in their environment or in the services delivered to them in order to improve their health. Table 16.3 suggests community action solutions to the health concerns listed. Often community action looks to authorities outside the community to take action to provide community rights. The health worker may adopt a community development role and encourage members of the community to do such things as write to their councillors and MPs; write to the press; picket, lobby and march to obtain the changes they want. The community action worker will help the community acquire the relevant skills and use all the ways of influencing policy makers described in Chapter 8. There are many examples of community action leading to the closure of polluting industrial processes, abandonment of plans to build roads through residential areas, installation of traffic lights and zebra crossings, or provision of health services (Sutcliffe 1994). Sadly it is harder to think of examples of employment being created by this type of community action. Accounts of community development projects improving health are given in Rosenthal (1983) and Butler and Cass (1993).

Community action is most effective when pressure on others to respect the community's rights is coupled with the determination of the community to help themselves. Thus the reasonable demand that police should take action against drug dealers will be of little use unless the community also tries to reduce the demand for drugs. Demands for the enforcement of by-laws on dog fouling imply that dog owners within the community will also take action to ensure that their pets are not contributing to the problem.

SUMMARY POINTS

People live in communities. Therefore health promotion activities should take place in communities and be relevant to life in the community.

Nurses and other health promoters have to co-operate. Community health events are one setting in which this can be done.

Staff working in people's homes should:

- ☐ recognise the many opportunities for health promotion
- ☐ remember that the client's priorities may not be the same as their own
- ☐ not raise unrealistic expectations
- ☐ develop positive, trusting relationships with their clients
- ☐ adapt advice and skills teaching to reflect the needs and unique situations of the client
- ☐ remember the needs of informal carers

The community can access health promotion and health education through many channels:

- ☐ clinics and health centres
- ☐ drop-in centres, health shops and help-lines
- ☐ schools and youth clubs
- ☐ libraries
- ☐ chemists' shops

There are many resources such as tenants and similar community groups that can be mobilised for health in any community. Community development emphasises self-help and combined action to improve the health of the community.

REFERENCES

Bowling A. (1992). Setting priorities in health: the Oregon experiment. *Nursing Standard* **6** (No. 38), 28–30.

Bowling A., Jacobson B. and Southgate L. (1993). Explorations in consultation of the public and health professionals on priority setting in an inner London health district. *Social Sciences and Medicine* **37**, 851–857.

Butler P. and Cass S. (1993). *Case studies of community development for health.* Blackburn: Centre for Development and Innovation in Health.

Cassidy J. (1994). Joining forces. *Nursing Times* **90** (No. 2), 16–17.

Dalziel Y. (1992) Breaking down the barriers. *Health Visitor* **65**, 228–229.

DoH (Department of Health) (1993). *Targeting practice: the contribution of nurses, midwives and health visitors.* The Health of the Nation. London: HMSO.

Evans P. (1993). Back to basics. *Nursing Times* **89** (No. 48), 48–50.

Fawcett H. (1993). Heartfelt advice. *Nursing Times* **89** (No. 47), 36–38.

Gane S. (1994). Time for a change. *Nursing Times* **90** (No. 4), 37–38.

Graham H. (1992). Informal care: problem or solution? *Health Visitor* **65**, 444–445.

Hick A. (1991). Pick it up with the shopping. *Health Services Journal* **101** (14 March), 24–25.

Hunt S. (1990). Building alliances: professional and political issues in community participation. *Health Promotion International* **5**, 179–186.

Magill-Cuerden J. (1993). The midwife's key role throughout pregnancy. *Modern Midwife* **3** (No. 6), 16–17.

Malin A. and May S. (1992). A health shop to meet public needs. *Professional Nurse* **7**, 392–394.

Manley G., Sheiham A. and Eadsforth W. (1994). Sugar coated care? *Nursing Times* **90** (No. 7), 34–35.

NAHAT (National Association of Health Authorities and Trusts) (1992). *Listening to local voices.* Birmingham: NAHAT.

Reid T. (1993). Partners in care. *Nursing Times* **89** (No. 33), 28–30.

Richardson N. (1993). Fit for the future. *Nursing Times* **89** (No. 44), 36–38.

Rosenthal H. (1983). Neighbourhood health projects – some new approaches to health and community work in parts of the UK. *Community Development Journal* **18**, 120–131.

Scally G. (1993). Teenage pregnancies: the challenge of prevention. *Midwives' Chronicle* **106**, 232–239.

Shepherd G. (1984). Institutional care and rehabilitation. New York: Longman.

Siney C. (1994). Team effort helps pregnant drug users. *Modern Midwifery* **4** (No. 2), 23–24.

Smith F. (1992). Community pharmacists and health promotion: a study of consultations between pharmacists and clients. *Health Promotion International* **7**, 249–255.

Spooner B. and Rudge G. (1993). Tasteful pictures. *Nursing Times* **89** (No. 33), 34–36.

Sutcliffe P. (1994). Ancoats: community health in action. *Health Visitor* **67** (No. 1), 30–32.

Thompson J. (1993). Supporting young mothers. *Nursing Times* **89** (No. 51), 64–67.

Todd J. (1993). The high street health scheme. Promoting health in the community pharmacy. *Health Education Journal* 52, 34–36.

Tyler C. (1993). Travellers tale. *Nursing Times* 89 (No. 33), 26–27.

Watt A. and Rodmell S. (1987). Community involvement in health promotion: progress or panacea. *Health Promotion* 2, 359–368.

White A.E. (1983). Teaching those in need in the community. Chapter 1 in Wilson-Barnett J. (ed.), *Patient teaching*. Edinburgh: Churchill Livingstone.

CHAPTER 17

Health promotion in the workplace

Margaret Bamford, PhD
Acting Director of Nursing Services, West Midlands Health

GOAL

To develop a greater understanding of the opportunities for health promotion in the workplace and the ways in which it can be delivered.

OBJECTIVES

- to appreciate the need for health promotion in the workplace
- to explain the purpose of occupational health services
- to describe the staffing of occupational service and the activities undertaken
- to understand the importance of controlling workplace hazards
- to appreciate that responsibility for workplace health must be shared between employers and employees
- to recognise the scope for extending workplace health promotion to non-occupation issues

THE NEED FOR WORKPLACE HEALTH PROMOTION

The nation relies on its workers to generate the wealth needed to provide health and social services. It therefore seems wise to pay particular attention to the health needs of this group by targeting health education and health promotion at the workplace. People at work:

- constitute nearly half the population of the United Kingdom
- cannot benefit from community-based health promotion activities in work hours
- sometimes have difficulty in getting to their general practitioner's services
- are a captive audience in the workplace for at least eight hours a day

For all these reasons it makes sense to use workplace health promotion to improve not only occupational health but also health in its widest sense. Ashton (1989) remarks: 'organisations, together with occupational health physicians and nurses, are in a unique position to influence the health of the workforce in this country [UK]'.

The working population is generally considered by health professionals and itself to be 'well'. In a recent survey (Bamford 1993), 92 per cent of a sample of people at work answered 'yes' when asked if they considered themselves to be healthy. People know how they feel, and are able to make judgments about their state of health. Workplace-based health promotion has to start from the premise that it is aimed chiefly at healthy people. It is intended to maintain health and to help workers make healthy choices so that they can continue in a state of health.

HEALTH FOR ALL BY THE YEAR 2000

The European targets for Health for All by the year 2000 included a section on targets for the workplace. Target number 25 states:

> By 1995, people of the Region should be effectively protected against work-related health risks. The achievement of this target will require the introduction of appropriate occupational health services to cover the needs of all workers: the development of health criteria for the protection of workers against biological, chemical and physical hazards; the implementation of technical and educational measures to reduce work-related risk factors; and the safeguarding of specially vulnerable groups of workers. (WHO 1985)

THE PURPOSE OF OCCUPATIONAL HEALTH SERVICES

Occupational health services are concerned with the effects of work on health and of health on work. The International Labour Organisation (ILO) defines occupational health services in the following convention:

> Occupational health services mean services entrusted with essentially preventive functions and responsibilities for advising the employer, the workers and their representatives in the undertaking on:
>
> (i) the requirements for establishing and maintaining a safe and healthy working environment which will facilitate optimal physical and mental health in relation to work;

(ii) the adaptation of work to the capabilities of workers in the light of their state of physical and mental health (Health and Safety Commission 1986).

The World Health Organisation (WHO) expands on this in its definition of the occupational health task as:

1. to identify and bring under control at the workplace all chemical, physical, mechanical, biological and psychosocial agents that are known to be or suspected of being hazardous;
2. to ensure that the physical and mental demands imposed on people at work by their respective jobs are properly matched with their individual anatomical, physiological and psychological capabilities, needs and limitations;
3. to provide effective measures to protect those who are especially vulnerable to adverse working conditions (WHO 1975).

HEALTH SERVICES FOR THE WORKPLACE

Health in the workplace is regulated by the Department of Employment and not the Department of Health. The Health and Safety Commission and its operational arm, the Health and Safety Executive, are the main agents enforcing health and safety at work. There is a minimum requirement that employers ensure the availability of first aiders (HMSO 1981), and allow workers access to staff of the Health and Safety Executive for certain prescribed medical examinations and screenings. However, there is no legal requirement for an employer to provide a health service in the workplace.

Occupational health services advise employees on health and work-related issues. Occupational health services also have the specific task of assisting managers to manage the organisation. Health supervision programmes are one of the main ways in which occupational health services protect the health of employees. The nature of the programme will depend on the particular problems of the organisation. Activities undertaken by occupational health services may include:

- health assessment before and during employment
- treatment of occupational and non-occupational problems
- counselling
- preventing occupational accidents and occupational disease
- workplace environment control

The occupational health service may also extend its role into general health promotion for employees.

THE OCCUPATIONAL HEALTH TEAM

The staffing of an occupational health service will depend on the size and complexity of the organisation. Most occupational health services will have full-time nurses. Other members of the team may include doctors, physiotherapists, safety engineers and occupational hygienists (to monitor and manage the environment). These others will have a variable input, depending on the breadth and range of activities. Physiotherapists are particularly likely to be included in the team in organisations where repetitive strain injury is a major concern. At one time, all organisations that used lead in any quantity would also have employed a dentist. This was because lead affects the gums of people who work with it, and damage could be prevented by regular inspections, and treatment.

HEALTH ASSESSMENT IN THE WORKPLACE

Pre-employment assessment is used to determine workers' suitability for the type of work proposed for them. It is also used to establish an individual benchmark before employment so that any later deterioration in a worker's state of health can be noticed. In occupational health it is more usual to pay attention to changes in a worker's health state than to set minimum levels. For example, in a worker exposed to noise one is more concerned to prevent deterioration of hearing than to set a general level of hearing below which action has to be taken. The pre-employment assessment may range from checking a self-completed health questionnaire through to a full medical examination.

Another form of health assessment which is now emerging in some organisations is that of checking for substance abuse. There are certain occupations in which workers must not drink alcohol or use other drugs in the time immediately before coming to work. These include public transport workers, drivers, people working on high scaffolds and people taking responsibility for other people's lives, such as doctors, nurses and teachers. This form of screening will probably become more widespread as the tests become more sophisticated.

TREATMENT SERVICES

Many occupational health services offer treatments, which deal not only with work-related conditions but also with non-occupational health conditions. Treatments could include such things as syringeing ears, suturing of lacerations, treatment of skin conditions, simple physiotherapy, treatment of minor injuries and treatment of coughs and colds. The agreement of the worker's family doctor has to be sought for anything other than urgent treatment.

Many services offer rehabilitation programmes. General rehabilitation after accident or illness is sometimes included in the programme. However, the main emphasis will be on rehabilitation specifically aimed at getting workers back to their job in the workplace. Examples of workers needing rehabilitation would be a man returning to work after suffering a myocardial infarction (heart attack), or a new mother returning to work following the birth of her first baby.

Occupational health services need to liaise with a whole range of other agencies in order to care for the employees. Sometimes the task is made difficult by other health professionals who do not understand the special relationships that exist in the workplace, and do not acknowledge the need to work together for the health of the people at work.

COUNSELLING

Many features of a person's life can affect their ability to function at work. People do not leave other aspects of their lives at home when they come to work. If they are tired, they will be tired at work. If they are unhappy, their unhappiness comes to work with them. Therefore counselling is an important part of the occupational health nurse's role. This may just be immediate 'first aid' counselling to establish the nature of the problem before moving the person on to more skilled counselling colleagues. Those who require counselling could include, for example, someone who has been recently bereaved, someone trying to battle with a drinking or other addiction problem or someone who has witnessed a fatal accident in the workplace. Counselling may also be used to help people cope with work-related stress.

OCCUPATIONAL HEALTH RECORDS

Keeping appropriate records is an important part of the work of an occupational health service. There are certain statutory records relating to accidents and dangerous occurrences in the workplace which must be kept. The Control of Substances Hazardous to Health Regulations (COSHH) require records to be kept of employees' exposure to specific substances, and the results of their health supervision in relation to that exposure (HMSO 1988). These regulations apply to workplaces which come under the Health and Safety at Work Act 1974 – in effect, all places where people work (HMSO 1970). National Health Service and other Crown premises are now covered by these regulations.

Discussion/Activity 17.1 Your occupational health service

Do you have access to an occupational health service? Who is available in that service for you to consult? What services are provided? Do you have access to an occupational health nurse and doctor? Does your organisation have access to an occupational hygienist? Is there a safety engineer? How would you get advice on issues related to health and safety at your workplace?

OCCUPATIONAL DISEASE AND OCCUPATIONAL ACCIDENTS

For a long time occupational health has emphasised safety and accident prevention rather than health promotion and disease prevention. However, workers are more likely to die of an occupational disease than from an occupational accident. In 1991, 538 people were killed in accidents in the workplace (Health and Safety Commission 1991). The precise number who die from occupational diseases each year is not known but has been estimated at 750 per year (Central Statistical Office 1987). A recent study (the Labour Force Survey) for the Health and Safety Executive showed that occupational incidents are grossly under-reported. The Reporting of Injuries, Diseases and Dangerous Occurrences Regulations 1985 (RIDDOR), requires that all injuries at work should be reported (Health and Safety Executive 1986) but it is possible that only a third of non-fatal injuries are reported. Other researchers feel that occupational disease is similarly under-reported. The total cost to society of workplace accidents and work-related ill health was estimated to be between £11 billion and £16 billion in 1992 (Health and Safety Commission 1993). This is a very large sum of money which could be used to promote health in the workplace or more generally in society.

SAFETY AT WORK

Much workplace health promotion has concentrated on prevention of accidents. Workers in hazardous industries will probably have been exposed to health education on workplace dangers. This education usually stresses compliance with safety measures, such as

Table 17.1 Hazardous substances listed in the Reporting of Injuries, Diseases and Dangerous Occurrences Regulations (RIDDOR)

acrylamide monomer
arsenic or one of its compounds
benzene or a homologue of benzene
beryllium or one of its compounds
cadmium or one of its compounds
carbon disulphide
diethylene dioxide (dioxin)
ethylene oxide
lead or one of its compounds
manganese or one of its compounds
mercury or one of its compounds
methyl bromide
nitrochlorobenzene, or a nitro- or amino- or chloro-derivative of benzene or of a homologue of benzene
oxides of nitrogen
phosphorus or one of its compounds

wearing protective clothing, using protective equipment and safe ways of working.

People who will be working with certain specified substances (see Table 17.1) prescribed in the RIDDOR regulations 1985, require special health surveillance (Health and Safety Executive 1986). There is a statutory requirement that they have a medical assessment before starting work and repeat assessments at prescribed intervals during their working year. The health assessment or medical examination is also an opportunity for health education. Those who work with hazardous substances must be instructed on how to handle them safely and on the use of protective clothing.

All workers need to understand the safe working practices that they must observe. Everyone working on dangerous processes or in dangerous settings must learn the ways of working that will protect them. This is important not only for the safety of the individual concerned, but also because unsafe working by one worker may endanger their work colleagues. In some situations unsafe working may also create risk for members of the public.

Occupational safety involves making sure that the equipment that people are using is safe, properly guarded and properly maintained. It also involves making sure that workers know how to work with the safety features provided.

ENVIRONMENTAL CONTROL

The employer has a responsibility to make the environment in which people work as safe as possible (see Table 17.2). Every

Table 17.2 Steps in environmental control

1. Assess all hazards in workplace.
2. Where possible, redesign workplace or job to remove hazard
   e.g. substitute a less harmful substance or practice
   store hazardous chemicals at a different site
   redesign shelving to eliminate need for high lifts.
3. Segregate the worker from the potential hazard
   e.g. total or partial enclosure of processes
   use ventilation systems to remove substances from breathing zone.
4. Provide safety equipment
   e.g. machine guards, noise baffles, etc.
5. Provide safety clothing – gloves, boots, goggles, overalls, etc.
6. Educate workforce about hazards and safe ways of working.

workplace must be assessed for hazards and then the hazards must be removed or minimised. Everything must be done to control dangerous activities and remove or control dangerous and noxious substances. There is no point in doing sophisticated health assessment procedures if the employee is then required to work in an unsafe environment. Protective clothing or equipment is not a substitute for environmental control. Indeed, protective clothing can contribute to accidents by limiting the worker's vision, hearing or mobility.

PARTNERSHIPS FOR HEALTH PROMOTION IN THE WORKPLACE

In occupational health as with health in other settings there is debate as to what extent the individual (in this instance, the worker) is responsible for their own health. In 1976, a government publication – 'Prevention and health: everybody's business' (DHSS 1976) – included this statement:

> To a large extent though, it is clear that the weight of responsibility for his own state of health lies on the shoulders of the individual himself.

While this may have reflected the attitudes of society at that time, the view on the links between health and behaviour is changing. Five years later the Black Report clearly showed that the behaviour of individuals could not explain the wide variations in health (Townsend and Davidson 1992).

At one time, it was similarly held that individual workers were responsible for the occupational accidents they suffered and the occupational diseases they contracted. Though comfortable for employers, this view is clearly wrong. One of the first to realise this was Sir Thomas Legge, the first medical inspector of factories. He resigned his post when the government of the day refused to ratify an international convention prohibiting the use of white lead for internal paintwork. He had a passion for the health of people at work and aptly summarised the balance of employers' and employees' responsibilities for workplace safety in this aphorism:

> unless and until the employer has done everything – and everything means a good deal – the workman can do next to nothing to protect himself, although he is naturally willing enough to do his share (Legge 1934, p. 3)

We have moved a long way from the philosophy which allows employers to disregard the safety of their workforce. The trade unions and employees' organisations have a long tradition of co-operation with employers' organisations in a partnership to manage workplace health and safety issues. Employees can contribute to safety at work by following safe working procedures and making use of protective equipment provided. However, it is the responsibility of management to make safety equipment available and to ensure that workers do observe safety procedures in the workplace. In most workplaces there is a partnership for safety between employer and employees.

STRESS

As organisations have controlled or removed physical dangers from the workplace they have been able to consider the broader issues affecting health. There is increased awareness of the effects of the working environment and work practices on the mental health of employees. Work gives people their place in society, it gives them a sense of purpose, and is often seen as a rewarding thing to do. Watson (1987) sees work as the 'Carrying out of tasks which enable people to make a living within the environment in which they find themselves'. Some jobs such as those in emergency services and health care, those requiring workers to deal with the public every day and those requiring people to work in isolation are stressful by their very nature. Some people thrive in these stressful jobs. For others the stress or pressure associated with work is too much, and they experience difficulty in coping with the demands of the job.

More and more people experience work-related stress. They may fear redundancy, or worry about not being able to keep up with the pace of work as they age or not being able to adjust to changes in the working environment. These feelings are not unknown among health care workers.

There are various ways in which damage to workers' health by stress can be reduced. When jobs are unavoidably stressful, occupational health staff can help workers tolerate work by counselling and by teaching them coping strategies. Better still, enlightened management can reduce anxiety and stress in the workplace by improving the job so it generates less stress. Ways of doing this include changing the organisation to reduce role ambiguity, increasing workers' participation in decision making, and increasing social support for staff (Argyle 1989: HEA 1992).

Discussion/Activity 17.2 Is your work stressful?

How do you feel about the work that you do? How do you recognise someone who is stressed? Are you stressed? Do you feel that the organisation cares about you? What could be done to reduce the stress? What strategies could help you cope with the stress better?

What is there about the way you do your work that might cause stress in others?

GENERAL HEALTH PROMOTION IN THE WORKPLACE

In the past the need to control the more obvious workplace hazards was so pressing that it was not possible to consider more general issues of health promotion. Now however workplace health promotion should be broadening its horizons. It should be concerned not only with the avoidance of occupational accidents and disease but also with the general health and well-being of the workers. Where they exist, occupational health services should take a lead in tackling not only specific organisational needs but also issues such as eating, smoking, drinking and exercise.

Widening the remit of occupational health services is not to reduce the importance of occupational health promotion and education, but to put it into place alongside those general health issues which are embodied in the Health of the Nation targets (DoH 1992). It is essential that in the enthusiasm to extend workplace health promotion, occupational accidents and occupational diseases are not forgotten. They are still a problem and new ones are still being identified.

The occupational health staff can contribute to these broader health programmes by advising on the development and implementation of health promotion policies in the organisation. Policies have to be realistic both in terms of costs to the company and as to what the employees could reasonably be expected to do.

BENEFITS TO EMPLOYER OF WORKPLACE HEALTH PROMOTION

Commercial organisations exist to make a profit not to provide welfare for their employees. Employers may therefore need to be persuaded that the introduction of health promotion activities to their workplace will increase or at least not decrease their ability to operate profitably.

The costs of ill health in the workforce to the employer are considerable. They include:

- costs of replacing staff lost by death or by retirement on health grounds
- costs of sick pay for short periods of sickness absence
- costs of disruption of production due to sickness absence
- costs of reduced productivity and impaired work performance from employees feeling unwell
- costs of management time in assessing ability of sick employees to continue work, negotiating retirement on health grounds, dismissal, etc.
- legal costs when employees allege that injuries and health problems are work-related

The benefits to the employer of workplace health promotion schemes are:

- reduction in costs of ill health listed above
- increased goodwill from employees
- increased production resulting from fitter employees
- improved image of organisation as a caring, socially responsible employer

Most employers recognise that their workforce is their greatest asset and they can see that broad health promotion in the workplace makes commercial sense as a way of protecting that asset.

EXPERIENCE WITH WORKPLACE HEALTH PROMOTION

Some of the most impressive initiatives in workplace health promotion have been taken in the USA. In part this may have been because many American companies include health insurance as a work benefit for their employees. The escalating costs of health care meant that many employers looked to find ways of reducing costs by keeping their employees well. To this end, many companies sought to encourage healthy lifestyles in their employees by

Table 17.3 Some UK companies with worksite health promotion programmes

1. British Steel PLC	7. Glaxo Pharmaceuticals UK Ltd	11. Nissan Motor Manufacturing (UK) Ltd
2. British Telecommunication PLC	8. IBM United Kingdom Ltd	12. Polaroid (UK) Ltd
3. Cadbury Schweppes PLC	9. Kelloggs Company of Great Britain Ltd	13. Post Office
4. Courtaulds PLC	10 Marks & Spencer PLC	14. Price Waterhouse
5. Du Pont (UK) Ltd		15. Rank Xerox (UK) Ltd
6. Ford Motor Co. Ltd		16. Shell UK Ltd
		17. Thomas Cook Group Ltd

providing health promotion in the workplace. Controlled studies (Bly, Jones and Richardson 1986) suggest this was effective.

Although many UK companies do not have the same financial incentive, many are now introducing similar workplace health promotion schemes. Table 17.3 lists some of the UK companies which already have worksite health promotion policies. Recently the Health Education Authority surveyed major employers, employers' associations, trade unions and organisations with interest in workplace health promotion. The report (Webb *et al.* 1988) found wide variation among organisations but identified certain common themes. Alcohol, stress and nutrition programmes were found to equal or outnumber programmes on the traditional occupational health issues of safety, noise and dusts. Many firms were planning further health promotion activities such as stop-smoking programmes and well-woman or well-man screening. General welfare advice programmes were becoming less common.

HEALTHY EATING PROGRAMMES

People are becoming more aware of their diet and how it affects their health. The occupational health nurses can build on this interest, reinforce people's positive feelings about healthy eating and give them reliable nutritional information. Routine health assessments can be used to give healthy eating advice. This is a particularly favourable setting for health promotion since the nurse and employee are together without interruption in a one-to-one relationship, totally focused on the individual.

There is also the opportunity for site-wide campaigns to educate people about healthy-eating issues. This may be by means of posters and notices in strategic places in the workplace. Special leaflets could be placed in wage packets, or circulated to individuals at their work station. In some companies, there will be opportunities for seminars and formal teaching sessions during induction programmes, or other workplace gatherings.

Workplace promotion of healthy eating will not be effective unless the healthy choices are available in the staff restaurants. The menus offered must make it easy for the staff to put into practice the behavioural changes advocated.

NO-SMOKING POLICIES

Many workplaces now have a no-smoking policy which either restricts smoking to a designated area or bans smoking anywhere on the premises. No-smoking policies need to be fully negotiated with the staff and carefully introduced (HEA 1987), paying full attention to employment law (Howard 1990). When the policy is introduced, people who do smoke should be offered help to cut down or stop their smoking (Norris 1991). Where occupational health staff are involved in helping people stop smoking, they must set an example by not smoking themselves.

More people are becoming aware of the effects of passive smoking, and are not prepared to tolerate other people's behaviour affecting their health. Some organisations have a no-smoking policy not for health reasons, but in order to protect the product, such as food, or because the product they deal with is particularly flammable or explosive. In these circumstances, the occupational health staff can build on this workplace requirement to encourage employees to stop smoking altogether.

SENSIBLE-DRINKING PROGRAMMES

Workplace sensible-drinking policies have presented some difficulties (HEA 1989). A sensible-drinking policy has to cover:

- management and disciplinary aspects to ensure that drinking does not interfere with workers' ability to work
- general health education to encourage people to avoid drinking behaviour that will damage their health
- personnel and occupational health aspects for early detection of people who are damaging their health and to offer help

There are various difficulties that may be encountered. Some workplaces have social clubs which depend on alcohol sales for their continuation. Alcohol workplace policies will not succeed unless they are seen to be equitable and to apply to all. There may be particular resistance from senior managers who, because of working lunches, social gatherings in the workplace, seminars, workshops and conferences, feel they cannot avoid heavy drinking. Practices such as providing drinks cabinets in senior managers' offices so that they can offer 'hospitality' to visitors have to be challenged.

Workers should not be carrying out their work when their judgment is impaired by alcohol. This applies to all work, not just driving, work with machines and work in dangerous situations. Management action, backed up by health education, is required to persuade people that drinking is not acceptable in the work setting even though it is a reasonable social activity in outside work.

EXERCISE FOR THE WORKFORCE

There has been considerable interest in worksite promotion of exercise, and many different arrangements have been tried. Historically, many large employers provided recreation facilities for their employees and encouraged them to take part in sport. These facilities would include pitches for team games, usually attached to a sports or social club. With the reduction in numbers of employees, and the greater distances that people now travel to get to work, these facilities have to some extent disappeared. They have been replaced with more sophisticated arrangements such as membership of a local gym at subsidised rates or on-site gym provision together with professional supervision. Evidence is emerging that those people who take regular exercise and are fit seem to have fewer periods of absenteeism, and a greater sense of job satisfaction (Shephard 1983; Shephard 1989; Ashton 1989). The Japanese have led the field in this area, and at one time were thought to be strange for doing so. In many Japanese companies, the day starts with group exercises which are repeated at set periods during the day. All people in the organisation take part.

In the past the involvement of occupational health professionals has sometimes been limited to the treatment of sports injuries. However, they should be advising people about appropriate types and levels of exercise and motivating them to be more active physically. In situations where exercise or sports facilities are less readily accessible, the occupational health staff can point out the health benefits of walking, simple stretching motions or perhaps swimming. The health message needs to be made clear: exercise need not involve expensive equipment, paying for lessons, or doing inappropriate things in the name of health. Exercise needs to be matched to the person's existing health and capabilities.

HEALTH PROMOTION IN SMALLER FIRMS

Firms may be classed as large (more than 500 employees), medium (50 to 500 employees) and small (less than 50 employees). Most health promotion in the workplace takes place within larger organisations which have had occupational health services for many years. People working in medium and small organisations often do not have access to occupational health personnel although they may be more at risk of occupational health problems (Schilling 1989). Most smaller firms do not have the management infrastructure, systems or expertise to undertake meaningful regulation of workplace safety. Many of the very small firms of five or more people are primarily concerned with surviving. They would have difficulty in arranging basic health and safety in the workplace let alone providing more general health promotion. The problem of providing health promotion can be understood when it is realised that the majority of employees in the UK work for small firms.

'HEALTH AT WORK IN THE NHS'

The government is actively targeting its own workplaces as a focus for health promotion and health education. Obviously the NHS ought to be an exemplary employer for health in the workplace. The Health Education Authority is taking a lead role in promoting the 'Health at Work in the NHS' programme aims. There is a twelve-point plan for making NHS workplaces healthier (HEA/NHS Management Executive 1992):

1. Raise awareness of health at work and healthy living.
2. Introduce a smoking policy, to provide smoking venues, stop sales of tobacco on NHS premises.
3. Provide and promote healthy choices for food.
4. Promote sensible drinking and provide support for problem drinkers.
5. Introduce physical activity programmes.
6. Promote positive mental health.
7. Encourage positive attitudes to sex.
8. Provide opportunities for all staff to have health checks and attend screenings, and appropriate follow-ups.
9. Explore changes that can be made within the work situation (this relates to environmental issues, not ergonomic issues).
10. Review health, hygiene and monitoring systems.
11. Develop management practices and monitoring systems.
12. Design a training strategy to support health initiatives and reinforce health-promoting behaviour.

Discussion/Activity 17.3 Health promotion in your workplace

Does the organisation you work for take steps to promote your health? What steps could it reasonably take? (Look at Table 14.1 for some suggestions.) What are the barriers to it being more proactive? Is there anything you can do to make your workplace healthier?

SUMMARY POINTS

There is both need and opportunity to do health promotion in the workplace.

Occupational health services exist to advise management and workers on:

- ☐ control of workplace hazards
- ☐ matching demands of job to capacity of worker
- ☐ protection of vulnerable workers

Occupational health services undertake:

- ☐ health assessment
- ☐ treatment of occupational and non-occupational conditions
- ☐ counselling
- ☐ prevention of occupational accidents and disease
- ☐ workplace environmental control

They also have opportunity to undertake broader health promotion.

Employers have a duty to do all in their power to prevent occupational accidents and disease. Employees should co-operate in making the workplace safe.

Work-related stress is a problem that can be reduced by appropriate action.

Organisations are increasingly providing workplace health promotion activities that are not specifically related to occupational hazards. These activities include:

- ☐ healthier eating programmes
- ☐ no-smoking policies
- ☐ sensible-drinking programmes
- ☐ opportunities for exercise

There are difficulties in providing health promotion in smaller firms.

The 'Health at Work in the NHS' programme seeks to make the NHS a healthy workplace.

REFERENCES

Argyle M. (1989). Stress, health and mental health. Chapter 10 in *The sociology of work* (new edition). London: Penguin.

Ashton D. (1989). *The corporate health care revolution*. London: Routledge and Kegan Paul.

Bamford M. (1993). Aspects of health amongst employed population. Doctoral Thesis, University of Aston in Birmingham.

Bly J.L., Jones R.C. and Richardson J.E. (1986). Impact of worksite health promotion on health care costs and utilisation. Evaluation of Johnson and Johnson's Live for Life programme. *Journal of American Medical Association* **256**, 3235–3240.

Central Statistical Office (1987). *Annual abstract of statistics: industrial diseases and fatal injuries at work*. London: HMSO.

DHSS (Department of Health and Social Security) (1976). *Prevention and health: everybody's business*. London: HMSO.

DoH (Department of Health) (1992). *The Health of the Nation: a strategy for health in England*. London: HMSO.

HEA (Health Education Authority) (1987). *Smoking policies at work*. London: HEA.

HEA (Health Education Authority) (1989). *Guidelines for local authorities in the development, implementation and evaluation of an alcohol policy for their staff*. London: HEA.

HEA (Health Education Authority) (1992). *Action on stress at work*. London: HEA.

HEA/NHS Management Executive (1992). *Health at work in the NHS*. London: HEA.

Health and Safety Commission (1986). *International Labour Organisation, Convention 161 and Recommendation 171 on Occupational Health Services. A Consultative Document*. London: HMSO/HSE.

Health and Safety Commission (1991). *Annual Report 1990/91*. London: HMSO.

Health and Safety Commission (1993). *Annual Report 1992/93*. London: HMSO.

Health and Safety Executive (1986). *Reporting of Injuries, Diseases and Dangerous Occurrences Regulations* 1985. London: HMSO.

HMSO (1974). *Health and Safety at Work Act 1974*. London : HMSO.

HMSO (1981). *The First Aid at Work Regulations 1981*. London: HMSO.

HMSO (1988). *Control of Substances Hazardous to Health Regulations 1988*. London: HMSO.

Howard G. (1990). The legal issues of smoking at work. *Environmental Health* **98**, 276–280.

Legge T.M. (1934). *Industrial maladies*. Oxford: Oxford University Press.

Norris A. (1991). How can you help employees give up? *Occupational Health* **43**, 303–305.

Schilling R.S.F. (1989). *Occupational health practice*. London: Butterworth.

Shephard R.J. (1983). Employees' health and fitness: the state of the art. *Preventive Medicine* **12**, 644–653.

Shephard R.J. (1989). Current perspectives on the economics of fitness and sport with particular reference to worksite programmes. *Sports Medicine* **7**, 286–309.

Townsend P. and Davidson N. (1992). *The Black Report on inequalities in health*. London: Penguin.

Watson T.J. (1987). *Sociology, work and industry* (2nd edition). London: Routledge.

Webb T., Schilling R., Jacobson B. and Babb P. (1988). *Health at work?* Research Report No. 22. London: Health Education Authority.

WHO (World Health Organisation) (1975). *Environmental and health monitoring in occupational health*. Technical Report No. 535. Geneva: WHO.

WHO (1985). *Targets for Health for All.* Copenhagen: WHO.

CHAPTER 18

Health promotion in the healthy city

GOAL

To appreciate the opportunities for health promotion in the context of healthy cities.

OBJECTIVES

- to describe the history and origins of the Healthy City movement
- to understand the organisational basis for a healthy city
- to make a community diagnosis
- to appreciate the need for participation in a healthy city
- to understand the potential of multidisciplinary and interagency working

ORIGINS OF THE HEALTHY CITY MOVEMENT

The rhetoric of Health for All is splendid (see Chapter 1, page 14). Who could object to such a concept? The difficulty is that Health for All is too big an idea to grasp. It has to be broken down into bite-size chunks to make it work. The Healthy City movement is one attempt to translate the idea of Health for All into reality.

People think of themselves as being part of the small geographical area or group in which they live. They can think about improving the health of a village or town or city. By the year 2000, three-quarters of Europeans will live in cities or large towns (Ashton 1992), so improving the health of cities would make a very significant impact on the health of the population. City dwellers identify with the city in which they live and think of themselves as 'Londoners', 'Brummies', 'Scousers' or in similar terms. There is also an administrative structure through which the city can be influenced. For all these reasons, working to improve the health of cities seemed a practical and worthwhile way of approaching Health for All.

The European region of WHO started the first Healthy City project in 1987. At that time there were 11 European cities involved, two of which – Bloomsbury/Camden and Liverpool – were in England. The cities varied widely in size, population characteristics, health problems and many other respects. The largest had populations of more than a million and the smallest a population of less than 100,000. They ranged from prosperous and elegant to poverty-stricken and run-down. What they had in common was a commitment to work towards giving their citizens the benefit of Health for All. The project was immediately a huge success and other European cities quickly asked to be recognised by WHO as 'healthy cities'. The project was expanded to include 24 and then 30 cities (see Figure 18.1). Thereafter WHO felt that there were enough cities in the project though further cities were invited to join national Healthy City networks. Now WHO is giving priority to developing the healthy city idea in countries adjusting to the post-Communist period in Eastern Europe (Kickbush 1989; Tsouros 1992).

The healthy city idea has also been taken up on other continents. Cities in the very different settings of North America, South America, Australasia and Asia are now working out what it means to be a 'healthy city' (Ashton 1992).

THE HEALTHY CITY PROCESS

Though every healthy city finds different ways of moving towards Health for All (HFA) goals, there are certain steps that are common to all:

- There is high-level political commitment to the health of the city.
- They accept the HFA principles of equity, empowerment, participation multiagency interdisciplinary working and emphasis on primary care.
- Administrative structures reflect the commitment to health and multiagency working.
- A community diagnosis is made in order to assess the health needs of the city.
- There is a widespread debate about how to make the city healthier.

Healthy city working therefore has two components:

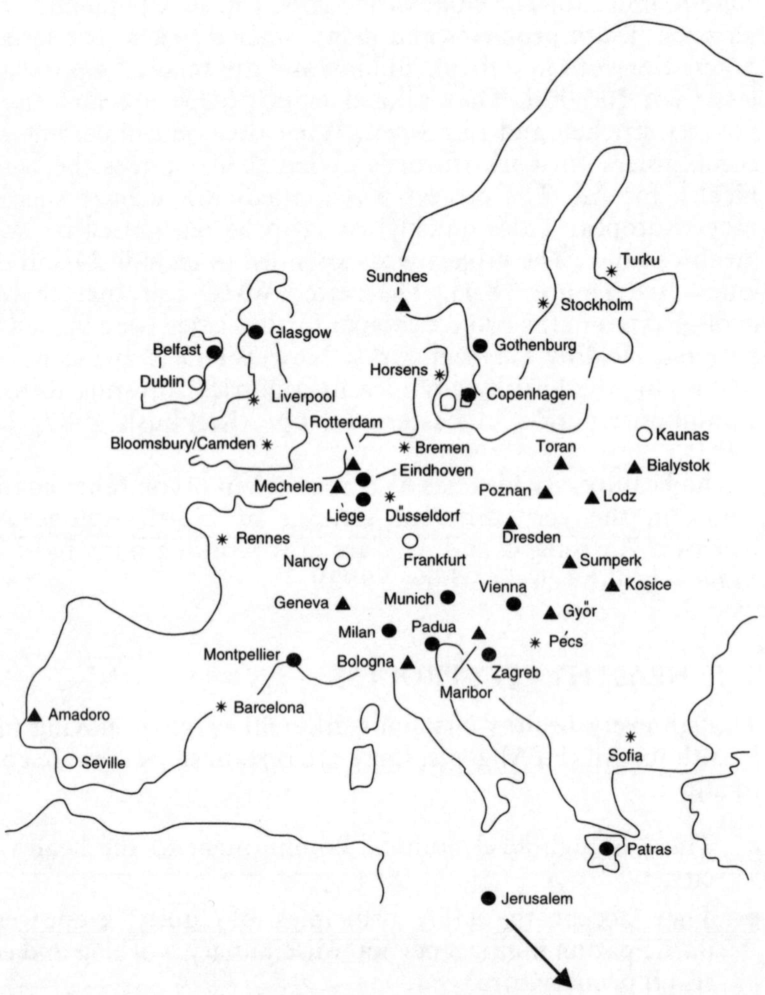

Figure 18.1 WHO Healthy Cities in Europe
The first 11 cities to become Healthy Cities in 1987 are marked with a asterisk. Those joining later are marked with a closed circle (1988) or an open circle (1989).
Source World Health Organisation, WHO Regional Office for Europe, Copenhagen

1. a top-down approach from city authorities
2. a bottom-up approach from citizens

These two themes will be discussed separately below but a successful healthy city programme requires that they should be closely interwoven.

THE COMMUNITY DIAGNOSIS

An early step in the process of becoming a healthy city is to draw together all existing information on the health of the city (Garretson, Van Gilst and Van Oers 1991; Cernick and Wearne 1992). This will include data on:

- population and births
- deaths
- disease – hospital admissions, infectious diseases, etc.
- social problems – crime, vandalism, family disputes, etc.
- economic health – unemployment, rent arrears, benefits, etc.
- health of the environment – housing, pollution, transport, etc.
- health-related lifestyle – smoking, diet, exercise, drinking, etc.
- participation – tenant groups, social clubs, religious groups, etc.
- health resources – clinics, hospitals, etc.
- education resources

These data should be collected in a way that makes it possible to identify inequalities among geographical areas such as electoral wards or housing estates and among ethnic groups.

Some of this information will be readily available, though usually it is lying in separate departments and may not have been drawn together before. Other bits of information will not be available, in which case one should simply note their absence. The information gathering needs to be done quickly so that it provides a basis for action rather than being a cause of delay. The information can be refined later on (see Chapter 9, pages 145–150). Photography can add to the community diagnosis – pictures convey impressions of the quality of life in a way that statistics cannot (Harrison 1994).

USING THE COMMUNITY DIAGNOSIS

The information from the community diagnosis will be used for several purposes:

- as a basis for policy making
- to justify resource requests
- to get local people interested and involved in their own health
- as a baseline against which later progress can be monitored

The information will need to be presented in different ways for different audiences. Council and health authority committees will want papers and reports. Seminars and workshops can be organised for interested groups. Newsletters and posters highlighting key findings can be circulated. Exhibitions and displays can be set up in libraries, shopping centres and other public places. Press releases and press briefings may also help disseminate the information. The press is always interested in health statistics, because they know their readers will also be interested.

Participation is a key Health for All principle and it follows that every effort should be made to ensure that the information from the community diagnosis is available not only to local and health authority employees but to every citizen (Binysh *et al.* 1989; Halliday and Adams 1992). As the community diagnosis develops, participation becomes even more important. City residents will not only want to see the information collected but also have a part in deciding what further information should be collected. The residents will also be needed to act as informants for much of the information (lifestyle and health worries, for example) and may also act as data collectors and interviewers. The community diagnosis can only be really successful when the citizens participate in all aspects.

The style in which the information is presented will depend on the audience. It must always be done in a way that is both easily understood and scientifically honest. Maps with different shadings, bar charts, pie diagrams and trend lines all help to communicate information. These pictures may concentrate on making comparisons between places (see Figure 18.2). How does the death rate in our city compare with the national average? Which ward in the city has the highest accident rate? Which ward has the lowest and how big is the difference?

When sharing information it is important to help people interpret the information. In particular one must give an idea of how much certainty can be attached to the information (usually by giving 95 per cent confidence limits) and whether apparent differences are likely to be real. For example, if people are told that the death rate from road traffic accidents in under fives last year was 1.23 per thousand in ward A and 4.76 in ward B, they might conclude that ward B has the greater problem. But if they also know that there was one road accident death in ward A and two deaths in ward B they will realise that we cannot be very sure that ward B is more dangerous than ward A.

Discussion/Activity 18.1 Making a community diagnosis

Think about the city or area in which you work. What information ought to go into a community diagnosis for that city or area? Where would you get the information? What do you think are the priorities for improving the health of the community?

HEALTHY CITY STRUCTURES

A healthy city will show its commitment to health by having an executive committee on which senior council members and members of other authorities such as the health authority make decisions about healthy city strategy. A technical committee of officers (paid employees of city council or health authority are referred to as officers) will have responsibility for advising the executive committee and implementing their strategic decisions. A small secretariat to prepare for meetings and chase up action after meetings is highly desirable.

There is an uncomfortable paradox in healthy city structures. The Healthy City movement must be closely integrated with city bureaucratic structures so that it is able to influence them but also sufficiently apart from them to be able to challenge aspects of city policy when necessary (Baum 1993).

HEALTHY CITY POLICY

Being a healthy city has to influence all aspects of the city function. Progress towards improving the health of the city should be on the performance review of its senior officers. The health implications of every council decision should be considered. Many councils have a standing order that all papers for council committees must consider the implications for women, ethnic minorities and people with disabilities. Implications for health could be added to this list. This does not mean that health should be the dominant factor in every council decision. There will be many times when other considerations have to override health considerations but the decision-making mechanisms should ensure that health is not simply overlooked.

It ought to be unnecessary to say that in a healthy city health authorities should also follow healthy policy. There will however be some aspects of health service operation which do not conform to the highest standards of health care or health promotion. Health authori-

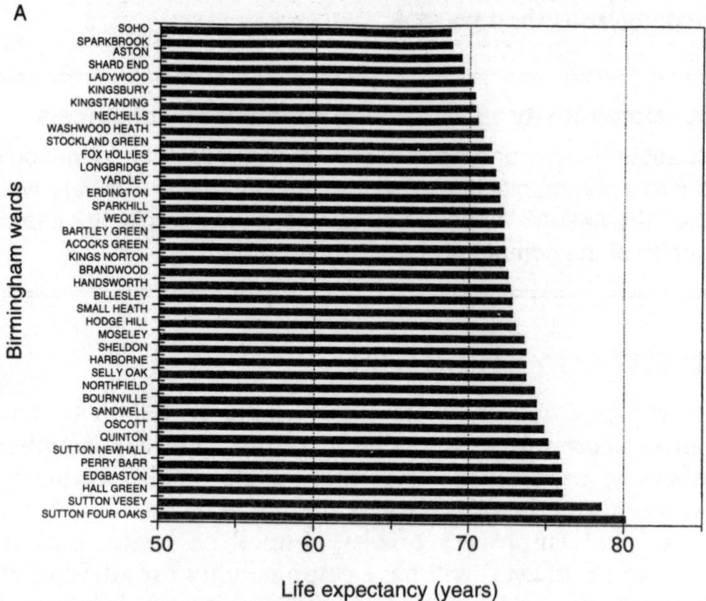

Figure 18.2 Inequalities in health in Birmingham
This is an example of how information on health inequalities can be presented in a community diagnosis.

18.2A shows differences in life expectancy in different wards of the city. Note the wide difference of 12 years between the best and the worst. (Life expectancy has been calculated by applying national age-specific death rates adjusted by the ward SMR to a notional population.)

ties need to commit themselves to Health for All principles and make sure that healthy city goals are reflected in all their activities.

HEALTHY CITY ENVIRONMENT

The environment of a healthy city should support health. Housing, transport, industry, parks and leisure facilities must all be examined in this light. Health of the environment covers big issues such as industrial pollution, traffic nuisance and quality of municipal housing (Krogh 1989). It also covers small issues such as litter, graffiti and dog excrement.

Removing all environmental features damaging to health will probably cost billions and it is therefore totally impractical. However, getting health on the agenda should ensure that the environment does not deteriorate further and marginal improvement may be possible. Many environmental improvements such as clearing dumped rubbish, greening empty urban spaces or putting safer

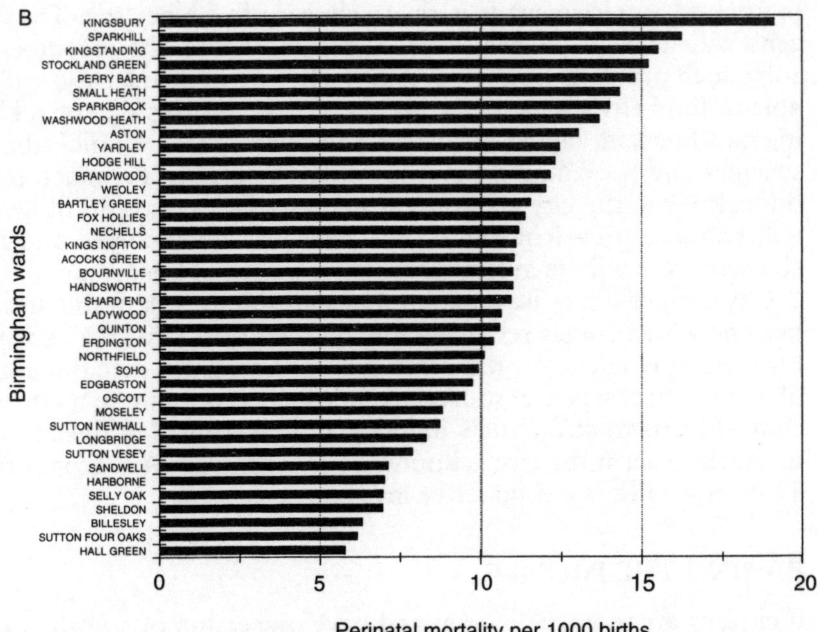

Figure 18.2 (*continued*)

18.2B shows perinatal mortality rates in different wards. Perinatal mortality is still births plus deaths in first week of life. Note the wide differences between wards. These figures have to be interpreted with care since they are based on relatively few still births and deaths and the 95 per cent confidence limits (indicating the range in which the true value could lie) will be wide. For example, the 95 per cent confidence limits for Sutton Four Oaks are 2.4–10.0 per 1000 and for Sparkbrook 10.3–17.7 per 1000.

surfaces (wood chippings) under play equipment (NCPRU 1992) are relatively cheap. In many cases residents will want to undertake the work themselves and only require minimum support. Careful rethinking of transport and traffic systems is one way in which many cities could drastically improve the quality of their environment and gain economic and social benefit (Friends of the Earth 1992).

The healthy city is an ecologically sound city. Waste management and recycling conserve non-renewable resources. Energy conservation minimises the harmful effect on the environment of the city. The healthy city is a self-sustaining city (Morris 1987).

THE CITY ECONOMY

The economic health of the city influences all other aspects of health. In a city with a booming economy and high levels of prosperity and employment it is relatively easy to be healthy. The citizens will have fewer health problems as well as the resources to solve such problems as they do have. The city exchequer too will be able to fund environmental schemes such as refurbishing or replacing bad housing, laying out parks and open spaces, traffic-calming schemes and providing good transport. The problem is much more difficult when the city economy is depressed. Disease and ill health will be more prevalent among the poor and unemployed and few city resources will be available for environmental upgrading.

City councils may be tempted to see health as a desirable luxury but one which comes relatively low on the priority list for expenditure. Healthy cities, on the other hand, understand that the health of their citizens is a resource from which economic growth will come. Efforts to attract new industry and investment to the city will be much easier if the city is known as a healthy city. Far from being a luxury, health is a productive investment.

RAISING THE PROFILE

If citizens are to participate in and have ownership of a healthy city initiative they need first to know about the initiative and second to see that progress is being made. However, healthy cities do not change overnight. Budgets will be small and there is a real difficulty in delivering change.

One way of making people feel something is happening is 'badge engineering' – changing the labels attached to pre-existing activity. Many of the city's activities will have been health promoting before the city politicians declared it a healthy city. There are probably programmes for housing improvements, pedestrianisation of roads, improvements to parks, upgrading of exercise facilities and opening of new health facilities. These can be linked with the healthy city aspirations and listed as health-promoting activities. This may sound cynical and pointless but it focuses attention on health and reminds people of progress made. Success breeds success.

EQUITY AND THE HEALTHY CITY

The section on community diagnosis stressed the need to highlight inequalities within the city. Identification of health inequalities is a first step towards reducing them. Healthy city principles suggest that communities and areas of the city with poorest health should have priority for investment and services (Draper 1989; Whitehead and Dahlgren 1991). If community health services are to be increased, the deprived areas should have priority. If community health services have to be cut, then deprived areas should be protected. Areas with poor health should have priority for investment in new health buildings. Similar considerations ought to guide decisions on investment in housing and school buildings and staff. Few would argue with these positive statements but unfortunately high priority for deprived areas also implies low priority for prosperous areas. Residents, councillors and health staff working in areas given low priority may find the principle of equity less attractive.

INTERAGENCY WORKING

Cities are served by a wide variety of agencies: the council and its departments, health services, police, fire service, non-statutory agencies, and so on. None of these – and certainly not the health service – can promote health in the city by itself. Just about every issue requires co-ordinated action by several agencies. The theory of interagency working is fine. The practice is more difficult. Each agency tends to guard its own patch and budgets. All are very willing to advise other agencies on what they should be doing but are reluctant to allow any interference in their own workings (Nocom *et al.* 1993). These difficulties can with effort be overcome. At a personal level, staff of each agency must make an effort to understand the problems faced by staff in other agencies and recognise their skills. At a policy level, there must be a real commitment to take into account the views of other agencies when resources are being allocated. Interagency working requires all the skills of influence discussed in Chapter 8. It requires people to show toleration and patience and to work at building trust. If health care workers do these things they will find that multidisciplinary and interagency working not only achieves far more than working alone but also is great fun.

Discussion/Activity 18.2 Interagency working

Make a list of the different agencies with which you (i.e. your professional group) come into contact in your work. How successful is co-operation between you?

What are the things you dislike about working with them? How could they alter their working practices to make things go better?

What are the things about your working practice that workers in other agencies find difficult? How could you alter your working practice to make things go better?

What general principles about interagency working have you discovered in this activity?

COMMERCE AND INDUSTRY

Commerce and industry should contribute to the healthy city in many ways. Much of this will be enlightened self-interest. As employers they can look to improve the health and welfare of their workforce. As owners of premises they can do their bit to make the city a greener, more pleasant environment. Retailers of products such as food, toys, home appliances, and sports goods can ensure health aspects are tied into their marketing strategy. Commerce may also help more directly by sponsoring events, giving prizes and so on. Healthy city planning and decision making can also benefit from the business and organisational skills of those who work in commerce and industry.

MAKING SERVICES FOR HEALTH ACCESSIBLE

Citizens need a wide variety of services to protect their health. Some of these are provided by the city council and some by health authorities. These services should be provided as close to people's homes as possible. A service which is two bus journeys away is not accessible to a mother with two toddlers and no car, or to a person who has difficulty walking 200 metres. The healthy city will therefore try and 'outpost' as many services as possible. City councils may set up neighbourhood offices which can answer queries about housing, education, social services, environmental services or the business of any council department. Computerised record systems, faxes and telephones mean that staff in the neighbourhood office can rapidly obtain information or expert advice from the main department, which may be several miles away.

Health services too must think how they can bring services closer to the patient. Local health centres already provide primary care. The move to midwife-led services is bringing antenatal care further into the community (DoH 1993). Progress has been made in moving care for some common conditions such as diabetes, asthma and hypertension away from the hospital with consultants visiting local health centres (Bailey, Black and Wilkin 1994). Of course, quality of care must not be compromised and many services cannot be delivered outside the hospital but in the healthy city health workers are continually looking for ways of bringing their services closer to patients' homes.

THE CITY AS AN EMPLOYER

Healthy cities should have healthy workplaces and healthy workforces. The city council and health authorities are likely to be among the larger employers in the city and starting here will make a significant contribution. They gain the advantages of a healthy workforce and can also offer their experience as an example and model for other large employers.

PARTICIPATION

So far the description of healthy cities has concentrated on council and health authority action. This is often necessary to make things happen but a top-down system must be complemented by strenuous efforts to involve citizens in the decision making of the healthy city. There must be an effort to find out the health concerns of the 'person in the street', their priorities and the solutions they want (Adams 1989; Bracht and Tsouros 1990).

There are many channels for community participation. Local politicians have been elected to represent people and will be in touch with the anxieties and aspirations of their constituents. Trade unions and residents' groups are other channels through which citizens can make their views known. Self-appointed or elected leaders of ethnic minority communities, religious groups and other citizen groups may also be willing and able to represent the views of their constituents. All these channels should be used both to encourage debate and to foster participation. It is also desirable to try to approach some citizens directly since their views may not always be adequately reflected by their representatives. For example, in some ethnic groups the spokespeople are usually male and may not adequately describe the health worries of female members of their community.

Participation may be sought by making visits to politicians and community leaders, by being invited to group meetings, by calling meetings or by inviting people to write in with their ideas. It is no easy matter to stimulate productive debate within a community (Richardson 1983). All the skills of community development discussed in Chapter 16 will be needed to empower people to participate. It may be that people are too polite to identify problems in health services or they may be so angry about some event (such as the closure of a hospital or the building of a new road) that they are unwilling to consider any wider health agenda. Discussion will probably need to be seeded by a presentation of some possible problems but this must be done in a way that does not limit the agenda. Health care workers should try to be seen as resources to help people make progress towards a healthy city rather than people who give instructions. The community architecture movement has shown how people can participate in creating their own environment (Wates and Knevitt 1987). Getting meaningful participation is not easy but the goal of a healthy city cannot be achieved without it.

LEVELS OF CITIZEN PARTICIPATION

There is a whole range of citizen participation (see Figure 18.3) (Arnstein 1969). At the lowest level are manipulation and therapy, where the health care worker or council official retains complete control and there is no participation. At the other extreme, citizens take complete control and the role of the health care worker or council official is to be an assistant or helper. In between are various degrees of shared power. In a healthy city, working arrangements are toward the citizen control end of the scale.

HEALTHY LIFESTYLE FOR CITIZENS

The city environment is important but ability to change it will be limited. Citizens of the healthy city will have healthy lifestyles: they will eat healthily, drink sensibly, take exercise, not smoke, and so on. Healthy city activities will therefore probably include health education to promote healthy lifestyles. Information and advice will be available through health centres, libraries and other places. Publicity events can raise awareness and prepare the ground for health education activities organised by health care workers and others (Fryer 1988). The most important strategy for promotion of healthy lifestyles is to ensure that the city environment favours them. Thus city-owned advertisement hoardings would not carry

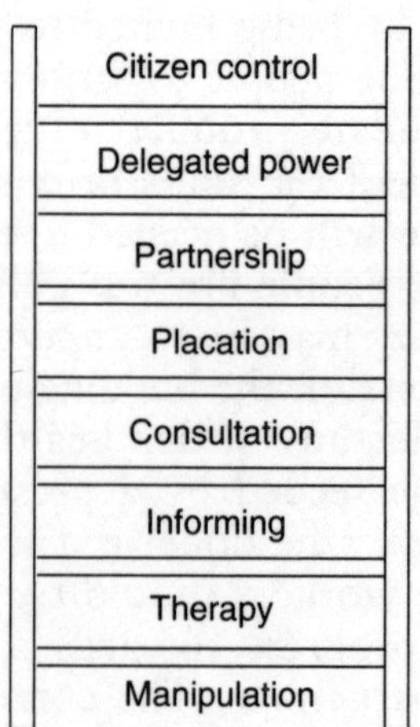

Figure 18.3 Ladder of citizen participation

cigarette advertisements, public buildings would be no-smoking areas, and laws forbidding cigarette sales to young people would be enforced. A good selection of the sorts of foods needed to make a healthy diet would be available in the shops people used; city, health authority and other catering would offer healthy choices, and so on.

HEALTH ACTION AREAS

There is a danger that the healthy city vision may seem too big. There is an argument for concentrating resources on a small area where it is possible to make a big difference rather than spread them diffusely throughout the city. This concentration of effort can also be part of the drive for equity. With small patches it is easier to get real community involvement, with residents' groups, social clubs, religious groups, schools and health services all taking part.

THE HEALTH EVENT

A healthy city venture depends on getting the support of all sorts of people across the city (see the section on commitment planning in Chapter 8). One way of doing this is to organise a health event. The target group might be city councillors, headteachers, leaders of industry or some other group whose support is needed. The aim is to expose them to an event which persuades them that the healthy city initiative is worth their support and gives them information on how they could help it.

The event must be enjoyable and informative. It should be held in a prestigious and pleasant venue (such as the council house or town hall) at a time convenient for the group. There will probably be some very short talks to indicate what the event is about and what action it is hoped people will take after attending the event. Displays around the meeting room staffed by people with appropriate knowledge can inform them about aspects of healthy cities (including highlights of the community diagnosis). An information pack can reinforce the points made and give people attending something to refresh their memories afterwards.

Offering a personal health check (similar to the MOT described in Chapter 15) can be very effective in motivating people attending these events and interesting them in the health of the city through getting them to think about their own health. If this is done it is essential that there is medical back-up so that anyone in whom health problems are identified can be offered proper counselling and follow-up. A buffet meal will help to put people in a co-operative frame of mind.

The sort of event described requires considerable resources. If it cannot be done well it is better not to do it at all. A badly organised event with insufficient staff and scrappy displays will reinforce all the wrong attitudes. On the other hand, if it is done well an event of this type can gain critical support and make all sorts of things possible.

SOCIAL HEALTH IN THE CITY

The real difference between healthy and unhealthy cities is their social structure. A city whose people are at ease with themselves will be healthy. Where there is social strife, no amount of environmental manipulation or lifestyle counselling will make the city healthy. Education, prevention of crime, stopping racial discrimination, good neighbourliness, good parenting and social well-being are all part of the healthy city vision. These things are difficult to promote directly but will be favoured by the process of working together and by participation and empowerment, as discussed above.

EXTENDING THE CONCEPT

Health of people in cities is important but so is the health of people outside cities. The principles of healthy cities have now been extended to other settings. Rural counties, regions and other groupings are trying to promote health using policy and participation and building on local identity.

A VISION

The Healthy City movement is driven by a vision (Hancock 1992). Cities (and other human communities) should be places in which people can realise their full potential. The city environment should foster physical, mental and social health and the citizens should protect and enrich that environment.

This vision cannot be brought about by any one person or group of persons. It will only happen when very many citizens share the vision and believe it can be made to happen. Healthy City movements can do three things:

1. They can be the grit in the system which irritates until city and health officials and others stop doing things harmful to health and instead produce the pearl of health.
2. They can be the oil which soothes inter-professional and inter-agency frictions and allows all to work together for the health of the city.

3. They can be the dye which permeates every city policy and every individual action with the aim of promoting health.

HEALTH WORKERS AND THE HEALTHY CITY

The role of the health worker has not been picked out in each section of this chapter. It must be obvious that health workers can and should support the healthy city in many ways:

- contributing special knowledge of health to the community diagnosis
- identifying health-damaging features of the environment
- identifying inequities in health distribution
- making a reality of multidisciplinary interagency working
- restructuring health services so they can be delivered closer to where the patient lives
- acting as advocate for the community and fostering participation
- sharing the vision of health

Discussion/Activity 18.3 Your vision of a healthy city

Think about the city or area in which you work. If you could solve all its problems and make everything right, what would the city or area be like? How can you set about sharing your vision with others?

SUMMARY POINTS

The Healthy City movement began with 11 European cities and has very rapidly grown to involve hundreds of cities in all parts of the world.

Healthy cities:

- ☐ make a high level political commitment to health
- ☐ seek to put Health for All principles into practice
- ☐ have structures that support multiagency working
- ☐ make a community diagnosis
- ☐ involve their citizens in a debate on the health of the city

The community diagnosis highlights health problems and inequalities of health. The information in the community diagnosis is widely shared. Citizens have a part in deciding what information to collect and in collecting it.

City council and health authorities should consider the health implications of all policy decisions they make. The city council should endeavour to build a health-promoting environment.

The principle of increasing equity will guide distribution of health and other resources in the healthy city. The different agencies within the city will develop ways of working together to deliver health care more effectively. Services for health are structured so that care can be delivered as close as possible to the client's home.

Participation is key to the working of the healthy city. At all stages efforts are made to ensure that the citizen is informed and involved in the decision making. All available channels are used to seek the citizens views and involve them.

Citizens are encouraged to adopt healthy lifestyles both through health education and by producing an environment in the city that supports healthy lifestyles.

REFERENCES

Adams L. (1989). Healthy cities, healthy participation. *Health Education Journal* **48**, 179–182.

Arnstein S. (1969). A ladder of citizen participation. *American Institute of Planners Journal* 5, 216–224.

Ashton J. (1992). *Healthy cities*. Milton Keynes: Open University Press.

Bailey J.J., Black M.E. and Wilkin D. (1994). Specialist outreach clinics in general practice. *British Medical Journal* **308**, 1083–1086.

Baum F.E. (1993). Healthy cities and change: social movement or bureaucratic tool? *Health Promotion International* 8, 31–40.

Binysh K., Chishty V., Pollock G. and Middleton J. (1989). The health of Coventry: use of a health profile to stimulate community health promotion. *Health Education Journal* 48, 94–96.

Bracht N.N. and Tsouros A. (1990). Principles and strategies of effective community participation. *Health Promotion International* 5, 199–208.

Cernick K. and Wearne M. (1992). Using community health profiles to improve service provision. *Health Visitor* **65**, 343–345.

DoH (Department of Health) (1993). *Changing childbirth: report of expert maternity group*. London: HMSO.

Draper R. (1989). Making equity policy. *Health Promotion International* **4**, 91–95.

Friends of the Earth (1992). *Less traffic, better towns*. London: Friends of the Earth.

Fryer P. (1988). A healthy city strategy three years on: the case of Oxford City Council. *Health Promotion International* 3, 213–218.

Garrettson H.F.L., Van Gilst C.H. and Van Oers H.A.M (1991). Collecting health information at a local level. *Health Promotion International* 6, 121–133.

Halliday M. and Adams L. (1992). Healthy Sheffield; the consultation experiment. *Health Education Journal* **51**, 43–46.

Hancock T. (1992). The healthy city: utopias and realities. Chapter 2 in Ashton (1992).

Harrison J. (1994). Every picture tells the story. *Health Visitor* 67, 66–67.
Kickbush I. (1989). Healthy cities: a working project and a growing movement. *Health Promotion* 4, 77–82.
Krogh L. (1989). Trends in town planning in the 1980s: equity and healthy planning. *Health Promotion International* 4, 97–101.
Morris D. (1987). Healthy cities: self-reliant cities. *Health Promotion International* 2, 169–176.
NCPRU (National Children's Play and Recreation Unit) (1992). *Playground Safety Guidelines*. London: HMSO.
Nocom A., Small N., Ferguson B. and Watt A. (1993). Made in heaven. *Health Services Journal* 103 (2 December), 24–26.
Richardson A. (1983). *Concepts in social policy 1: participation*. London: Routledge and Kegan Paul.
Tsouros A.D. (1992). *Healthy Cities: a project becomes a movement*. Copenhagen: WHO.
Wates N. and Knevitt C. (1987). *Community architecture: how people are creating their own environment*. London: Penguin.
Whitehead M. and Dahlgren G. (1991). What can be done about inequalities in health? *Lancet* 338, 1059–1062.

CHAPTER 19

Working with national campaigns

Dr Jacky Chambers
Director of Public Health, Health Education Authority

GOAL

To understand the aims of national health education campaigns and be able to organise linked activities at a local level.

OBJECTIVES

- to appreciate the importance of health education campaigns – what they can and cannot achieve
- to describe examples of current national campaigns
- to plan practical linked local-level activities
- to identify simple ways to measure success

INTRODUCTION

One way of communicating directly with thousands of people simultaneously is to use the mass media, i.e. television, radio, cinema and print media (e.g. newspapers, magazines, etc.). Over the past twenty years, the publicity created by organised health education campaigns has had a major impact on public knowledge, attitudes and behaviour (Pasick and Wallack 1988).

THE MAIN FUNCTIONS OF A HEALTH EDUCATION CAMPAIGN

Campaigns can be used to communicate directly with the public for a variety of purposes, including:

- to provide basic information (e.g. about a new vaccine or screening programme)
- to increase awareness and concern about an important health problem (e.g. heart disease)

- to motivate people to take action or not to behave in a certain way (e.g. fasten seat belt, use a condom, not to drink and drive)
- to demonstrate visually how to do something (e.g. prepare a baby's feed, take your pulse rate)

THEORETICAL BASIS FOR THE DEVELOPMENT OF A MASS-MEDIA CAMPAIGN

The preparation of a health education campaign draws on a number of disciplines (Whitehead and Tones 1991):

- epidemiology
- social sciences
- marketing and management

Epidemiology is needed to define and prioritise the populations or target audiences to whom the health education messages will mainly be directed, i.e. market segmentation. For example, epidemiological analysis shows incidence of skin cancer (malignant melanoma) and exposure to sun are greatest in children, adolescents and young adults (16–35 years), so these groups might be chosen as the target for a skin cancer prevention campaign.

Social sciences include psychology, sociology and anthropology. These disciplines give an insight into the existing beliefs, cultures and social structures which influence perception of and response to the message. In particular, theories of behavioural change such as the health belief model, which promotes both the idea that one is susceptible to a health problem and the benefits of taking action (see the section on the health belief model in Chapter 7), or Bandura's socio-cognitive theory, which includes the notion of self-efficacy or the belief in one's own capacity to effect change (see the section on socio-cognitive theory in Chapter 7) commonly underlie the construction of a particular message.

Marketing and management theories ensure that the most effective methods and techniques are used to influence or 'sell' new ideas and attitudes, and to model new behaviours (this process is sometimes described as social marketing) (Hastings and Hayward 1991). Theories of social and organisational change may be used to support campaigns which involve working with and getting the support of other sectors such as schools, local government workplaces and health care services.

STAGES IN THE DEVELOPMENT OF A CAMPAIGN

Once the overall aims and target group(s) for a campaign have been agreed, a number of stages then follow. The example of skin cancer will be used to illustrate these stages.

Stage 1 Initial formative research aims to find out the current beliefs of young women (who were believed to be the group most at risk) about the importance, benefits and risks of sunbathing; what they are currently doing to protect themselves against exposure; what they already know about skin cancer and what causes it; their skin types and methods of protection; when, where and how they sunbathe; and what might increase their motivation to protect themselves.

Stage 2 A clear, concise statement of the communication objectives is prepared. This statement becomes the communications brief for an advertising, public relations or publicity media plan. In the example of skin cancer, the communication objectives might be:

- to highlight the risks of sunbathing and reinforce individuals' intentions to protect themselves
- to counter existing beliefs that you need to get burnt to have a suntan
- to promote recognition of suncream protection factors in relation to skin type

Stage 3 The creative design stage involves constructing various images, words and sounds which together make up the 'message'. The specialist skills of a public relations firm, advertising agency or journalist will be required to do this effectively. They will produce a range of options from which the final creative design for the campaign will be chosen.

Stage 4 Pre-testing the campaign message involves checking the comprehensibility, acceptability and appropriateness of the message with the target audience using various qualitative research techniques such as focus groups, observational studies, intercept surveys, and interviews. The creative materials are usually shown in rough and responses analysed. A final decision is then made on a particular creative design or set of designs.

Stage 5 Distribution, dissemination and promotion of the message are the last stage. The channels for promoting a particular message are chosen so that they can reach the target audience most effectively. For example, radio might be chosen as the optimum method for reaching certain ethnic minority populations, cinema for young people, and morning television for mothers of young children. The timing, frequency and duration of a particular message are important factors. In general, the more exposure there is to a particular message, the more awareness of the message there will be in the target population. However awareness, understanding and impact of a particular campaign can vary considerably. The salience of the message, the presence or otherwise of complementary or negative publicity and local reinforcement of the messages with posters or leaflets can all influence how effective a particular campaign will be.

EVALUATION

Campaigns are often evaluated using before and after ('pre and post') studies in which data relating to the knowledge, attitudes and actions of the target audience are collected through telephone surveys, face-to-face interviews, shoppers' exit surveys, etc. Sampling of national campaigns needs to be representative, taken from various points across the country and large enough to detect small changes in prevalence of behaviour. Sample sizes of about 1000 are commonplace.

CAMPAIGN ELEMENTS

A national campaign will often use many different media forms to achieve a particular objective. Campaigns are distinguished from *ad hoc* publicity by the following characteristics:

- The target audience is carefully defined (e.g. smokers who wish to give up, first-time parents).
- There is a simple theme or message which can be clearly understood.
- The media are chosen with a particular target audience in mind (e.g. cinema, women's magazines).
- Campaigns are often planned so that maximum publicity occurs at a particular time (e.g. No Smoking Day) or over a defined period.
- Reinforcement may be provided by offering a telephone helpline, booklets, suggestions about who else to contact, etc.
- They often have a unique identity (i.e. logo) to increase recognition and visibility of the campaign.
- They can provide opportunities for active participation through special events, health fairs or organised displays.

- They are sometimes associated with sponsorship or other commercial involvement.

The most successful campaigns are likely to be those which have a simple distinct message which is properly understood by the target audience. Other features of successful campaigns are inclusion of recommendations for positive steps which can be taken and widespread publicity over a sustained period which reaches large numbers of people.

It is important to be realistic about what a single campaign can achieve. The most immediate effect of a health education campaign is to raise awareness and create interest in a particular health issue. Occasionally, this interest may lead a highly motivated individual to take action – for example, to change the sleeping position of their infant or to visit their general practitioner for a vaccination. It is unrealistic to expect a single campaign to have an impact on complex behaviour patterns such as eating or smoking which have been established over long periods of time (Redman, Spencer and Sanson-Fisher 1990).

Most of the successes in changing behaviour during recent years, in this country and in others, have occurred as a result of the cumulative interaction of mass-media campaigns with other factors such as legislation, price rises, and the personal advice and influence of friends, relatives and health professionals (Flay 1987; Pierce, Macaskill and Hill 1990).

RECENT EXAMPLES OF PUBLIC EDUCATION CAMPAIGNS

No Smoking Day

No Smoking Day is the leading smoking cessation campaign in the United Kingdom when for one day in March (just after the Chancellor's budget!), smokers are encouraged to try to stop for part or all of that day. It has been running since 1984, has a current annual budget of about £400,000 and is organised by a coalition of about thirty statutory and voluntary bodies.

The campaign objectives are:

- to encourage and assist smokers to give up for one day (or longer)
- to bring the Day to the public's attention
- to involve as many people and organisations as possible in smoking education

Paid-for advertising directed at smokers is not an option with the available budget. The campaign plan is therefore based on two elements: public relations activities and giving support to local activities.

Public relations activities usually involve creating stories for the national media by providing new information about smoking, organising a press launch three or four weeks before the Day itself and supporting the actual Day by having a well-known political figure or celebrity take part, and preparing video film and interviews for use on radio and TV networks.

The success of the campaign depends very heavily on people organising activities and taking part at a local level. Supporting these local organisers is essential. Local organisers of No Smoking Day activities come from a whole range of different professions, including primary health care and hospital staff, occupational health personnel, teachers and environmental health officers.

Health promotion units funded by district health authorities also have a major role in supporting and co-ordinating these activities at local level. This includes achieving local media coverage and providing contact with the public through stalls, exhibitions and competitions as well as supplying materials for use in workplaces, schools and other community settings.

The achievements of No Smoking Day

An annual survey of public awareness and smoker participation shows that about nine out of ten smokers are aware of No Smoking Day (see Table 19.1).

On the Day itself, around 15% of smokers try to quit or cut down. After three months, the majority of those who tried to give up on the Day will have gone back to their normal smoking behaviour, but about 0.5% (or about 50 000 smokers) are still not smoking at that time and about 2.7% say they have reduced their consumption (see Figure 19.1) (McGuire 1992).

Around 10 000 local organisers are registered to take part in the No Smoking Day campaign.

Table 19.1 Prompted awareness of No Smoking Day

	Percentage aware of Day*	
Year	**All adults**	**Smokers**
1986	79	85
1987	85	88
1988	92	94
1989	91	95
1990	92	96
1991	85	91

*Percentage of people who said they had been aware of No Smoking Day after being reminded about it.

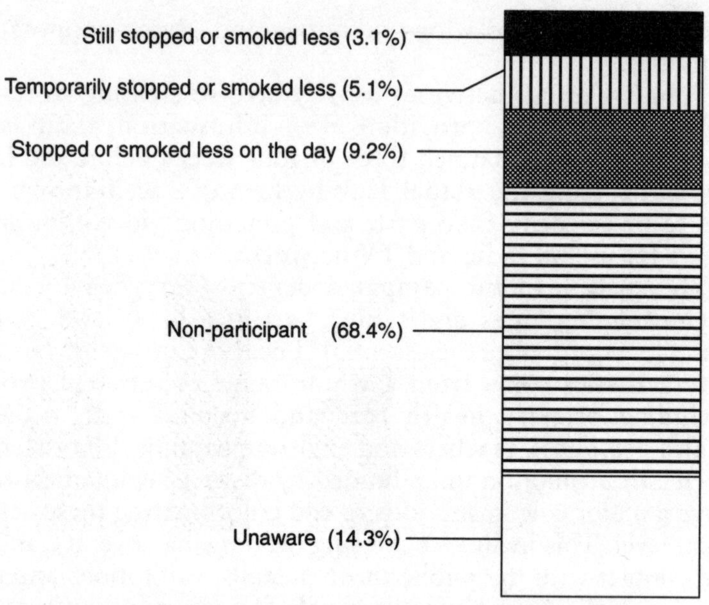

Figure 19.1 Responses of smokers to No Smoking Day 1989
Showing the percentage of smokers who were unaware of No Smoking Day, aware but did not participate (non-participant) and those who stopped or smoked less on the day, temporarily stopped or have still stopped or smoked less after three months. Results are based on a sample of 10 133 smokers.
Source Data from McGuire C. (1992), *Pausing for breath: a review of No Smoking Day research 1984 to 1991*; London: HEA.

Drinkwise

Drinkwise Day is an annual event run along similar lines to No Smoking Day. Its aim is to promote sensible drinking and encourage people to think about their levels of consumption. It has been running for four years and normally take place in June.

The key messages are:

- drink sensibly
- be aware
- know your weekly limits when you drink

Five thousand local groups and organisations take part in Drinkwise Day, which receives widespread coverage in the national press, TV and radio. As a result:

- awareness of the term 'unit' has risen from 55% in 1989 to 75% in 1992

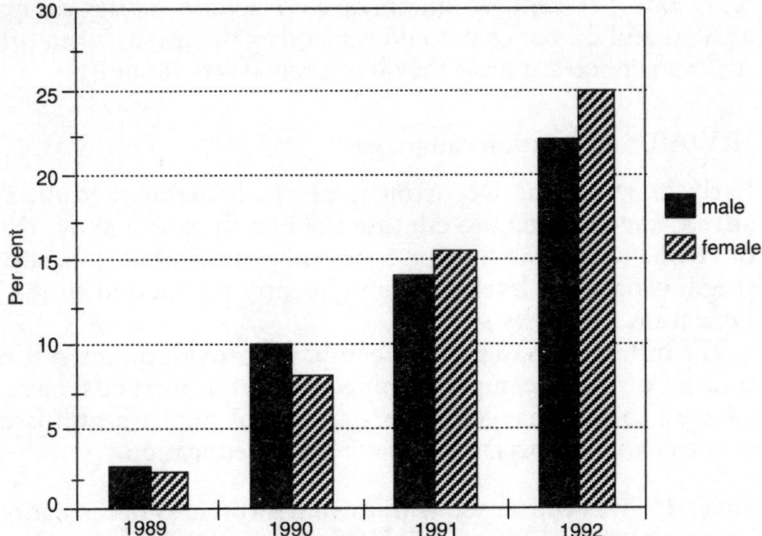

Figure 19.2 Increasing knowledge of safe drinking limits
Repeated surveys show an increase in the percentage of men and women who can identify the safe limit for weekly alcohol consumption (21 units per week for men, 14 for women). The 1989 survey was before Drinkwise Day and the other surveys after Drinkwise. Of course many other factors as well as Drinkwise Day will have influenced this change in knowledge.
Sources *Drinkwise Campaign Reports 1991* and *1992*; London: HEA.

- knowledge of the weekly recommended limits for men and women has risen to around 25% of women and 22% of men (see Figure 19.2).

Food for the Heart campaign

Food for the Heart was a national campaign to promote healthier eating. Every year (1989–93) major food retailers (including the top seven supermarket chains), trade associations, national and local health educators took part in a month-long campaign to raise awareness of the risks of heart disease and promote awareness of healthy eating to the general public. Use was made of both the media and 'in store' promotions, with leaflets, shelf banner cards, special displays and demonstrations.

The key messages were:

- eat less fat, particularly saturated fat
- eat more fibre-rich starchy foods
- simple dietary changes can significantly reduce the risk of coronary heart disease

Sixty one per cent of shoppers were aware of the campaign in general and 21 per cent could remember the leaflet when prompted (i.e. remembered it after they had been asked about it).

HIV/AIDS prevention campaigns

Early in 1986, the Department of Health embarked on a major advertising campaign to educate the British people about the threat of AIDS. Responsibility for continuing this public education campaign at national level was subsequently transferred to the Health Education Authority in 1987.

The different phases of this campaign provide an interesting illustration of how campaign objectives and methods have to be adapted to our changed understanding of public health issues and to the changing social context for public education.

Phase 1 was concerned with raising awareness in the entire population about the dangers of AIDS and presenting facts about how HIV can and cannot be transmitted. Campaign messages included 'Don't die of ignorance'; the tone was alarmist and gloomy; and the methods included TV, cinema, magazines, billboards.

Phase 2 was concerned with informing young people about the risks of HIV infection, how to protect themselves against infection and encouraging them to take responsibility for the practice of safer sex.

Phase 3 was concerned with risk reduction in particular target groups, such as gay men, women and holiday makers. Campaign messages included 'Don't go too far without one' and 'You're as safe as you want to be'; the tone was more lighthearted.

Phase 4 began in 1989, when it had become increasingly obvious that the scale of the epidemic amongst heterosexuals was far less than originally estimated. The press began to question the validity of this campaign, accusing health educators and the government of deliberately misleading the public into a false sense of panic and being sexual killjoys. The planned objectives had to be changed to confirm the existence of heterosexual transmission using 'experts' such as the Chief Medical Officer, and the personal testimonies of people who had become infected with HIV through heterosexual intercourse.

Phase 5 was concerned to maintain general awareness of HIV infection but also to create a climate in which the older generation can talk about condoms, where young people feel more positive about condom use and accept them as an everyday precaution against infection ('condom normalisation').

Cinema and television featured two characters, Mrs Dawson (who made condoms) and Mr Brewster (an old soldier who had used a very primitive condom forty years ago), talking about condoms in a humorous or lighthearted way. There were also campaigns aimed at helping young women raise the subject of safer sex with their partners and encouraging holiday or business travellers to take condoms with them.

Phase 6 Plans for this phase of the national campaign have begun to reflect the broader targets for sexual health set out in the Health of the Nation. It aims to address the risks of infection from other sexually transmitted diseases as well as HIV by encouraging young people to negotiate safer sex in different situations and demonstrating how this can be done.

This move toward a 'skills enhancing' approach means that the methods adopted will have to change again. They will shift towards greater use of magazine and editorial features in the print media, more coverage by national and local radio, more use of posters, billboards and possibly cinema. Local personnel will also need to become more actively involved in giving advice and support.

Achievements of the HIV/AIDS campaign

The initial fear-inducing campaigns had an immediate and rapid effect on condom sales in the UK. Within three years of the start of the national campaign, volume of sales had increased by 15%, later settling down to a slower rate of growth of around 2–3% per annum.

Annual tracking surveys of the campaign (British Market Research Bureau 1987–89) also confirm that amongst young adults (aged 16–34) reported condom use on the last occasion of sexual intercourse has shown a consistent upward trend over the past three years (see Figure 19.3).

GETTING INVOLVED IN LOCAL ACTIVITIES

Taking part in national and local campaigns is not only important for their overall success, it can also be interesting and fun. Here are some practical ideas about what to do:

- displays and stalls
- sponsored events and competitions
- local publicity

DISPLAYS AND STALLS

Displays can range from a covered table to a more elaborate arrangement of posters, leaflets, display boards and booths. As well

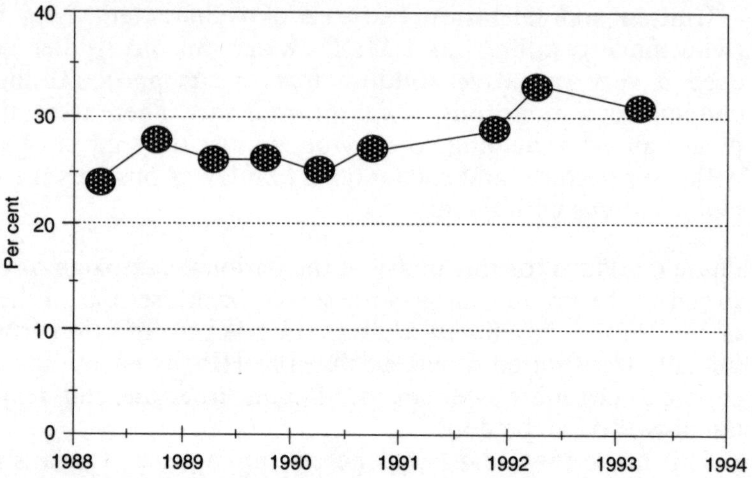

Figure 19.3 Trends in reported use of condoms
Repeated surveys of young adults (aged 16–34) show that the percentage of those who are sexually active who report using a condom on the last occasion of sexual intercourse has risen fairly steadily.
Source British Market Research Bureau (1987–89); London: HEA.

as creating displays in the health centre, school or hospital where you work, think about nearby facilities:

- the window or floor space of a local store, bookshop or post office
- the local pharmacy could organise a special display of smoking cessation aids, condoms, suncreams and associated leaflets

Running a stall in the local shopping centre, market or high street is a good way of taking a campaign deep into the heart of a community. Possible ways of attracting attention include:

- providing information that people can take away
- quizzes, tests (e.g. breathalysers, step test) or questionnaires that get people into conversation about their health
- give-aways such as balloons, badges and stickers, and taster foods

SPONSORED EVENTS AND COMPETITIONS

Numerous events can be organised as part of a local campaign. These can be used to generate publicity as well as actively involve local people. Ideas include:

- running a prize draw
- sponsoring individuals or organisations to achieve a particular target (e.g. loose 10 lb in weight, stop smoking for 48 hours, walk or cycle 4 miles)
- organise a competition of children's drawings or photos depicting the campaign theme

LOCAL PUBLICITY

The key to getting good media coverage is to create 'news' which is fresh and interesting. To do this you need to:

- give your story an angle that makes it more newsworthy and exciting
- direct your story to the publication or programme you are targeting
- write a good press release – concentrate on the five Ws: WHAT is happening, WHO is involved, WHERE, WHEN and WHY is it happening?
- include a simple quote from local people
- provide photographs or opportunities for photographs

EVALUATING LOCAL ACTIVITIES

Here is a simple checklist for assessing what has been achieved by a local activity as part of a national campaign:

- Were people aware of the campaign? Did they show interest and ask for more information as a result of your activities? How many people did you make contact with during the campaign period?
- Who else got involved? Were they the people you expected or did you discover new allies? Did you/they get any positive feedback from unexpected quarters?
- What did those who took part think about the campaign? Do they want to try it again next year?
- Did you get any media coverage? If yes, how good was it and how long did it last?
- How much did you spend and was it worth it in relation to what you think was achieved?

SUMMARY POINTS

National campaigns may aim to:

- ☐ provide basic information
- ☐ increase awareness
- ☐ motivate people to act
- ☐ demonstrate skills

Preparation of a national campaign is based on the disciplines of epidemiology, social sciences, marketing and management.

Development of a campaign involves identifying target groups, setting communication objectives, creative design of materials and dissemination. Evaluation must also be planned.

It is realistic to expect a campaign to raise awareness and possibly motivate a few individuals. It is unrealistic to expect change in deeply ingrained behaviours.

Recent example of campaigns are:

- ☐ No Smoking Day
- ☐ Drinkwise
- ☐ Food for the Heart
- ☐ HIV/AIDS prevention campaign

Most national campaigns rely heavily on support from local activities such as:

- ☐ displays and stalls
- ☐ sponsored events and competitions
- ☐ local publicity

REFERENCES

British Market Research Bureau (1987–89). *AIDS strategic monitor*. Health Education Authority.

Flay B.R. (1987). Mass media and smoking cessation: a critical review. *American Journal of Public Health* 77, 153–160.

Hastings G. and Hayward A. (1991). Social marketing and communication in health promotion. *Health Promotion International* 6, 135–147.

McGuire C. (1992). *Pausing for breath: a review of No Smoking Day research 1984 to 1991*. London: Health Education Authority.

Pasick R. and Wallack L. (1988) Mass media in health promotion: a compilation of expert opinion. *International Quarterly of Community Health Education* 9, 89–110.

Pierce J., Macaskill P. and Hill D. (1990). Long term effectiveness of mass media led anti smoking campaigns in Australia. *American Journal of Public Health* 80, 565–569.

Redman R., Spencer A. and Sanson-Fisher R. (1990). Role of mass media in changing health related behaviour. *Health Promotion International* 5, 85–102.

Whitehead M. and Tones K. (1991). Notes on the planning and implementation of health education strategies. Chapter 2 in *Avoiding the pitfalls*. London: Health Education Authority.

Index